Advanced Materials for Biomedical Applications

This textbook discusses the synthesis, processing, design, simulation, and characterization of biomaterials for biomedical applications. It synergizes exploration related to various properties and functionalities in the biomedical field through extensive theoretical and experimental modeling. It further presents advanced integrated design and nonlinear simulation problems occurring in the biomedical engineering field. It will serve as an ideal reference text for senior undergraduate and graduate students, and academic researchers in fields including biomedical engineering, mechanical engineering, materials science, ergonomics, and human factors.

This book

- Employs a problem-solution approach, where, in each chapter, a specific biomedical engineering problem is raised and its numerical and experimental solutions are presented.
- Covers recent developments in biomaterials such as OPMF/KGG biocomposites, PEEK-based biomaterials, PF/KGG biocomposites, oil palm mesocarp fiber/KGG biocomposite, and polymeric resorbable materials for orthopedic, dentistry, and shoulder arthroplasty applications.
- Discusses mechanical performance and corrosive analysis of biomaterials for biomedical applications in detail.
- Presents advanced integrated design and nonlinear simulation problems occurring in the biomedical engineering field.
- Presents biodegradable polymers for various biomedical applications over the last decade owing to their non-corrosion in the body, biocompatibility, and superior strength in growing state.
- Synergizes exploration related to various properties and functionalities in the biomedical field through extensive theoretical and experimental modeling.

Advances in Manufacturing, Design and Computational Intelligence Techniques

Series Editor:
Ashwani Kumar

Advanced Materials for Biomedical Applications
Ashwani Kumar, Yatika Gori, Avinash Kumar,
Chandan Swaroop Meena, and Nitesh Dutt

For more information about this series, please visit: https://www.routledge.com/Advances-In-Manufacturing-Design-andComputational-Intelligence-Techniques/book-series/%20CRCAIMDCIT

Advanced Materials for Biomedical Applications

Edited by
Ashwani Kumar, Yatika Gori, Avinash Kumar,
Chandan Swaroop Meena, and Nitesh Dutt

CRC Press
Taylor & Francis Group
Boca Raton London New York

CRC Press is an imprint of the
Taylor & Francis Group, an **informa** business

First edition published 2023
by CRC Press
6000 Broken Sound Parkway NW, Suite 300, Boca Raton, FL 33487-2742

and by CRC Press
4 Park Square, Milton Park, Abingdon, Oxon, OX14 4RN

CRC Press is an imprint of Taylor & Francis Group, LLC

ISBN: 9781032356068 (hbk)
ISBN: 9781032356075 (pbk)
ISBN: 9781003344810 (ebk)

DOI: 10.1201/9781003344810

Typeset in Sabon
by codeMantra

"This book is dedicated to all engineers, researchers, and academicians".

Contents

Preface

Advanced Materials for Biomedical Applications consists of the synthesis, processing, design, simulation, and characterization of biomaterials for biomedical applications. Advanced materials for biomedical applications are the central theme of the book. Biomaterials are used in bone plates, joint replacement, bone cement, surgical sutures, clips and staples to close wounds, pins and screws to stabilize fractures, surgical mesh, breast implants, artificial ligaments and tendons, dental implants for teeth stabilization, blood vessel prostheses, heart valves, vascular grafts, stents, nerve conduits, skin repair devices, intraocular lenses in eye surgery, contact lenses, drug delivery systems, etc. There is a huge demand for biomedical fixations devices and implants. The resorbable material plays a vital role in developing and mimicking the bone. From the industry point of view, many processing techniques are researched in the biomedical domain in a very cost-effective way. Many conventional metals such as SS304, titanium alloys, and magnesium alloys have many biomedical limitations. So, there is a need of the hour to introduce new materials and their manufacturing techniques to the medical world. This book content is helpful to practitioners in fields of orthopedic, dental, and cardiology departments.

Chapters 1 and 2 provide details about the recent developments in biomaterials and their broad applications. **Chapter 1** deals with future trends in next-generation smart materials for biomedical applications. Smart materials may now provide wonderful capabilities such as controlled treatments by fine-tuning certain stimulus agents to improve therapeutic efficiency. Dual- or multistimuli-responsive smart materials, which may activate several functionalities on a single smart nanomaterial, have lately received increased attention in order to enhance illness diagnostics. In addition, **Chapter 2** deals with biological implants and surgical tool materials. A vast range of medical, assistive, and surgical instruments have been developed to improve human life. The aging population, accidents, and sports-related injuries are driving the ever-increasing need for ortho-, dental, cardiologic, ophthalmic, and IVD equipment, as well as enhanced diagnostic tests, in the worldwide medical device market.

Chapters 3 and 4 highlight two specific areas of biomedicine, i.e., shoulder arthroplasty and dentistry applications. **Chapter 3** deals with shoulder arthroplasty. Shoulder arthroplasty is the main treatment option for patients with osteoarthritis. Most of these patients are associated with bone loss at the posterior side of the glenoid, making the glenoid become retroverted. The retroverted glenoid induces posterior humeral head subluxation. This chapter aims to introduce the concept of total shoulder arthroplasty, including the material used for implant fabrication and clinical complications, especially regarding the management of retroverted glenoid. **Chapter 4** deals with dentistry applications. This chapter presents the study of fabrication of the mandible with 3D printing. Its comparative cost estimation was made and analyzed with quality function deployment.

The next four Chapters 5–8 deal with PEEK- and KGG-based advanced biomaterials and their dielectric, mechanical, and thermal properties by conducting different experiments. **Chapter 5** presents study of PEEK-based biomaterials. This chapter deeply illustrates the embedded strange character of the polymer PEEK (polyether ether ketone). Generally, the PEEK is a high-performance semi-crystalline thermoplastic polymer and it is a part of the PAEK (polyaryletherketone) family. PEEK polymer property to create good bonding character while being added with fortified material makes it suitable for multiple applications. Especially in the biomedical field, PEEK-based polymer composites are considered an advanced biomaterial used in various medical implants such as orthopedic implants, spinal implants, facial and cranial implants, cardiac implants, and dental prosthesis. **Chapter 6** examines the dielectric properties of OPMF/KGG biocomposites. This chapter presents the experimental results of KGG biocomposites. The results indicate that 10% of treated fiber content with 12 mm fiber length performs better than other weight fractions of the untreated composites. A higher compatibility of OPMF with the KGG matrix was observed with the scanning electron microscope. In continuation, **Chapter 7** deals with the physical properties of coir fiber/KGG biocomposites. Coir fibers are hydrophilic because of the presence of water delicate parts, which will in general deliver a helpless similarity when restricting with Kondagogu gum (KGG). The composites treated with coir fibers give better results than neat resin and raw fiber composites. In **Chapter 8**, the authors examine the thermal properties of PF/KGG biocomposites. The mechanical and thermal characteristics of the developed composites are evaluated and presented. The tensile test results suggest a slight increase in tensile strength with the increase in fiber weight percentage when contrasted with pure resin and other composites. Overall, Palmyra fiber-reinforced biocomposites with 15 wt. % fiber loading have better properties than other composites. In addition, scanning electron microscope (SEM) is used for observing the interfacial bonding in fractured tensile surfaces.

New studies on posture analysis, needle insertion, and isolation of circulating tumor cells are presented in Chapters 9–11.

In **Chapter 9,** the study provides a reference range for COP in two axes, namely the A/P direction and the M/L direction. Posture and stability during upright standing is possible through a combination of mechanical, sensory, and motor processing strategies. Postural stability can be defined as the ability to control the velocity and amplitude of the center of gravity's (COG) displacement while quiet standing. The stability is higher when the COG displacement's amplitudes and velocities are smaller.

Chapter 10 presents the human-robot interaction in the healthcare sector. **In this chapter,** a novel analytical model, including a perceptual filter that considers human perception thresholds during needle-tissue interactions (perceptually reduced model, PRM), was developed. The first stage of the experiment is to verify the effect of PRM, and the second stage is to compare the PRM and the physical phantom tissue (PPT). Twenty participants volunteered for the two stages of the Turing test experiment. The results of the first stage show that the participants were fooled in differentiating the PRM and the model without perceptual filter, and the second stage shows that the participants tend to perceive the PPT as the PRM for around 50% of the trials. In conclusion, it is observed that the PRM is perceptually similar to the model without filter and the PPT with reasonable accuracy.

Chapter 11 deals with the methods of isolation of CTCs in microfluidic channels based on chemical, physical, and electrical characteristics of CTCs. This chapter includes a detailed description of affinity-based and label-free strategies for the isolation of CTCs. The affinity of surface proteins on the CTCs and other blood cells toward the antibodies coated on microfluidic channels is the basic principle of affinity-based strategies.

Chapter 12 addresses the current status of advanced abrasive-based nano-finishing processes along with their operating parameters for biomedical implant applications.

Chapters 13–15 deal with advanced KGG biocomposites, FGM, and polymeric resorbable materials for orthopedic applications.

Chapter 13 deals with OPMF/KGG biocomposites. OPMF/KGG biocomposites with treated fiber have strong dynamic and thermal characteristics as a whole. Therefore, the OPMF/KGG biocomposites may be effectively used as a primary packaging material in future on the basis of these observations. New biocomposites, FGM, and new Ti alloys-based biomaterials are used for orthopedic fracture healing in **Chapter 14.** Metal internal fixation for orthopedic fracture fixations has been explained in **Chapter 15.** These metal fixations have many limitations such as stress shielding, leaching of ions, corrosion, and stress palpability. It is also observed that in the case of metallic fixation devices, the underlying bone gets damaged and many factors also arise. The biodegradable polymers for various biomedical applications over the last decade owing to their non-corrosion in the body, biocompatibility, and superior strength have been in growing state. Chapters 1–15 presented in this book make it an ideal book for upper-level undergraduate and graduate students, engineers, technologists, doctors, and researchers working in the area of biomedical engineering and manufacturing techniques.

Editors
Dr. Ashwani Kumar
Yatika Gori
Dr. Avinash Kumar
Dr. Chandan Swaroop Meena
Dr. Nitesh Dutt

AIM AND SCOPE OF BOOK

The book *Advanced Materials for Biomedical Applications* provides essential knowledge about the synthesis of biomedical products, their development, nanomaterial properties, fabrication processes, and design techniques for different applications, as well as process design and optimization. This book is focused on the materials and related manufacturing techniques for biomedical applications. Further, this book encourages readers to discover and convert newly reported technologies into products and services for the future development of biomedical applications. This is an ideal book for upper-level undergraduate and graduate students, engineers, technologists, doctors, and researchers working in the area of biomedical engineering and manufacturing techniques.

The book *Advanced Materials for Biomedical Applications* sheds light on new-generation biomaterials, i.e., PEEK and KGG. The main aim of this book is to inventory the latest achievements in the research and development of modern biomaterials, synthesis routes, and their processing that are used in modern medicine, fracture fixations, and biomedical applications. This book has 15 chapters dealing with the recent developments in biomaterials and their application in dentistry, orthopedics, shoulder arthroplasty, and isolation of circulating tumor cells. Case studies of needle insertion and posture analysis are also explained in this book.

PEEK- and KGG-based advanced biomaterials and their dielectric, mechanical, and thermal properties are presented in different chapters. Different important experimental results about KGG biocomposites, FGM, and polymeric resorbable materials for orthopedic applications are explained in this book. There is a huge demand for biomaterials in internal fixation devices, joint replacement, fracture fixation, bone plates, bone cement, surgical sutures, and clips and staples having broader applications in dentistry, cardiology, and wound healing. This book has the potential to reach audience such as researchers, postgraduate students, practitioners and academicians conducting research in biomedical fields.

Acknowledgments

We express our gratitude to CRC Press (Taylor & Francis Group) and the editorial team for their suggestions and support during the completion of this book. We are grateful to all contributors and reviewers for their illuminating views on each book chapter presented in this book *Advanced Materials for Biomedical Applications*.

Editors

Dr. Ashwani Kumar earned a PhD in Mechanical Engineering in the area of Mechanical Vibration and Design. Since December 2013 he has been a senior lecturer of mechanical engineering (Gazetted Officer Group B) at the Technical Education Department, Kanpur, Uttar Pradesh (under Government of Uttar Pradesh), India. He worked as an assistant professor in the Department of Mechanical Engineering, Graphic Era University, Dehradun, India, from July 2010 to November 2013. He has twelve years of research and academic experience in mechanical and materials engineering. He is series editor of the book series *Advances in Manufacturing, Design and Computational Intelligence Techniques* published by CRC Press, Taylor & Francis Group. He is an associate editor for the International Journal of Mathematical, Engineering and Management Sciences (IJMEMS) Indexed in ESCI/ Scopus and DOAJ. He is an editorial board member of 4 international journals and is a review board member of 20 prestigious (indexed in SCI/SCIE/Scopus) international journals with high impact factor, i.e., Applied Acoustics, Measurement, JESTEC, AJSE, SV-JME, and LAJSS. In addition, he has published 90 research articles in journals, book chapters, and conferences. He has authored/co-authored-cum-edited 20 books of Mechanical and Materials Engineering. He is associated with international conferences as invited speaker/advisory board member/review board member. He has delivered many invited talks in webinars, FDPs, and workshops. Dr. Ashwani Kumar was awarded Best Teacher for excellence in academic and research. He successfully guided 12 B.Tech., M.Tech., and Ph.D. students for their theses. In administration, he is working as a coordinator for AICTE, E.O.A., Nodal officer for PMKVY-TI Scheme (Government of India), and internal coordinator for CDTP scheme (Government of Uttar Pradesh). He is currently involved in the research areas of AI & ML in mechanical engineering, advanced materials & manufacturing techniques, renewable energy harvesting, heavy vehicle dynamics, and sustainable transportation.

Yatika Gori is pursuing her PhD in Tribology and working as an assistant professor in the Department of Mechanical Engineering, Graphic Era University, Dehradun, Uttarakhand, India. She has more than 8 years of research and academic experience. She is working in the areas of FEA, crack propagation, welding, and tribology. She has published 18 research articles in international journals. Her recent article, published in Tribology International, obtained an impact factor of 4.872. She is a core team member of NAAC and NBA accreditation work in the Mechanical Engineering Department. She is an editor of two international books. She is an editor of two international books on mechanical and materials engineering published by CRC Press, Taylor & Francis Group.

Dr. Avinash Kumar is an assistant professor in the Department of Mechanical Engineering at the Indian Institute of Information Technology, Design and Manufacturing (IIITDM) Kancheepuram, Chennai (an institute of national importance under Ministry of Education, Government of India). His research interests include micro-/nanofabrication, laser machining, and surface engineering for microfluidics and MEMS/micro-/bio-devices. He has published more than 10 articles in international journals, 4 book chapters, and 7 international conference papers. His Google Scholar ID is eiJd-MdoAAAAJ, ORCID ID is 0000-0002-8071-5748, Scopus ID is 56564412000, and Web of Science Researcher ID is P-6124-2018. He is a reviewer in ASME Journal of Solar Energy Engineering, Journal of Engineering Applications of Computational Fluid Mechanics, ASME Journal of Heat Transfer, Journal of Physics of Fluids, among others. Dr. Avinash Kumar worked as a Post-Doctoral Fellow at the Indian Institute of Technology Kanpur until 2019. His post-PhD research experience includes Early Post-Doctoral Fellow in the Department of Mechanical Engineering, Indian Institute of Technology Delhi. He also worked as an assistant professor (TEQIP faculty) in a World Bank and MHRD (Government of India) project (NPIU) for a semester (2018) at theTHDC Institute of Hydropower Engineering & Technology, Tehri, Uttarakhand. He earned his PhD from the Department of Mechanical Engineering, Indian Institute of Technology Delhi, in 2018. He earned a Bachelor of Engineering in Mechanical Engineering from Rajiv Gandhi Proudyogiki Vishwavidyalaya, Bhopal, in 2010 and MTech degree in Mechanical Engineering from the Indian Institute of Technology Kanpur, India, in 2012. He was a research associate at the Bio-MEMS and Micro-fluidics Laboratory, Indian Institute of Technology Kanpur, India, from August 2012 to November 2012. He worked as a research associate with Prof. G. K. Ananthsuresh and Prof. Ashitava Ghoshal in Robert Bosch Centre for Cyber-Physical Systems, Mechanical Engineering Department, Indian Institute of Science Bangalore, for a year (2013). He qualified in Indian Engineering Services in 2010. He qualified in GATE-2010 with 98.20% in 2010. His PhD thesis was nominated for the best thesis award by the foreign and Indian examiner. He was selected in India-Sri Lanka Youth Exchange Program 2017, organized by the Ministry of Youth Affairs and Sports, Government of India. He was awarded DST-International Travel Fellowship in 2018 to visit Hawaii, the USA. He is currently working on various research projects by CSIR and DST-GOI. He has coordinated and organized many conferences and workshops at IIITDM Kancheepuram, Chennai, IIT Delhi, IIT Kanpur, and AIIMS Delhi. He has delivered many talks in webinars, faculty development programs, and workshops in the institutes. He has examined many MTech and PhD students at SRM University, Chennai. He has guided more than 10 BTech, M.Tech, and PhD students for their thesis.

Dr. Chandan Swaroop Meena is a scientist in the Building Energy Efficiency Department and assistant professor in the Academy of Scientific & Innovative Research (AcSIR) at CSIR-Central Building Research Institute, Roorkee (Ministry of Science and Technology, Government of India). He earned his PhD in thermal engineering from IIT Roorkee and did his MTech in thermal engineering from NIT Kurukshetra. He does research in solar energy utilization techniques, geothermal systems, building energy efficiency, two-phase flow, and heat transfer. He is a Life Member of Indian Society of Heat and Mass Transfer (ISHMT), Life Member of India Building Congress (IBC), and Life Member of The Institution of Engineers India (IEI). He has published 29 research articles in reputed journals and international conferences. He is associated with international conferences as invited speaker/ advisory board member/ review board member. He has delivered many invited talks in webinars, FDPs, and workshops.

Dr. Nitesh Dutt is an assistant professor in the Department of Mechanical Engineering, College of Engineering Roorkee, Uttarakhand, India. He has more than 7 years of teaching experience. He earned his bachelor's degree in Mechanical Engineering, and his master's degree and PhD from IIT Roorkee. He has published more than 11 research articles in international journals and conferences. His main areas of research are nuclear engineering, heat and mass transfer, thermodynamics, fluid mechanics, refrigeration and air conditioning, and computational fluid dynamics (CFD). He is an editor of two international books on mechanical and materials engineering published by CRC Press, Taylor & Francis Group.

Contributors

Adharsh Raj M. K
Department of Biotechnology and Medical Engineering
National Institute of Technology
Rourkela, India

P. Anil Kumar
Kakatiya Institute of Technology and Science
Warangal, India

Anju R. Babu
Department of Biotechnology and Medical Engineering
National Institute of Technology
Rourkela, India

Bansod Sneha Bharat
Department of Biotechnology and Medical Engineering
National Institute of Technology
Rourkela, India

Anil Kumar Birru
Department of mechanical Engineering
National Institute of Technology
Manipur, India

Sanjay Kumar Chak
Division of Manufacturing Processes and Automation Engineering
Netaji Subhas Institute of Technology (NSIT)
New Delhi, India

Prasun Chakraborti
Department of Mechanical Engineering
National Institute of Technology
Agartala, India

Gourhari Chakraborty
Department of Mechanical Engineering
National Institute of Technology
Andhra Pradesh, India

Anka Datta
Department of Mechanical Engineering
Indian Institute of Information Technology Design & Manufacturing
Chennai, India

Nitesh Dutt
Department of Mechanical Engineering
College of Engineering
Roorkee, India

Arun Kumar Singh Gangwar
Department of Mechanical Engineering
Technical Education Department
Kanpur, India

Yatika Gori
Department of Mechanical Engineering
Graphic Era University
Dehradun, India

Ravali Gourishetti
Indian Institute of Technology Madras
Chennai, India

Satoshi Ito
International Joint Department of Integrated Mechanical Engineering
    between IITG and Gifu University
Graduate School of Engineering
Gifu University
Gifu, Japan

P. Jawahar
Department of Mechanical Engineering
National Institute of Technology
Agartala, India

Subramani Kanagaraj
Department of Mechanical Engineering
Indian Institute of Technology
Guwahati, India

Amandeep Kaur
Conservative Dentistry and Endodontics
Department Dental College
RIMS
Imphal, India

M. Keerthika
Mechanical Engineering Department
Kakatiya Institute of Technology and Science
Warangal, India

Khundrakpam Nimo Singh
Department of Mechanical Engineering
National Institute of Technology
Imphal, India

Abhishek Kumar
Department of Mechanical Engineering
University of California
Merced, California

Ashwani Kumar
Department of Mechanical Engineering
Technical Education Department Uttar Pradesh Kanpur
India

Avinash Kumar
Department of Mechanical Engineering
Indian Institute of Information Technology Design & Manufacturing
Chennai, India

Chinu Kumari
Division of Manufacturing Processes and Automation Engineering
Netaji Subhas Institute of Technology (NSIT)
New Delhi, India

M. Manivannan
Department of Applied Mechanics
Indian Institute of Technology Madras
Chennai, India

Chandan Swaroop Meena
CSIR-Central Building Research Institute
Roorkee, India

Vamsi Krishna Pasam
Department of Mechanical Engineering
National Institute of Technology
Warangal, India

Arbind Prasad
Department of Mechanical Engineering
Katihar Engineering College
(under Department of Science and Technology,
Govt. of Bihar)
Katihar, India

K. Punnam Chander
Mechanical Engineering Department
Kakatiya Institute of Technology and Science
Warangal, India

K. Raja Narender Reddy
Mechanical Engineering Department
Kakatiya Institute of Technology and Science
Warangal, India

R. Sai Kumar
Mechanical Engineering Department
Kakatiya Institute of Technology and Science
Warangal, India

Arnab Sarmah
Department of Mechanical Engineering
Indian Institute of Technology
Guwahati, India
And
International Joint Department of Integrated Mechanical Engineering
    between IITG and Gifu University
Graduate School of Engineering
Gifu University
Gifu, Japan

S. Sathishkumar
Department of Mechanical Engineering
National Institute of Technology
Agartala, India

Varun Pratap Singh
Department of Mechanical Engineering
School of Engineering
University of Petroleum and Energy Studies
Dehradun, India

V. Srikanth
Mechanical Engineering Department
Kakatiya Institute of Technology and Science
Warangal, India

Chamaiporn Sukjamsri
Department of Biomedical Engineering
Srinakharinwirot University
Nakhon Nayok, Thailand

Chapter 1

Recent advancements and future trends in next-generation materials for biomedical applications

Avinash Kumar and Anka Datta
Indian Institute of Information Technology Design & Manufacturing Kanchipuram Chennai

Ashwani Kumar
Technical Education Department Uttar Pradesh Kanpur

Abhishek Kumar
University of California Merced

CONTENTS

DOI: 10.1201/9781003344810-1

1.1 INTRODUCTION

Smart materials have the capability to alter some of their properties in reaction to a variation in their immediate surroundings. Currently, smart materials are receiving a lot of consideration in the biomedical field owing to their potential use in a wide variety of biological devices (Greco & Mattoli, 2012). These smart materials have lighter weight, longer life, and corrosion resistance properties, which makes them a suitable candidate for biomedical applications. Smart materials can detect defects and fractures by altering their characteristics, making them helpful as a diagnostic tool.

Shape memory alloys and polymers are some of the varieties of smart materials that can change their physical shape in response to temperature variations. Other smart materials such as micro- or nanostructured block copolymers can change their surface properties from hydrophilic to hydrophobic and conversely due to temperature changes. Some varieties of cross-linked polymers (CLPs) can self-heal themselves from the damage caused by mechanical stresses just by re-establishing their cleaved chemical bonds. Piezoelectric materials are also a type of smart materials that can transform mechanical deformation to electrical potential and vice versa. Smart hydrogels are other types of novel materials that can swell/deswell in response to pH changes. These all smart materials are widely used in drug transfer systems due to their capabilities to respond to external stimuli. The examples shown above demonstrate the enormous capability of smart materials in biomedical applications (Greco & Mattoli, 2012; Kumar Natarajan, 2019; Teotia et al., 2015; Kumar et al., 2015; Kumar et al., 2014a). The aim of this chapter is to briefly discuss the current state of the smart materials in biomedical applications and their future scope in the biomedical application field. Biomaterials are commonly used in orthopaedic and dental applications, for example joint replacement, bone plates, vascular grafts, bone cement, heart valves, clips and staples to close wounds, dental implants for teeth stabilisation, artificial ligaments and tendons, stents, and lenses in eye surgery.

Biomaterials can be produced from nature or synthesised in the laboratory utilising a wide variety of materials such as metals, polymers, ceramics, and composites. They are often adapted for biomedical applications. In this chapter, readers will gain in-depth knowledge of advanced materials such as titanium (Ti), titanium alloys (Ti alloys), stainless steel, cobalt-chromium alloys (Co-Cr alloys), and composite materials for biomedical applications such as joint replacements, bone plates, artificial ligaments and tendons, bone cement, hip implants, and dental implants for tooth fixation.

1.2 NEED OF SMART MATERIALS IN BIOMEDICAL APPLICATIONS

Nowadays, smart materials (SMs) are mainly specified by their adaptability in response to environmental condition changes. Temperature, magnetic

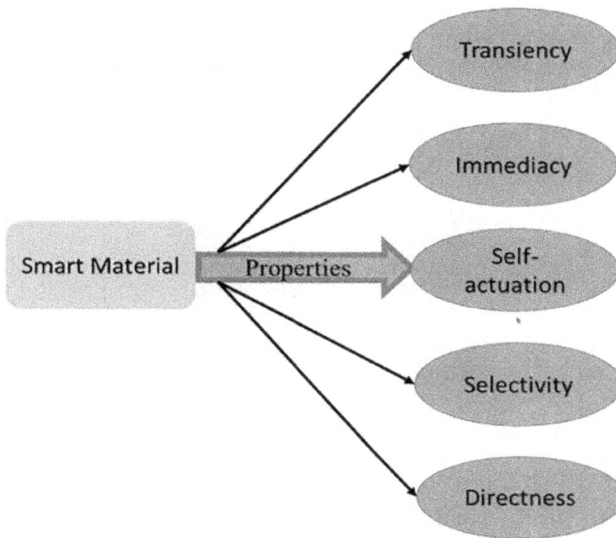

Figure 1.1 Properties of smart materials.

field, electric current, mechanical stress and strain, and hydrostatic pressure may all affect the size, colour, moisture content, odour, and viscosity of flow. As a result, the aforementioned characteristics may be used to satisfy the application of smart materials as sensors, actuators, and drug carriers in biomedical area (QADER et al., 2019). Figure 1.1 shows the various properties of smart materials.

Currently, in microtechnologies such as microelectromechanical system (MEMS) and nanoelectromechanical system (NEMS), scientists are using smart materials to enable unique functions such as sensing qualities (Liu, 2007). They may also offer novel approaches for powering and controlling the movement of micro-objects. The necessity for the fine-tuning of smart materials' physico-chemical characteristics and functions, as well as their adaptability to diverse work environments, is important in these micro-world applications.

In piezoelectric materials, due to the fact that this action also occurs in reverse, a voltage across the sample produces tension within the sample. Thus, well-engineered structures consisting of these materials may be made to bend, expand, or compress in response to an applied voltage (Kumar Natarajan, 2019). Polymer materials are increasingly being used instead of more common inorganic materials, such as semiconductors, to make small electronic and optical devices such as displays, transistors, and photovoltaic devices, which are smaller and more powerful (Greco & Mattoli, 2012).

In another example, the development of microactuating devices, which can be used for things such as wirelessly moving micro-objects, measuring local pressure, and pumping fluids in microfluidics, often requires elastic or compliant materials that can bend a lot and keep their shape even when they're bent. Because of the necessity for such a tough material, many polymers (particularly elastomers) are suitable options (Jeong & Gutowska, 2002; Kumar et al., 2007).

1.3 TYPES OF SMART MATERIALS

Smart materials' properties can be changed significantly by external factors. Smart materials have a built-in intrinsic sensor or actuator and a control mechanism that help these materials to respond to a stimulus in the exact way and in the accurate time and to return to their original state when the stimulus is gone. To keep the discussion limited here, we are addressing the categorisation of those smart materials that are more promising for the biomedical area.

1.3.1 Piezoelectric materials

Piezoelectric materials can generate electricity when they are pressurised. These are the ideal materials for all types of electro-mechanical transduction applications. In biomedical applications, piezoelectric materials are very important (Greco & Mattoli, 2012). They produce mechanical strain when electromotive force is applied on the surface of a piezoelectric material. As a result, the structure built by this material has the ability to bend, expand, and compress (Bahl et al., 2020; Mekhzoum et al., 2020; QADER et al., 2019). Figure 1.2 shows the phenomenon of piezoelectric effect in materials.

Piezoelectric materials are small and lightweight. They are high efficiency materials that scale well when shrunk. Piezoelectric materials can be used as a transducer between electric potential and frequency. And, they can also display their simultaneous actuator/sensor activity (Bahl et al., 2020;

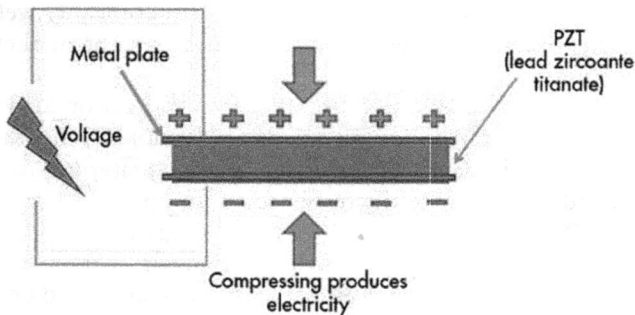

Figure 1.2 Piezoelectric effect. (Adapted with permission from Kumar Natarajan, 2019.)

Table 1.1 Types of piezoelectric materials

Types of piezoelectric materials	Examples
Natural crystals	Quart, Rochelle salt, ammonium phosphate
Liquid crystals	
Noncrystalline materials	Glass rubber, paraffin
Textures	Bone, wood
Synthetic piezoelectric materials	
Piezoceramics	Lead zirconate titanate, barium titanate, lead nibolate, zirconate titanate
Crystalline materials	Ammonium dihydrogen phosphate
Piezoelectric polymer	Polyvinylidene fluoride

Source: Adapted with permission from Mekhzoum et al. (2020).

Greco & Mattoli, 2012; Mekhzoum et al., 2020; QADER et al., 2019). Different kinds of piezoelectric materials are shown in Table 1.1.

1.3.2 Shape memory alloys

Shape memory alloys (SMAs) and shape memory polymers (SMPs) are examples of thermo-responsive materials. Heating may distort them and then restore them to their normal shape. When heated, metallic materials such as CuAlNi, NiTi, and NiTiCu can recover from distortion and restore themselves to their previous form. In general, the martensitic form is the more stable form at low temperatures and exhibits a pseudo-plastic behaviour, whereas the austenite form is the more stable form at high temperatures and exhibits super-elastic behaviour (Greco & Mattoli, 2012; Mekhzoum et al., 2020). Figure 1.3 shows the shape memory effect (SME) in biomaterials.

The SMA most often utilised in biomedical applications is called Nitinol (a 50/50 alloy of nickel and titanium). Nitinol, developed in 1962, quickly gained popularity because of its excellent mechanical characteristics and biocompatibility. Nitinol can be easily deformed mechanically. It can restore thermal stress up to 8% in martensitic phase. In austenitic phase, it shows elastic behaviour with flexibility 10%–20% more than the stainless steel. SMAs are used as a guiding wire for catheters inserted into arteries and veins and also for minimally invasive biopsy operations (Bahl et al., 2020; Greco & Mattoli, 2012; QADER et al., 2019). Figure 1.4 shows a stent and vena cava filter (VCF) made of Nitinol.

1.3.3 Magnetostrictive materials

Magnetostrictive materials may be magnetised or deformed in reaction to a magnetic field by applying stress. They are also known as the transducer.

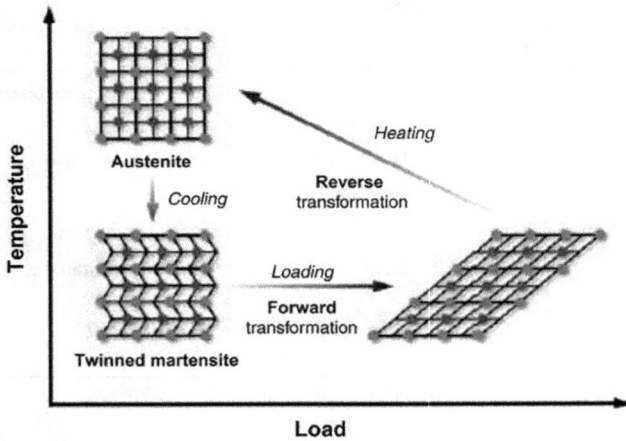

Figure 1.3 Shape memory effect. (Adapted with permission from Mekhzoum et al., 2020.)

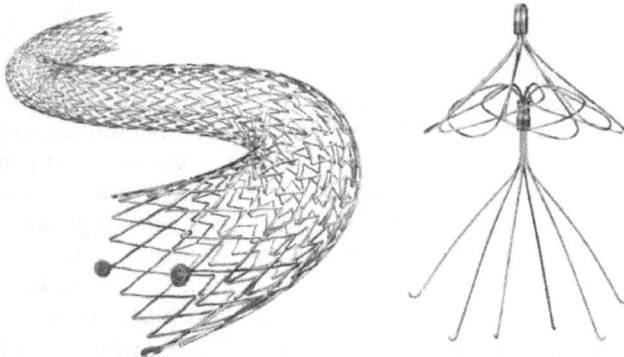

Figure 1.4 Stent and vena cava filter (VCF) made of Nitinol. (Adapted with permission from Kumar Natarajan, 2019.)

Due to magnetisation, a change in length may occur. Workability, good chemical stability, high Curie temperature, moderate saturation magnetisation, and high coercivity are some of the mechanical features of magnetostrictive materials (Keswani et al., 2019; QADER et al., 2019; Wahi et al., 2019). Cobalt ferrite has a high saturation magnetostriction. Due to the lack of earth natural essentials, it is an excellent alternative to Terfenol-D (Olabi & Grunwald, 2008). With the help of magnetic annealing, the magnetic properties of magnetostrictive materials can be changed (Lo et al., 2005; Wang et al., 2016). Table 1.2 shows the comparison and uses of smart materials.

Table 1.2 Applications of smart materials

Types of smart material	Advantage	Disadvantage	Use in biomedical application
Piezoelectric	• High-frequency response • Structure is simple	• Wear and heat generation • Difficult to manufacture	• Wrist pulse • Joint movement • Hand motion • Breathing • Heartbeat and respiration detection • Tissue engineering
Shape memory alloy	• Elastic behaviour • High fatigue behaviour • High strength • Corrosion resistance	• High cycle fatigue • Complicated design and high weight • Expensive	• Stent grafts • Inferior vena cava filters • Orthopaedics
Magnetostrictive	• Higher energy density • Intrinsic robustness	• Increase the complexity of the system • Less accuracy	• Biomonitoring systems • Pacemaker • Cardioverter-defibrillator • Hearing aid • Retinal implants

Source: Adapted from Bahl et al. (2020); Morgan (2004); Rasouli & Phee (2014); Zaszczyńska et al. (2020).

1.3.4 Responsive polymer gels

Polymer gels are another intriguing class of smart materials with a wide variety of biomedical uses because of their reactivity to temperature or chemical stimuli. A polymer gel is a soft, moist, elastic substance made up of a network of CLP chains that encloses a fluid (Kumar et al., 2016). Hydrogels are the most significant of these types in terms of biological uses (Greco & Mattoli, 2012). Both chemical and physical cross-linking approaches have been used to create hydrogels. The cross-linked polymeric network of covalently cross-linked thermo-responsive hydrogels swells reversibly as a function of temperature stimuli (Teotia et al., 2015). People are currently using hydrogel in a variety of biomedical applications such as actuators, sensors, chemical valves, and smart scaffolds (Greco & Mattoli, 2012).

1.4 RECENT ADVANCEMENTS IN MATERIALS FOR BIOMEDICAL APPLICATIONS

Cherkasov et al. (2020) developed a class of ultrasensitive smart nanoagents using a blend of gold nanoparticles and a low-energy polymer framework.

It features an input-dependent switchable on/off affinity for a target tissue. Smart materials which can flip between distinct states in response to chemical triggers are in great demand in biomedicine, where accurate diagnoses and treatment need unique responsiveness to biomarkers. The suggested approach involves coating the surface of a nanoparticle-based medication with a custom-designed extensible polymer chain and an input-switchable structure that changes the availability of the terminal receptor for product standardisation. The notion was implemented using a DNA model, which resulted in nanoagents with input-dependent cell-targeting abilities and responsiveness to as little as 30 fM DNA input in an experiment lasting 15 minutes. The suggested strategy has the potential to accelerate the growth of next-generation theranostic drugs and ultrasensitive nanosensors for step diagnostics.

Erdem et al. (2021) investigated COVID-19 diagnosis using smart materials with embedded sensor technology. Today, real-time reverse transcriptase (RT)-PCR test is a gold standard technique for accurate diagnosis of this disease. The shortcomings of this test, such as long test times, high costs, and the requirement for highly trained workers, have significantly prompted the use of sensor systems in clinical diagnostics. They state in their study that integrating smart materials into sensor technologies enables them to maximise their analytical properties, such as sensitivity, linear dynamic range, and specificity.

Tang et al. (2020) prepared bio-piezoelectric composites for biomedical applications using graphene/barium titanate/polymethyl methacrylate. One of the most successful approaches to increase the osteoinductivity of biomaterials such as polymethyl methacrylate (PMMA) bone cement is to incorporate $BaTiO_3$ (BT) particles. Their aim was to assess how piezoelectric properties of a composite matching with human bones can be found under the assumption of adequate mechanical properties. They observed that graphene improves the piezoelectric coefficient by enhancing the conduction and dielectric properties of the composites. The compressive strength of the above-mentioned composites that meet the standards for bone implant materials increased from 83.5 to 89.5 MPa with the addition of 0.5 volume percent graphene. G/BT/PMMA bio-piezoelectric composites have zero cytotoxicity, and the surface of the composite's graphene can also help in cell adhesion and propagation.

Chiu et al. (2021) studied the improvement of the SME in the β-Ti alloy for biomedical applications by including chromium. The effects of addition concentrations of Cr and Sn on the cold workability, phase constituents, mechanical properties, super-elasticity, and SME of β-Ti alloy were investigated. They discovered that a Ti–6Cr–3Sn alloy with excellent ultimate tensile strength, 40% ductility, 91% SME, and great shape recovery after reducing external stress could be a viable material for biomedical devices.

Additionally, metal ion cross-linked hydrogels have garnered considerable attention because of their unique properties, which include self-healing, quick recovery, biocompatibility, and good mechanical capabilities along with multistimuli sensitivity. As a result, researchers began to use chemical cross-links and metal ions to improve cross-linking density and provide hydrogels greater functional capabilities. The utilisation of synthetic metal ions provides not only cross-linking and durability, but also several benefits for the body's biological functioning. In biological systems, metal ions have a range of roles, including protein complexes, nucleic acid structure, electron transfer, charge balancing, oxidative catalysis, alkaline catalysis, bone structure, and DNA. So, in many aspects, employing these metal ions in tissue regeneration and biomaterials might be beneficial to the cells (Janarthanan & Noh, 2021).

1.5 APPLICATIONS OF NEXT-GENERATION MATERIALS IN BIOMEDICINE

Recent advances in smart materials have put a lot of emphasis on smart materials that respond to two or more different types of stimuli for more effective treatments (Thangudu, 2020). Multistimuli-responsive smart materials are better than single-stimulus-responsive smart materials because they have more functions and can be controlled more precisely through other parameters. As a result, several dual-stimuli- and multistimuli-sensitive smart nanomaterials have effectively been used in a range of biological applications with favourable treatment interventions (Genchi et al., 2017; Thangudu, 2020). Figure 1.5 shows the schematic diagram of numerous multifunctional nanostructures and their responsive stimuli, and Table 1.3 shows a list of few multistimuli-responsive smart materials and their uses in biomedical applications.

The removal and build-up of nanoparticles in non-targeted regions such as kidney and liver are the key issues in disease diagnosis. It is mostly owing to the fact that some nanomaterials are unable to penetrate biological barriers effectively. In future, smart nanomaterials have a lot of potential due to their flexibility, effectiveness, and multistimuli-responsive properties.

Recent advancements in next-generation materials in biomedicine, based on the area of application, is classified as follows.

1.5.1 Advanced materials for biomedical implants and surgical tools

Since the beginning of time, humans have been enticed to live a long life and have made attempts to create effective medications, equipment, and treatments that add to their comfort (Sharma & Khurana, 2018). A vast range of medical, assistive, and surgical instruments have been developed to improve human life. Materials that interact with living organisms are

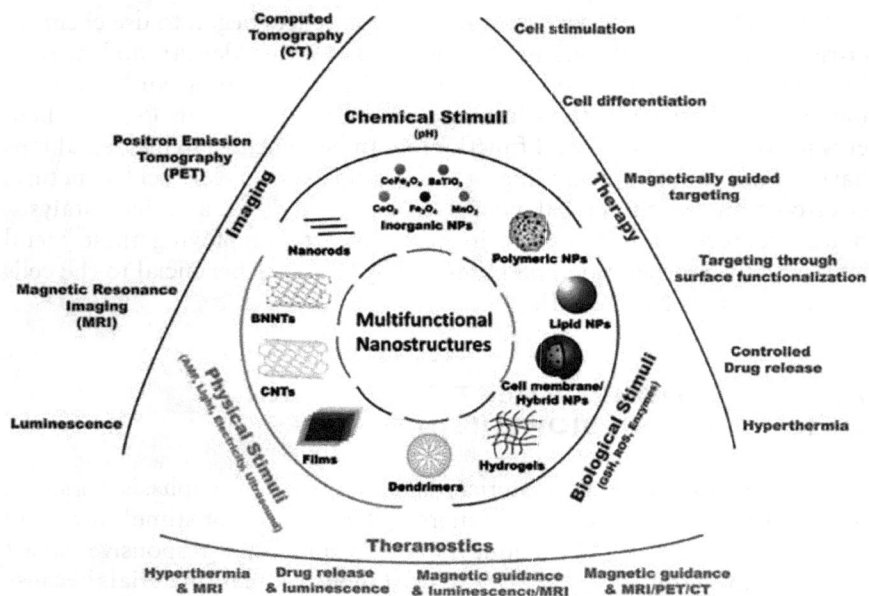

Figure 1.5 Schematic diagram of different multifunctional nanostructures and their response to different stimuli. (Adapted with permission from Genchi et al., 2017.)

Table 1.3 Multistimuli-responsive smart materials and their uses in biomedical applications

Multistimuli-responsive smart material	Application
PLA-g-P(NIPAAm-coMAA)	Drug carrier and release
DS-g-PEG/CRGD nanoparticles	Nucleus-targeted drug delivery
Fe3O4-capped MSNs	Drug delivery
DNA-capped MSNs	Controlled drug delivery
Azo-PDMAEMA	Controlled drug release
PMAAS-S@Fe_3O_4 microcontainers	Drug carrier, hyperthermia, imaging
P(NIPAAm-co-MAA)-coated magnetic MSNs	Drug delivery system
S-NPs@DOX	Drug delivery system
MFNPs	Targeting, drug delivery, MR imaging
rGO-PDA nanosheets	Drug supply and phototherapy

Source: Adapted with permission from Thangudu (2020).

known as biomaterials. Biomaterials are seldom utilised alone in medical applications, but are often incorporated into devices or implants (Valiulis, 2007). Various types of biomaterials are used as a medical device to improve the health condition of the patients. The biomaterials are mostly made of metallic materials, nanomaterials, biomaterials, ceramics, polymers, hybrid materials, and functionally graded materials (Valiulis, 2007).

Shape memory, which is one of the examples of properties of smart materials, is the ability to change the physical form in response to temperature changes and to subsequently return to the original shape when the temperature change is reversed. Some types of CLPs can repair themselves by resetting broken chemical bonds. Smart hydrogels, which can expand and contract with changes in pH, are used in many drug delivery systems. All these kinds of materials are used in biological implants and surgical tools (Greco & Mattoli, 2012).

Implants have changed substantially in recent decades with an emphasis on bioactive materials and osteogenesis. The newest approaches and tactics to strengthen and maintain the bone and implant attachment, as well as its interaction with the living system, have enabled new technologies to regulate and adjust microlevel surface features. The clinical prognosis of patients might be dramatically impacted if the implant covering delaminates from the implant surface. Establishing a uniform coating on the surface of the implant manufactured using metallic additives is difficult due to its peculiar topography. Hence, new coating processes are required for highly specialised topographical geometric implants to enhance the corrosion protection and to consequently increase the load bearing strength of the artificial components or joints. In future, we should expect to see innovative composite biomaterials that improve patient satisfaction (Hong et al. (2022). However, strong collaboration between surgeons, biologists, and engineers is required to meet the challenges in biomedical applications.

1.5.2 Advancements in shoulder arthroplasty

Total shoulder arthroplasty is recommended for people who have very bad glenohumeral osteoarthritis, which can cause a lot of wear on the back of the shoulder (Kersten et al., 2015). Glenoid bone loss and retroversion complicate and impair initial shoulder arthroplasty. Eccentric reaming, bone transplants, and reverse arthroplasty have all been utilised to treat bone loss and retroversion, but there is still no consented treatment (Ghoraishian et al., 2019; McFarland et al., 2016). Polymer designs for the back are now available in full-wedged, partially, and stepped configurations. Biomechanical and computational modelling findings support the use of enhanced implants to address glenoid retroversion greater than 15°. At the moment, the majority of clinical trials are retrospective case series. Currently, there is no consensus that one commercially available design is preferable than another. Individualisation of component type based on glenoid shape has been recommended by certain authors, although data demonstrating that these suggestions enhance the results are not available (Kersten et al., 2015).

1.5.3 Advancements in OPMF/KGG biocomposites for biomedical applications

In the last few years, there has been a big drop in petroleum resources and people are worried about the use of conventional polymers. This has led people around the world to start using natural fibres and biopolymers in many products. Oil palm is one of Malaysia's and Indonesia's most important crops. It's an excellent source of lignocellulosic fibres for biocomposites. The cellulose present in the oil palm fibres (OPFs) improves the strength of the composites (Asyraf et al., 2022; Srikanth et al., 2021). Natural gums are mostly derived from a variety of plants found in India's forests. Kondagogu gum, also known as "Cochlospermum gossypium," is a recently discovered gum. Oil palm mesocarp fibre (OPMF) is derived from locally accessible palm fruits in a similar way. The KGG matrix is primarily used in the preparation of OPMF-reinforced composites (Vinod et al., 2008). Srikanth et al. (2021) examined the mechanical and thermal characteristics of the alkali-treated OPMF/KGG composites. Thermographic study reveals that mass degradation causes less weight loss in treated laminates than in untreated laminates. Additionally, at a temperature of 149°C, differential thermal analysis (DTA) showed a weight loss difference of 0.53% with respect to time.

1.5.4 Advancements in coir fibre/KGG biocomposites

In tropical areas, coconuts (Cocos nucifera) are widely farmed. Coir fibre-reinforced biocomposites made from coconut husk are gaining popularity due to a growing market need for environmentally friendly materials that are biodegradable and recyclable. Coconut husks and shells are often discarded as garbage, although they may be used as important raw materials for the development of environmentally beneficial biocomposite products. Coir fibres are robust and rigid, which makes them ideal for use in biocomposite materials as reinforcement. However, due to the inhomogeneous coir material features, the resultant biocomposites exhibit a wide range of performance characteristics. Fibre-reinforced composites made of coir perform better mechanically, thermally, and physically than those made of synthetic fibres. Pre-treating the surfaces of coir fibre improves the mechanical properties of coconut fibre-reinforced composites (Hasan et al., 2021). Jayavani et al. (2016) investigated the effects of substances such as silane, alkali, sodium periodate coupled with p-aminophenol and urea, hydrogen peroxide, sodium hypochlorite, benzene diazonium salt, and maleated coupling agent on coir fibre composites. Coir fibre has a low cellulose concentration when compared to other natural fibres. However, chemical treatments and interface alteration can improve its mechanical, thermal, and other properties.

1.5.5 Advancements in microfluidics for isolation of tumour cells

Circulating tumour cells play a big part in cancer spread and may be used to predict how well cancer is isolated and found. Many microfluidic systems have been developed as a result of advancements in the area of miniaturisation during the previous decade. Microfluidic systems can be used to study cell biology in a controlled environment, which led to the rapid development of microfluidic isolation of circulating tumour cells. The magnetophoresis method is currently widely used to isolate circulating tumour cells. This is because magnets can provide forces from a distance (Luo & He, 2020).

In microfluid systems, fluids are pumped into very tiny polymeric channels in very small volumes. These amounts can be micro-, nano-, or picolitres. These channels are built into small chips. A variety of special structures in the chips, such as pump, valve, and channel, allow the chips to accept different types of fluids into the channels. The chips are mostly made of crystals, silicone, or elastomers (Sahmani et al., 2016). Limited purity and low efficacy are some of the drawbacks of magnetic isolation technology (MIT) based on a microfluidic system. In order to advance the field of circulating tumour cells (CTCs), new methods must be implemented to improve efficiency and achieve more pure populace with more cell viability for future study. The best CTC isolation device should be able to capture a large range of cell populations, sustain cellular activities in the chip circuits, and allow further cell analysis (Luo & He, 2020).

1.5.6 Advancements in finishing processes of biomedical tools and implants

Polishing, removing molten layers, and completing complicated forms on the workpiece's exterior surfaces are done using abrasive flow finishing. Abrasive flow finishing procedures offer a broad variety of applications and may be employed as a finishing solution on any shop floor (Das et al., 2020). Advanced finishing procedures are divided into two categories: those that require magnetic fields and those that do not. Magnetic abrasive finishing (MAF) and magnetorheological finishing (MRF) fall under the first category, whereas abrasive flow machining (AFM) falls under the second. The choice of polishing particle is critical for ultra-fine finishing (UFF) of complicated free-form products (Azami et al., 2020).

1.5.7 Advancements in biomaterials for femur bone fracture and healing

The only bone at the thigh region is the femur bone. Femurs interact with the tibiae's distal ends at the knee. The position of the femur bone, called the "shaft", is said to be the most balanced in the entire bone. The femur is the most distal bone of the leg in animals that are capable of walking or running. During typical weightlifting activities, this femur bone is responsible for the bulk of the body weight (Aftab et al., 2021; Kumar et al., 2014b; Gangwar et al., 2019; Gangwar et al., 2021). Femur fractures happen when it is acted upon by a large value of applied force, such as when someone falls from high places or has an infection in the bone.

Fractures of the femur that are small, short fissures in the bone normally do not need surgery, but if the bone is broken, damaged, or completely displaced, the bone needs to be treated with prosthetic implants to make it look and work better. Fracture management products include wire, needles, screws, and plates as well as spine fixation devices and artificial tendons, for persons who have fractured bones (Kirthana et al., 2020). Different types of prosthetic plates that have been used since the beginning of implant surgery are compression plates (CP), dynamic compression plates (DCP), limited contact dynamic compression plates (LCDCP), and locking compression plates (LCP) (Igna & Schuszler, 1980; Malekani et al., 2012; Mehmood et al., 2014; Nag & Banerjee, 2012; Kumar et al., 2022).

Normally, smart metals, smart polymers, smart composites, and smart ceramics are utilised to create these prosthetic plates. Titanium (Ti) is also used as a prosthetic implant since it is more robust and lighter than stainless steel. PMMA, polylactic acid, and polyglycolic acid (PGA) are examples of polymers and composites used for femur bone healing application. The bioceramics category includes alumina and hydroxyapatite (HA) (Kirthana et al., 2020).

1.5.8 Advancements in biopolymer and biocomposites for orthopaedic and other biomedical applications

Biodegradable polymers and composites have witnessed a substantial growth in use for biomedical applications over the last two decades, since these materials not only have adequate physical and mechanical qualities, but also have the potential to be removed from the body. As a result, biodegradable polymers are excellent biomaterials for tissue regeneration because they allow host tissue infiltration during deterioration. Surgical aids, controlled and local medication delivery devices, and tissue engineering scaffolds are all made of biodegradable polymers. Biodegradable polymers are mainly synthetic and natural polymers. Synthetic polymers include Poly(α-esters), polyfumarates, polyurethanes, polyanhydrides, and polyphosphates, and natural polymers include protein-based polymers, polysaccharide-based polymers, and natural polyesters.

1.6 CONCLUSIONS

It is evident that smart materials offer many functional advantages over conventional implantable alloys. Smart materials have lighter weight, longer life, and corrosion resistance as compared to conventional materials. Smart materials can change their characteristics in response to the changes in external stimuli such as temperature, pH, vibration, and magnetic field. In this chapter, we discussed the various types of smart materials, their specific properties, and their advantages and disadvantages and also discussed the current applications of smart materials in the biomedical industry. Nowadays, scientists are working to increase the capability of smart materials in biomedical applications, especially that of the multistimuli-responsive smart materials in which a single material would be able to respond to changes in various parameters in the environment. Finally, we hope that the insights in this chapter will aid in better understanding the capabilities of various types of smart nanomaterials and in the development of a more sophisticated smart material framework for future biological applications aimed at improving human health.

REFERENCES

Aftab, S. G., Faisal, A., Hussain, H., Sreedhara, B., Babu, N. R., & Praveen, B. A. (2021). Structural analysis of human femur bone to select an alternative composite material. *Materials Today: Proceedings*. https://doi.org/10.1016/J. MATPR.2021.08.197.

Asyraf, M. R. M., Ishak, M. R., Syamsir, A., Nurazzi, N. M., Sabaruddin, F. A., Shazleen, S. S., Norrrahim, M. N. F., Rafidah, M., Ilyas, R. A., Rashid, M. Z. A., & Razman, M. R. (2022). Mechanical properties of oil palm fibre-reinforced polymer composites: A review. *Journal of Materials Research and Technology, 17*, 33–65. https://doi.org/10.1016/J.JMRT.2021.12.122.

Azami, A., Azizi, A., Khoshanjam, A., & Hadad, M. (2020). A new approach for nanofinishing of complicated-surfaces using rotational abrasive finishing process. *Materials and Manufacturing Processes, 35*(8), 940–950. https://doi.org /10.1080/10426914.2020.1750631.

Bahl, S., Nagar, H., Singh, I., & Sehgal, S. (2020). Smart materials types, properties and applications: A review. *Materials Today: Proceedings, 28*, 1302–1306. https://doi.org/10.1016/J.MATPR.2020.04.505.

Cherkasov, V. R., Mochalova, E. N., Babenyshev, A. V., Vasilyeva, A. V., Nikitin, P. I., & Nikitin, M. P. (2020). Nanoparticle beacons: Supersensitive smart materials with on/off-switchable affinity to biomedical targets. *ACS Nano, 14*(2), 1792–1803. https://doi.org/10.1021/ACSNANO.9B07569/SUPPL_FILE/ NN9B07569_SI_001.PDF.

Chiu, W. T., Wakabayashi, K., Umise, A., Tahara, M., Inamura, T., & Hosoda, H. (2021). Enhancement of the shape memory effect by the introductions of Cr and Sn into the β–Ti alloy towards the biomedical applications. *Journal of Alloys and Compounds, 875*, 160088. https://doi.org/10.1016/J. JALLCOM.2021.160088.

Das, S., Kibria, G., Doloi, B., & Bhattacharyya, B. (Eds.). (2020). *Advances in Abrasive Based Machining and Finishing Processes*. https://doi.org/10.1007/978-3-030-43312-3.

Erdem, Ö., Derin, E., Sagdic, K., Yilmaz, E. G., & Inci, F. (2021). Smart materials-integrated sensor technologies for COVID-19 diagnosis. *Emergent Materials*, 4(1), 169–185. https://doi.org/10.1007/S42247-020-00150-W/TABLES/1.

Gangwar, A. K. S., Rao, P. S., Kumar, A., & Patil, P.P. (2019). Design and analysis of femur bone: BioMechanical aspects. *Journal of Critical Reviews*, 6(4), 133–139.

Gangwar, A. K. S., Rao, P. S., & Kumar, A. (2021). Bio-mechanical design and analysis of femur bone. *Materials Today: Proceedings*, 44(Part 1), 2179–2187. https://doi.org/10.1016/j.matpr.2020.12.282.

Genchi, G. G., Marino, A., Tapeinos, C., & Ciofani, G. (2017). Smart materials meet multifunctional biomedical devices: Current and prospective implications for nanomedicine. *Frontiers in Bioengineering and Biotechnology*, 5, 80. https://doi.org/10.3389/FBIOE.2017.00080/BIBTEX.

Ghoraishian, M., Abboud, J. A., Romeo, A. A., Williams, G. R., & Namdari, S. (2019). Augmented glenoid implants in anatomic total shoulder arthroplasty: Review of available implants and current literature. *Journal of Shoulder and Elbow Surgery*, 28(2), 387–395. https://doi.org/10.1016/J.JSE.2018.08.017.

Greco, F., & Mattoli, V. (2012). *Introduction to Active Smart Materials for Biomedical Applications*, pp. 1–27. https://doi.org/10.1007/978-3-642-28044-3_1.

Hasan, K. F., Horváth, P. G., Bak, M., & Alpár, T. (2021). A state-of-the-art review on coir fiber-reinforced biocomposites. *RSC Advances*, 11(18), 10548–10571. https://doi.org/10.1039/D1RA00231G.

Hong, Z., Hong, M., Wang, N., Ma, Y., Zhou, X., & Wang, W. (2022). A wearable-based posture recognition system with AI-assisted approach for healthcare IoT. *Future Generation Computer Systems*, 127, 286–296. https://doi.org/10.1016/J.FUTURE.2021.08.030.

Igna, C., & Schuszler, L. (1980). Current concepts of internal fixation of fractures. *Canadian Journal of Surgery*, 23(3), 213–214. https://doi.org/10.1016/0020-1383(81)90078-4.

Janarthanan, G., & Noh, I. (2021). Recent trends in metal ion based hydrogel biomaterials for tissue engineering and other biomedical applications. *Journal of Materials Science & Technology*, 63, 35–53. https://doi.org/10.1016/J.JMST.2020.02.052.

Jayavani, S., Deka, H., Varghese, T. O., & Nayak, S. K. (2016). Recent development and future trends in coir fiber-reinforced green polymer composites: Review and evaluation. *Polymer Composites*, 37(11), 3296–3309. https://doi.org/10.1002/PC.23529.

Jeong, B., & Gutowska, A. (2002). Lessons from nature: Stimuli-responsive polymers and their biomedical applications. *Trends in Biotechnology*, 20(7), 305–311. https://doi.org/10.1016/S0167-7799(02)01962-5.

Kersten, A. D., Flores-Hernandez, C., Hoenecke, H. R., & D'Lima, D. D. (2015). Posterior augmented glenoid designs preserve more bone in biconcave glenoids. *Journal of Shoulder and Elbow Surgery*, 24(7), 1135–1141. https://doi.org/10.1016/J.JSE.2014.12.007.

Keswani, B. C., Patil, S. I., Kolekar, Y. D., & Ramana, C. V. (2019). Improved magnetostrictive properties of cobalt ferrite ($CoFe_2O_4$) by Mn and Dy co-substitution for magneto-mechanical sensors. *Journal of Applied Physics*, 126(17), 174503. https://doi.org/10.1063/1.5114815.

Kirthana, S., Nagamallika, J. V. L., & Nizamuddin, M. K. (2020). A FEA on Assembled fractured human femur bone with and without HA coated prosthetic plate material. *Materials Today: Proceedings*, 22, 2890–2898. https://doi.org/10.1016/J.MATPR.2020.03.422.

Kumar, A., Srivastava, A., Galaev, I. Y., & Mattiasson, B. (2007). Smart polymers: Physical forms and bioengineering applications. *Progress in Polymer Science*, 32(10), 1205–1237. https://doi.org/10.1016/J.PROGPOLYMSCI.2007.05.003.

Kumar, A., Behmad, S. I., & Patil, P. (2014a). Vibration characterization and static analysis of cortical bone fracture based on finite element analysis. *Engineering and Automation Problems*, No. 3, 115–119.

Kumar, A., Jaiswal, H., Garg, T., & Patil, P. (2014b). Free vibration modes analysis of femur bone fracture using varying boundary conditions based on FEA. *Procedia Materials Science*, 6, 1593–1599. https://doi.org/10.1016/j.mspro.2014.07.142.

Kumar, A., Mamgain, D.P., Jaiswal, H., & Patil, P. (2015). Modal analysis of hand arm vibration (humerus bone) for biodynamic response using varying boundary conditions based on FEA. *Advances in Intelligent Systems and Computing*, 308, 169–176. https://doi.org/10.1007/978-81-322-2012-1_18.

Kumar, A., Datta, S., & Kalyanasundaram, D. (2016). Permeability and effective slip in confined flows transverse to wall slippage patterns. *Physics of Fluids*, 28(8), 082002. https://doi.org/10.1063/1.4959184.

Kumar, A., Gori, Y., Rana, S., Sharma, N.K., & Yadav, B. (2022). FEA of humerus bone fracture and healing. *Advanced Materials for Biomechanical Applications* (1st ed.) CRC Press. https://doi.org/10.1201/9781003286806.

Kumar Natarajan, S. (2019). Biomedical application of smart materials-An overview. *International Journal of Recent Research Aspects*, 6, 9–12.

Liu, C. (2007). Recent developments in polymer MEMS. *Advanced Materials*, 19(22), 3783–3790. https://doi.org/10.1002/ADMA.200701709.

Lo, C. C. H., Ring, A. P., Snyder, J. E., & Jiles, D. C. (2005). Improvement of magnetomechancial properties of cobalt ferrite by magnetic annealing. *IEEE Transactions on Magnetics*, 41(10), 3676–3678. https://doi.org/10.1109/TMAG.2005.854790.

Luo, L., & He, Y. (2020). Magnetically driven microfluidics for isolation of circulating tumor cells. *Cancer Medicine*, 9(12), 4207–4231. https://doi.org/10.1002/CAM4.3077.

Malekani, J., Schmutz, B., Gu, Y., Schuetz, M., & Yarlagadda, P. (2012). Orthopedic bone plates: Evolution in Structure, Implementation technique and biomaterial. *GSTF Journal of Engineering Technology*, 1(1). https://doi.org/10.5176/2251-3701_1.1.23.

McFarland, E. G., Huri, G., Hyun, Y. S., Petersen, S. A., & Srikumaran, U. (2016). Reverse total shoulder arthroplasty without bone-grafting for severe glenoid bone loss in patients with osteoarthritis and intact rotator cuff. *The Journal of Bone and Joint Surgery. American Volume*, 98(21), 1801–1807. https://doi.org/10.2106/JBJS.15.01181.

Mehmood, S., Ansari, U., Ali, M. N., & Rana, N. F. (2014). Internal fixation: An evolutionary appraisal of methods used for long bone fractures. *International Journal of Biomedical and Advance Research*, 5(3), 142–149. https://doi.org/10.7439/IJBAR.V5I3.627.

Mekhzoum, M. E. M., Qaiss, A. E. K., & Bouhfid, R. (2020). Introduction: Different types of smart materials and their practical applications. *Polymer Nanocomposite-Based Smart Materials*, pp. 1–19. https://doi.org/10.1016/B978-0-08-103013-4.00001-7.

Morgan, N. B. (2004). Medical shape memory alloy applications—the market and its products. *Materials Science and Engineering: A, 378*(1–2), 16–23. https://doi.org/10.1016/J.MSEA.2003.10.326.

Nag, S., & Banerjee, R. (2012). Fundamentals of medical impllant materials. *ASM International, 23*. www.asminternational.org.

Olabi, A. G., & Grunwald, A. (2008). Design and application of magnetostrictive materials. *Materials & Design, 29*(2), 469–483. https://doi.org/10.1016/J.MATDES.2006.12.016.

Qader, İ. N., Kök, M., Dagdelen, F., & Aydoğdu, Y. (2019). A review of smart materials: Researches and applications. *El-Cezeri, 6*(3), 755–788. https://doi.org/10.31202/ECJSE.562177.

Rasouli, M., & Phee, L. S. J. (2014). Energy sources and their development for application in medical devices. *Expert Review of Medical Devices, 7*(5), 693–709. https://doi.org/10.1586/ERD.10.20.

Sahmani, M., Vatanmakanian, M., Goudarzi, M., Mobarra, N., & Azad, M. (2016). Microchips and their significance in isolation of circulating tumor cells and monitoring of cancers. https://www.scopus.com/inward/record.uri?eid=2-s2.0-84965002258&partnerID=40&md5=e8b954b7727198bcd5 1696265313f397.

Sharma, M., & Khurana, S. M. P. (2018). Biomedical engineering: The recent trends. *Omics Technologies and Bio-Engineering: Volume 2: Towards Improving Quality of Life*, pp. 323–336. https://doi.org/10.1016/B978-0-12-815870-8.00017-6.

Srikanth, V., Narender Reddy, K. R., & Rao, D. K. N. (2021). Bio-composites: A study on behavior of oil palm mesocarp fiber reinforced Kgg. *IOP Conference Series: Materials Science and Engineering, 1123*(1), 012005. https://doi.org/10.1088/1757-899X/1123/1/012005.

Tang, Y., Chen, L., Duan, Z., Zhao, K., & Wu, Z. (2020). Graphene/barium titanate/polymethyl methacrylate bio-piezoelectric composites for biomedical application. *Ceramics International, 46*(5), 6567–6574. https://doi.org/10.1016/J.CERAMINT.2019.11.142.

Teotia, A. K., Sami, H., & Kumar, A. (2015). Thermo-responsive polymers: Structure and design of smart materials. *Switchable and Responsive Surfaces and Materials for Biomedical Applications*, pp. 3–43. https://doi.org/10.1016/B978-0-85709-713-2.00001-8.

Thangudu, S. (2020). Next generation nanomaterials: Smart nanomaterials, significance, and biomedical applications. *Applications of Nanomaterials in Human Health*, pp. 287–312. https://doi.org/10.1007/978-981-15-4802-4_15.

Valiulis, A. (2007). The advanced structural materials for living beings implants. *Journal of Vibroengineering, 9*, 323.

Vinod, V. T. P., Sashidhar, R. B., Sarma, V. U. M., & Vijaya Saradhi, U. V. R. (2008). Compositional analysis and rheological properties of gum kondagogu (Cochlospermum gossypium): A tree gum from India. *Journal of Agricultural and Food Chemistry, 56*(6), 2199–2207. https://doi.org/10.1021/JF072766P.

Wahi, S. K., Kumar, M., Santapuri, S., & Dapino, M. J. (2019). Computationally efficient locally linearized constitutive model for magnetostrictive materials. *Journal of Applied Physics*, *125*(21), 215108. https://doi.org/10.1063/1.5086953.

Wang, J., Gao, X., Yuan, C., Li, J., & Bao, X. (2016). Magnetostriction properties of oriented polycrystalline $CoFe_2O_4$. *Journal of Magnetism and Magnetic Materials*, *401*, 662–666. https://doi.org/10.1016/J.JMMM.2015.10.073.

Zaszczyńska, A., Gradys, A., & Sajkiewicz, P. (2020). Progress in the applications of smart piezoelectric materials for medical devices. *Polymers*, *12*(11), 2754. https://doi.org/10.3390/POLYM12112754.

Chapter 2

Advanced materials in biological implants and surgical tools

Anka Datta and Avinash Kumar

Indian Institute of Information Technology Design & Manufacturing Kanchipuram Chennai

Ashwani Kumar

Technical Education Department Uttar Pradesh Kanpur

Abhishek Kumar

University of California Merced

Varun Pratap Singh

University of Petroleum and Energy Studies Dehradun

CONTENTS

DOI: 10.1201/9781003344810-2

2.1 INTRODUCTION

Since the beginning of time, humans have been enticed to live a long life and have made attempts to create effective medications, equipment, and treatments that add to their comfort (Sharma & Khurana, 2018). A vast range of medical, assistive, and surgical instruments have been developed to improve human life. The medical device business has had rapid growth and high research activity during the last decade. By 2023, the bio-implant market is expected to develop at a compound annual growth rate (CAGR) of 8.6%. According to recent reports, the bio-implant industry is worth more than $100,000 million (Sumayli, 2021). Incorporating ideas from allied fields such as pharmaceutics, bioengineering, biotechnology, and chemistry has allowed researchers to build improved medical solutions that benefit patients. An ageing population, accidents, and sports-related injuries are driving the ever-increasing need for ortho-, dental, cardiology, ophthalmic, and IVD equipment, as well as enhanced diagnostic tests, in the worldwide medical device market (Munir et al., 2020; Wegner et al., 2014).

Materials that interact with living organisms are known as biomaterials. Biomaterials are seldom utilized alone in medical applications, but are often incorporated into devices or implants (Valiulis, 2007). Various types of biomaterials are used as a medical device to improve the health condition of the patients. The ancient Egyptians used animal sinew to make sutures for wound mending (Munir et al., 2020). The first generation of materials was created in the 1960s and 1970s for internal usage. The biomaterials are mostly made of metallics, nanomaterials, biomaterials, ceramics, polymers, hybrid materials, and functionally graded material (Valiulis, 2007).

The biological environment is harsh, and many materials may break down quickly or gradually. With time, implant materials may solubilize, crumble, become rubbery, or become stiff. Because of the potential uses in a broad variety of active structures and devices, remarkable advancements in nanoscience and nanotechnology have attracted a lot of attention in the biomedical field (Greco & Mattoli, 2012; Valiulis, 2007). Certain types of cross-linked polymers are capable of self-healing from mechanical damage by re-establishing cleaved chemical bonds. Smart hydrogels that can expand/contract in response to changes in pH are widely used in drug delivery systems. All these kinds of materials are used in biological implants and surgical tools (Greco & Mattoli, 2012). Biocompatibility and mechanical strength are critical requirements for any implanted biomaterial used in biomedical, orthopaedic, or dentistry applications. The biomaterial should not be poisonous to the host tissues and should not cause allergic or inflammatory responses (Prasadh et al., 2021). Surgical instruments used to cut soft biological tissues are needed to be sharp and wear-resistant. Tiny cutting edges are needed to optimize cutting performance, prevent tool failure, and extend tool life (Liu et al., 2021).

Bioactive materials are currently the focus of medical devices, which have changed substantially in the recent decades. With advances in technology, new materials are emerging that may replace present implant materials and help the future implant generations in mimicking the qualities, features, and function of actual bone (Bandopadhyay et al., 2019). Thus, the purpose of this analysis is to highlight the biomaterials that have been examined the most often and to emphasize their enormous potential in the fields of implantable devices and surgical equipment.

2.1.1 Implantable devices and surgical tools

A biomedical device is a device that is used to treat or restore function. Medical gadgets are designed to assist people in overcoming injuries and diseases, thereby increasing their quality of life. Before allowing their commercialization and clinical use, these medical devices should be shown safe and operative (Munir et al., 2020). In 2013, the worldwide market for implantable materials was estimated to be worth roughly $75.1 billion. Recent technologies, whether wearable or implanted, have shown promise in managing illnesses such as Alzheimer's, diabetes, orthopaedic disorders, and cardiovascular diseases via real-time parameter monitoring. Finally, implantable devices have accelerated the pace of research in areas where personalized or real-time diagnostics are required. Biomedical implants are a broad term that refers to a variety of medical remedies for different body ailments. Table 2.1 shows the various types of implantable devices and surgical tools.

2.1.1.1 Cardiovascular implants

Cardiovascular illnesses are the main cause of mortality, owing to congenital heart defects, a sedentary and unhealthy lifestyle, and an ageing population (Wegner et al., 2014). All these cardiovascular implantable devices help the patients to keep up their good health. Pacemaker is normally a small device that helps patients to control their heartbeats. After an atherosclerosis-related constriction, vascular stents are utilized to restore blood flow. Heart valves are used for aortic and mitral heart valves replacement. Defibrillators are used for controlling the heartbeats, and artificial hearts are used to mimic the ventricular movement by air-driven pump (Wegner et al., 2014).

2.1.1.2 Central and peripheral neural implants

The human nervous system can detect and react to changes in the body and its surroundings. The nervous system regulates variations in the internal

Table 2.1 Types of biological implants and surgical tools

Biological implants

Types	Devices
Cardiovascular implants	• Pacemakers • Vascular stents • Heart valves • Defibrillators • Artificial hearts
Central and peripheral neural implants	• Neural prostheses • Retinal prostheses • Cochlear prostheses
Orthopaedic implants	• Bone plates • Bone screws • Compression hip screws
Dental implants	• Screws • Veneers • Crowns

Surgical tools

Types	Use
Scalpels, needles, and drill bits	They are used to cut, separate, remove, or suture biological tissues

Source: Adapted from Arsiwala et al. (2014); Bandopadhyay et al. (2019); Munir et al. (2020); Okazaki (2019).

and external surroundings to preserve homeostasis (a state of relative body stability). The neurological system can be affected by hypoxia infections, stroke, poisoning, chronic degenerative sickness, and severe trauma. Injuries or chronic neurodegenerative diseases create some of the most serious nervous system problems and damage (Wegner et al., 2014). Neural prostheses are assistive devices that help people regain the abilities they have lost as a consequence of a neurological disease (Fekete & Pongrácz, 2017). Retinal implants are an innovative technique to restore vision in retinal disorders. Vision-restoring implants that interact with the retina have been created (Chuang et al., 2014). Cochlear implants seem to represent the first major step in the quest for a mechanical hearing aid for the severely deaf. Deaf people may now access a vast variety of information because of current implant improvements (House et al., 2016).

2.1.1.3 Orthopaedic implants

The major objective of orthopaedic implants is to offer mechanical stability in order to preserve optimum bone alignment and function during physiologic stress of bones and joints. Thus, the implants promote pain alleviation and more normal use of the wounded limb or body part, resulting in a faster return to function. Orthopaedic implants, for example, indirectly aid the biological components of bone repair by reducing undesired shear stress (Goodman et al., 2013; Kumar et al., 2015; Kumar et al., 2014a; Kumar et al., 2022). The bone plate's function is to maintain shattered bone segments in place when they are subjected to crucial compression forces, hence expediting healing (Benli et al., 2008). The function of bone screw is to provide rigid internal fixation to all types of fractures of the scaphoid (Goldhagen et al., 1994).

2.1.1.4 Dental implants

Tooth loss is quite prevalent and may occur as a consequence of illness or trauma; this necessitates the use of dental implants such as screws, veneers, and crowns to give support for tooth replacement (Gaviria et al., 2014). Figure 2.1 shows the various types of implantable devices in human body.

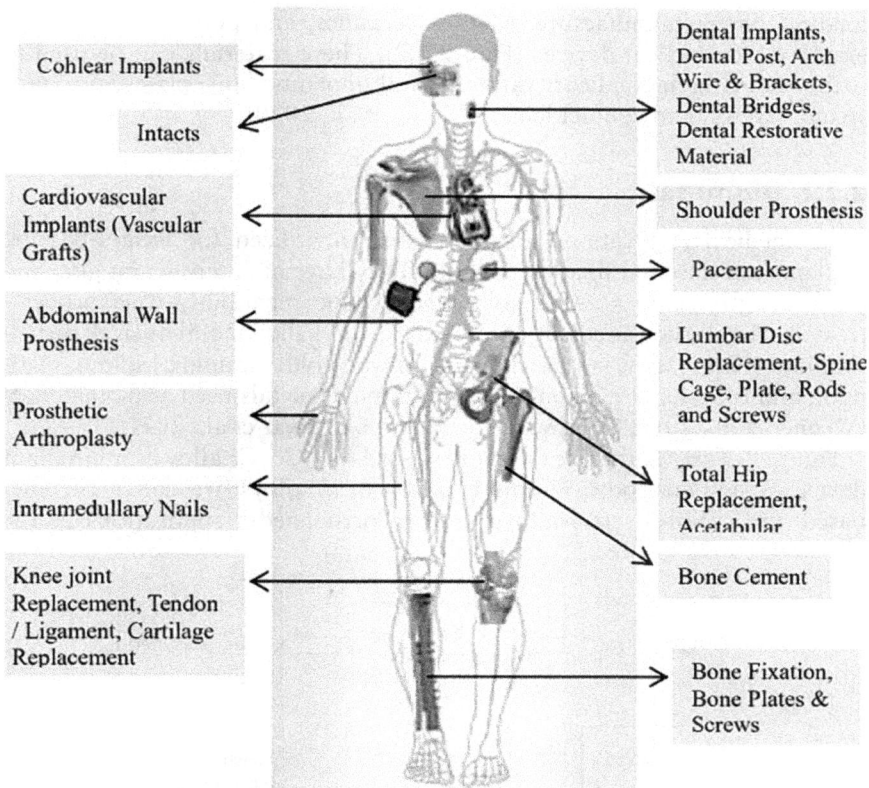

Figure 2.1 Different types of implants in human anatomy. (With permission from Patel & Gohil, 2012.)

2.2 BIOMATERIALS

Biomaterials have been used by ancient cultures. At the beginning of the 20th century, efforts towards implant manufacturing were minimal, since the medical industry was not dedicated to the use of metallic or non-metallic artificial components. Sir William Arbuthnot Lane, a British surgeon, working with Albin Lambotte, a Belgian surgeon, and Agnes Gwendoline Hunt, a British nurse, performed the first surgical treatment for the healing of long bone and joint fractures (Bandopadhyay et al., 2019). Modern synthetic materials, surgical procedures, and sterilizing processes have allowed biomaterials to be used in many novel ways.

However, understanding biomaterials is a multidisciplinary activity that combines numerous scientific fields such as biology, physics, biology, chemistry, and tissue engineering, material science engineering and manufacturing engineering. As illustrated in Figure 2.1, the discipline has developed significantly in recent decades as a result of substantial breakthroughs in regenerative medicine, tissue engineering, and their application to biomedical device manufacture. Metals, ceramics, and polymers can all be employed as medical devices (Figure 2.2). These materials can be used in orthopaedic implants, heart valves, dental implants, bone plates, coronary stents, screws, and contact lenses (Munir et al., 2020).

2.2.1 Biometals

In biomedical applications, metals are often utilized for weight-bearing implants and internal fixation systems. They have high tensile, fatigue, and yield strength qualities, as well as acceptable biocompatibility, when properly treated. Metals such as cobalt-chromium (Co-Cr) alloy, stainless steel, nickel-titanium (Ni-Ti) alloy, magnesium alloy, silver, gold, titanium, iridium, platinum, and tungsten are among the most popular metals used as biomaterials (Wegner et al., 2014; Gangwar et al., 2019; Gangwar et al., 2021).

Figure 2.3 shows the use of stainless steel and Co-Cr alloy as an implant device in human body. The first metal-based alloys are cobalt-chrome-based and stainless steel alloys used in orthopaedic applications in the

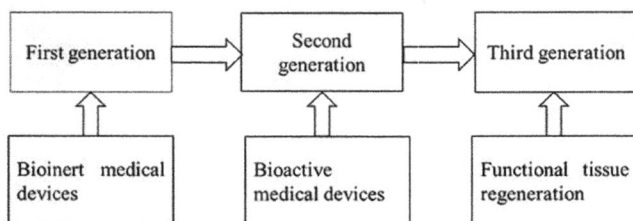

Figure 2.2 Evaluation of biomaterials. (Adapted from Munir et al., 2020.)

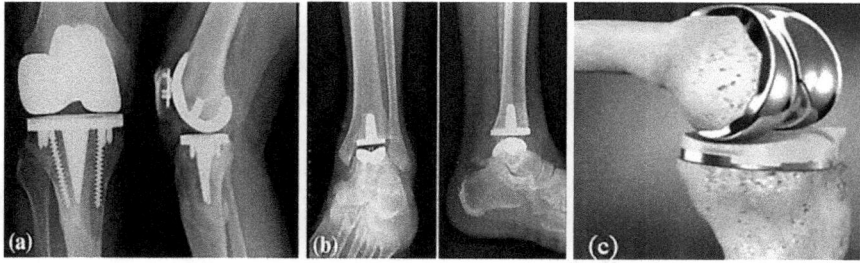

Figure 2.3 Stainless steel implants in (a) knee and (b) ankle. (c) Knee replacement made from CoCrMo alloy.

20th century. 316L stainless steel implants have previously proven to be effective. Because it is inexpensive, has been demonstrated to be safe, and has excellent mechanical qualities, 316L SS has been the most frequent alloy used in implantable devices until recently. Titanium (Ti) and Ti alloys were first employed in the 1940s, and Ni-Ti alloys were developed in the 1960s owing to their unique mechanical properties (Bandopadhyay et al., 2019). Table 2.2 shows the comparison of various mechanical properties of implant materials to natural bones.

Table 2.3 shows a comparison of different metals in biomedical applications. Stainless steel is resistant to fatigue and so suitable for biological tissues. 316L single-phase austenitic stainless steel (FCC) is the most often used stainless steel for medical implants (Rezaie et al., 1998). The cobalt-chromium alloys can be broken down into two main types: the CoCrMo alloy and Ni (2.5%). They have been employed in dentistry and the fabrication of prosthetic joints for a long period of time. The CoNiCrMo alloy and Mo (9%–11%)] have been used to make the stems of prostheses for joints that are heavily used, like in the hip and knee. The cobalt-based alloys are of excellent corrosion resistance even in a corrosive environment due to the formation of a passive film in the human body (Patel & Gohil, 2012). Titanium alloys for tibial tray and titanium-niobium nitride for femoral component are utilized owing to strong corrosion resistance, great biocompatibility, low density, and low elastic modulus (Pande & Dhatrak, 2021).

2.2.2 Bioceramics

Ceramics are non-metallic, inorganic materials that have a high strength of compressive nature and are biologically inert. As a result, their application in bulk is confined to functions that solely apply compressive stresses (Kamachi Mudali et al., 2003). Ceramic materials have a high degree of brittleness and hardness, excellent stiffness and strength, high resistance to wear and corrosion, and a low density (Patel & Gohil, 2012). They are electrical and thermal insulators. Ceramics are utilized in dentistry,

Table 2.2 Comparison of the properties of various biomaterials and natural bones

Properties	(NB) Natural bone	Stainless steel	Co-Cr alloy	Ti alloy	Mg	Mg alloy		XLPE	Hydroxyapatite
						Mg-6ZN	Mg-1Ca-Zn		
(ρ) Density (g/cm^3)	1.80–2.10	7.90–8.10	8.3–9.2	4.4–4.5	1.74–2.00	N/A	N/A	0.47–1.26	3.1
(E) Elastic modulus (GPa)	3.0–20	189–205	230	110–117	41–45	42.3	45.3	0.005–0.69	73–117
(σ) Yield strength (MPa)	130–180	170–310	450–1000	758–1117	65–100	169.5	67	20	600
(K_{Ic}) Fracture toughness (MPa m$^{0.5}$)	3.0–6.0	50–200	N/A	55–115	15–40	N/A	N/A	N/A	0.7

Source: Adapted from Prasadh et al. (2021);Valiulis (2007).

Table 2.3 Types of metals in biomedical applications

Type of material	Composition	Application
Stainless steel		
Martensitic	10.5%–18% Cr	Dental chisels, bone curettes, heart valves, orthodontic pliers and scalpels, chisels and gouges, and dental burs
Ferritic	11%–30% Cr	Guide pins, solid handles for instruments, and fasteners
Austenitic	16%–26% Cr	Knee implants, hypodermic needles, steam sterilizers, dental impression trays, guide pins, hip nails, hip implants and knee implants, and cannulae
Cobalt alloy		
F75	58%–70% Co, 26%–30% Cr	Bone plate used for fracture fixation, dental implants, maxillofacial implants
F799	58%–70% Co, 26%–30% Cr	Dental implants, surgical tools, bone replacement, hip and knee replacements
F562	35% Co, 20% Ni, 10% Mo	Dental root implant, pacer, and screws
F90	20% Cr, 15% W, 10% Ni	Dental and orthopaedic prosthesis and suture
Titanium alloy		
Ti–6Al–4V	90% Ti, 6% Al, 4% V	Total knee and hip joint replacements
Ti–6Al–7Nb	87% Ti, 6% Al, 7% niobium (Nb)	Fracture fixation plates, femoral hip stems, spinal components, dental implants, rods, nails, screws, and wire
Ti–13Nb–13Zr	72% Ti, 13.5% Nb, 13.5% Zr	Orthopaedic implants

Source: Adapted from Bandopadhyay et al. (2019); Patel & Gohil (2012); Rezaie et al. (1998).

orthopaedics, and medical sensors. Ceramics usually fail with little plastic deformation and are vulnerable to fractures or other flaws (Patel & Gohil, 2012; Rezaie et al., 1998). Table 2.4 shows the mechanical properties of various ceramics.

Ceramic materials were successfully used to replace the material used in hip prostheses (i.e. metallic femoral heads) (Figure 2.4). For many years, alumina has been employed because it is less susceptible to wear and friction, while zirconia's strength makes it ideal for medical uses with less wear (Gamble et al., 2017).

2.2.2.1 Alumina

The main sources of high-purity alumina are bauxite and natural corundum. The first ceramic that was used in the medical field was high-density,

Table 2.4 Mechanical properties of various ceramics

Ceramics types	Young's modulus (GPa)	Strength (MPa) (compressive nature)	Strength (MPa) (tensile nature)	Hardness (GPa)
Bio-inert				
Alumina (Al_2O_3)	380	4500	350	20–30
Zirconia (ZrO_2)	150–200	2000	200–500	10–30
Pyrolytic carbon	18–28	517	280–560	
Bioactive				
Bioglass and glass ceramics	22	500	56–83	3–9
Bioresorbable				
Calcium phosphate	40–117	510–896	69–193	< 1

Source: Adapted from Patel & Gohil (2012); Wegner et al. (2014).

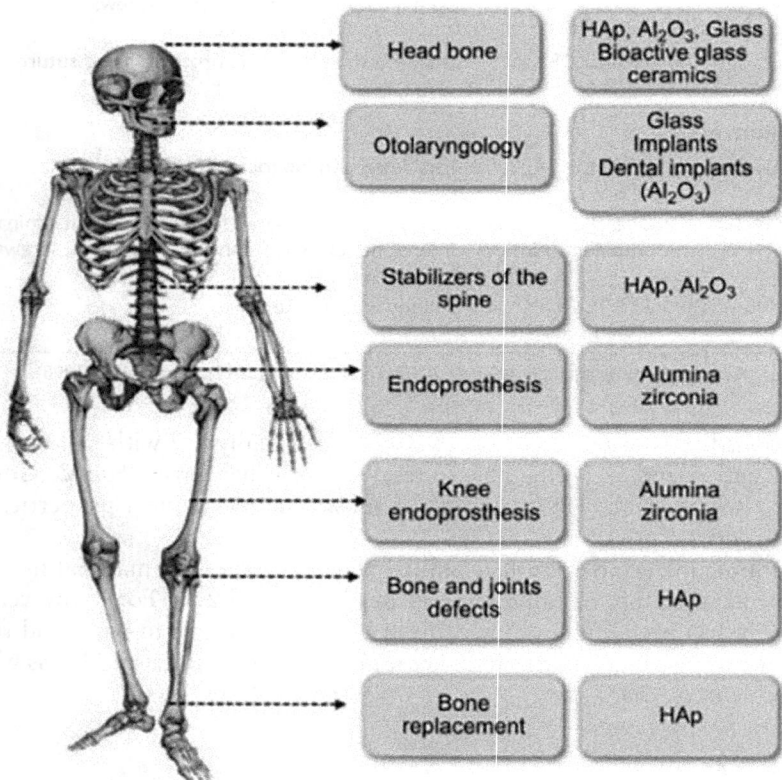

Figure 2.4 Application of a ceramic biomaterial in human body. (Adapted from Renugadevi et al., 2020.)

high-purity alumina (Patel & Gohil, 2012; Rezaie et al., 1998). Generally, alumina has a hardness of 20–30 GPa. Even though alumina is hard, it doesn't have much friction or wear, which are big benefits for replacing joints with alumina. An artificial joint or tooth made of alumina is a good choice because it is non-allergenic, is biocompatible, is non-sensitizing, and has good wear and friction properties. Alumina is a good choice for artificial joints and teeth because it has a lot more compressive strength than tensile strength (Rezaie et al., 1998).

2.2.2.2 Zirconia

Because of its strength and corrosion resistance, zirconia (ZrO_2) is a typical bio-inert ceramic used in hip and knee prostheses (Wegner et al., 2014). For its great toughness and mechanical strength, zirconia is a promising biomaterial. Ceramics are very biocompatible and may be used in huge implants like in hip joint replacement (Ibrahim et al., 2017; Patel & Gohil, 2012; Rezaie et al., 1998).

2.2.2.3 Pyrolytic carbon

Carbon is a very flexible element that may be found in a variety of forms. In addition to having a high degree of compatibility with bone and other tissues, the mechanical characteristics of carbon are quite comparable to those of bone, making it an excellent option for orthopaedic implants (Patel & Gohil, 2012).

2.2.2.4 Bioglass and glass ceramics

Bioglass ceramics have a capacity to form a direct chemical interaction with bones. Because of this quality, a vast range of bioglasses with varying proportions have been created as bone-replacing materials (Dimitriadis et al., 2021). Bioglass ceramics have extensively been utilized for the treatment of bone deformities. The porosity of bioglass is advantageous in terms of resorption and biological activity (Patel & Gohil, 2012).

2.2.2.5 Calcium phosphate

Calcium orthophosphates (CaPs) are the most widely explored biomaterials. CaPs are obtained in a variety of crystalline phases and chemical compositions. The most popular of these are β-tricalcium phosphate (β-TCP), hydroxyapatite (HA), and biphasic HA/TCP ceramics. The solubility of these CaPs in the biological environment rises when the concentration of β-TCP rises (i.e. β-TCP > biphasic CaP > HA) (Bianchi et al., 2014).

2.2.3 Biopolymers

Polymers are readily formed due to their malleable qualities, which include mechanical, electrical, chemical, and thermal capabilities. Additionally, their biocompatibility and ability to be combined with other materials to form composites make them an ideal material for biomedical applications (Kulshrestha & Mahapatro, 2008). Various types of polymers, including fibres, fabrics, rods, and viscoelastic liquids, are being studied for implant applications. Polymers have recently been implemented for hip socket replacement in orthopaedic implant applications (Kamachi Mudali et al., 2003). Different types of polymers used in biomedical applications and their mechanical properties are shown in Table 2.5.

2.3 SMART MATERIALS

Smart biomaterials have pushed the frontiers of current medicine. These biomaterials may function as an 'on–off' switch for many applications from nanometre to micrometre sizes due to their unique environmental responsiveness. These biomaterials might be used for complicated diagnostics and clinical therapies. The need for emergency medical treatment, personal protective equipment, medication, diagnostic kits, and vaccinations has skyrocketed since the COVID-19 epidemic caused global misery. To fulfil this growing need, a paradigm change from traditional biomaterials to intelligent systems is required (Amukarimi et al., 2021).

Shape memory alloys (SMAs) and polymers could change their shape and then revert to its original shape in response to temperature changes. Due

Table 2.5 Types of polymers used in biomedical applications and their mechanical properties

Polymers	Tensile strength S_{UTS} (MPa)	Young's modulus S_{UTS} (MPa)	Application
Poly(methyl methacrylate) (PMMA)	30.0	2.20	Bone cement
Nylon 6/6	76.0	2.80	Sutures, catheters, and dentures
Poly(ethylene terephthalate)	53.0	2.14	Blood vessels
Poly(lactic acid)	28.0–50.0	1.2–3.0	Sutures
Polypropylene	28.0–36.0	1.1–1.55	Suture materials
Polytetrafluoroethylene	17.0–28.0	0.50	Vascular grafts
Silicon rubber	2.80	Up to 10	Finger joints
Ultra-high molecular weight polyethylene (UHMWPE)	>35	4.0–12.0	Knee, hip, and shoulder joints

Source: Adapted from Klee & Höcker (2000); Patel & Gohil (2012); Rezaie et al. (1998); Shakiba et al.. (2021).

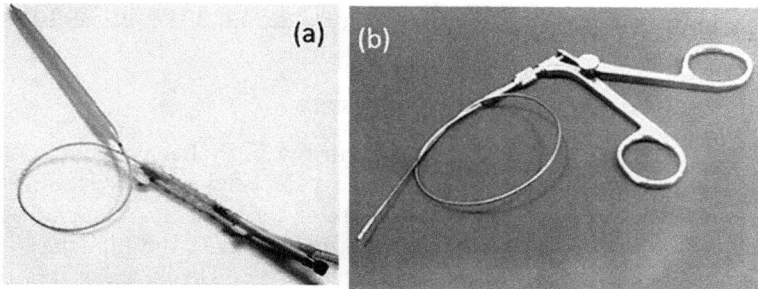

Figure 2.5 (a) Intra-aortic balloon pump; (b) Nitinol-based biopsy forceps. (Adapted with permission from Greco & Mattoli, 2012.)

to these qualities, SMAs may also function as actuators, changing their surface characteristics from hydrophobic to hydrophilic (and/or vice versa) in response to temperature changes (Schild, 1992). Some of cross-linked polymers that have the ability to self-heal their own system are all well-known examples of smart materials (Trask et al., 2007; Wu et al., 2008). Figure 2.5a and b shows the use of SMA in biomedical applications.

The SMA most often utilized in biomedical applications is called Nitinol (a 50/50 alloy of nickel and titanium). Mechanical qualities together with a resistance towards strong fatigue at high stresses make Nitinol material ideal for minimally invasive surgery, such as a guide wire for catheters inserted into arteries and veins (Greco & Mattoli, 2012).

2.4 PROPERTIES OF MATERIALS IN BIOMEDICAL APPLICATIONS

Biomaterials must possess unique features that can be modified to match the requirements of a certain application. For instance, a biomaterial must be biocompatible, be corrosion-resistant, be non-carcinogenic, and have a low wear and rating. However, other restrictions may apply depending on the application. At times, these criteria might be diametrically opposed (Hin, 2004).

2.4.1 Biocompatibility

The biocompatibility of a biomaterial is a critical prerequisite for its use. A biocompatible substance is one that performs in a given application while eliciting an adequate host reaction. In order to determine a material's biocompatibility, two important elements are considered necessary: the host responses generated through the material and the degradation of the material in the body environment. Often, both elements should be taken into account (Bandopadhyay et al., 2019; Boutrand, 2012; Eliaz, 2019).

2.4.2 Mechanical forces on implants

Usually, the devices that are implanted in the body has a lot of complex service conditions and high loads. They are exposed to both dynamic and static loads depending on the movements of the patients. The changes in load depend on the position in the walking cycle. At the hip, the load is approximately four times the weight of the body, and at the knee, it is about three times the weight. The number of loading and unloading cycles that happen over a certain amount of time is also important (Kamachi Mudali et al., 2003).

2.4.3 Sterilizability

Sterilization is required for the biomaterial. Gamma, gas, and steam autoclaving are all sterilization techniques. When exposed to high-energy radiation, such as gamma, certain polymers such as polyacetal depolymerize and release toxic formaldehyde gas. As a result, ETO sterilization is the optimal method for these polymers (Hin, 2004).

2.4.4 Biofunctionality

The material must perform according to its design specifications in applications such as fluid flow and blood control (e.g. artificial heart), electrical stimulation (e.g. pacemaker), light transmission (e.g. implanted lenses), space filling (e.g. aesthetic surgery), and sound transmission (e.g. cochlear implant) (Hin, 2004; Patel & Gohil, 2012).

2.4.5 Wear resistance

Implant loosening is caused due to high coefficient or a smaller amount of wear resistance (Alvarado et al., 2006; Okazaki & Gotoh, 2005). Friction-induced corrosion is a major concern because it releases non-compatible metallic ions. Mechanical loading can also cause corrosion fatigue and accelerated wear processes (Hin, 2004; Patel & Gohil, 2012). Figure 2.6 shows the wear of an implant material.

Figure 2.6 shows the bone resorption that causes the implant loosening due to the discharge of worn debris from the implant. The implant loosens as a result of this process, and it must be replaced. Furthermore, the presence of impurities near the contact, such as metal beads, hydroxyapatite produced from coating, and cement particles, aggravates the generation of wear debris (Geetha et al., 2009).

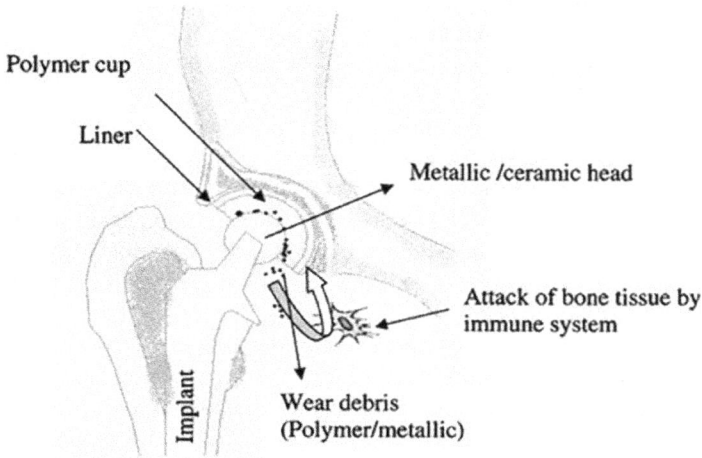

Polymer cup

Liner

Metallic /ceramic head

Attack of bone tissue by immune system

Implant

Wear debris
(Polymer/metallic)

Figure 2.6 Wears in implant devices. (With permission from Geetha et al., 2009.)

2.4.6 Manufacturability

Machinable, mouldable, and extrudable biomaterials are desirable. Modern manufacturing procedures are now required to provide the required quality in orthopaedic equipment (Hin, 2004; Patel & Gohil, 2012).

2.5 RECENT TRENDS IN BIO-IMPLANTS AND SURGICAL TOOLS

New technologies to regulate and change microlevel surface features have enabled new strategies and techniques to strengthen and interact with the biological system and sustain the bone, as well as implant attachment. New materials are emerging as a result of technological advancements that may eventually replace current implant materials and lead to implant generations that mimic the properties, features, and function of real bone (Bandopadhyay et al., 2019; Kumar et al., 2014b).

Tantalum (Ta) and niobium (Nb) are new materials that could be used to make new implants. In terms of biomedical applications, amorphous alloys are used because they have more strength, lower Young's moduli, and better corrosion resistance than the crystal alloys. $Pd_{78}Si_{16}Cu_{6-x}$, Zr-7.6Ni-12.3Cu-3.5Al, and Zr-11Ti-132Cu-10Ni-3.7Be are some examples of amorphous alloys (Okazaki, 2019). In order to make amorphous alloys that are safer for living bodies, it is required to alter the compositions (Okazaki, 2019). Nowadays, amorphous thin-film metallic glasses (TFMGs) are becoming a centre of attraction for the researches because they have the superior mechanical and biological properties that are suitable for the bio-implants and surgical tools. The current progress is going on in Fe-based, Ti-based, Zr-based, and Mg-based TFMGS for bio-implants and surgical tools (Rajan & Arockiarajan, 2021).

Mg and its alloys have recently gained favour as bio-implant materials due to their mechanical characteristics that are comparable to those of the human body, especially bone. In terms of bio-implant materials, Mg is much superior to other metals, as well as polymers and ceramics. As a consequence, research for biodegradable magnesium implants is now ongoing, and the findings should be fairly exciting sooner rather than later (Dutta et al., 2020).

Bioceramics, particularly calcium silicate-based compounds, have widely been used in orthopaedic and dental applications because of their excellent biocompatibility. Because of its more adjustable mechanical features and faster disintegration rate, akermanite (AK; $Ca_2MgSi_2O_7$), a bioceramic comprising Ca, Mg, and Si, has recently obtained a lot of interest. As a result, it's been hypothesized that this notion, as well as the introduction of akermanite bioceramic, might lead to substantial improvements in the area of bone tissue engineering in the near future (Zadehnajar et al., 2021).

Nowadays, bioceramics are also widely used for the treatment of osteomyelitis (OM). OM is a bone disease caused by bacteria named *Staphylococcus aureus*. OM is characterized by high recurrence and death rates. In the area of bone regeneration, CP is used as scaffolds, pastes, cement, and hydrogels, either alone or in composites with other polymers (Radwan et al., 2020). The transition to intelligent biomaterials will result in improved supervision and localization of treatments, which will result in cost-effective healthcare procedures and the development of novel biomaterials with multistimuli-responsive characteristics (Amukarimi et al., 2021).

Kaliaraj et al. (2021) developed a new bio-implant using surface coating. They used medical grade stainless steel (316L SS) for the surface modification. Nanocomposite coatings were developed using novel calcia-stabilized zirconia (CaSZ) and silver-CaSZ. Metals such as stainless steel, cobalt-chrome, titanium, and their alloys are now often used in implantology as prosthetic implant materials.

According to clinical data, prolonged exposure to metallic prosthetic materials causes localized corrosion in the human body. 316L SS prosthetic implants, in particular, are prone to failure due to the release of metallic ions into the adjacent tissues via crevice and pitting corrosion (Sivakumar et al., 1994; Sivakumar & Rajeswari, 1992). Surface modification techniques using oxides, nitrides, oxynitrides, ceramics, and ternary and multi-component materials have all been studied (Arunkumar et al., 2020; Hee et al., 2019; Kaliaraj et al., 2016; Zhao et al., 2011).

Among various coatings, ceramic materials are prominent because of their high biocompatibility. Antimicrobial compounds are added to ceramic coatings to enhance microbicidal activity in nearby tissues and reduce antibiotic consumption, which helps to prevent initial bacterial invasion (Kaliaraj et al., 2021).

Xu et al. (2021) also coated certain Ti6Al4V alloys with α-Ta5Si3 using the double cathode glow discharge process. Additionally, the coatings encouraged the creation of bone-like mineralized layers and improved the adherence, spreading, and proliferation of MC3T3-E1 cells. Ag alloying significantly enhanced the antibacterial ability of the α-Ta5Si3 coating against *Escherichia coli* (*E. coli*) and *Staphylococcus aureus* (*S. aureus*) strains, and the liberated Ag ions enhanced antibacterial performance.

People are also using laser texturing for enhancing the surface properties of the bio-implant and surgical tool operation (Kumar et al., 2018; Kumar Seth, 2012; Parihar et al., 2021). Laser surface texturing (LST) is the most revolutionary technique in this situation because it allows for fine control of surface topography, morphology, wettability, and chemistry, making it ideal for creating biocompatible, antimicrobial, and early bone-healing surfaces. Laser texturing materials can be used in orthopaedic and dental implants.

2.6 CONCLUSIONS AND FUTURE SCOPE

This chapter briefly summarized the various biomaterials and their applications in the biomedical industry. Implants have changed substantially in recent decades, with an emphasis on bioactive materials and osteogenesis. New advancements that allow for the control and modification of microscopic surface characteristics have allowed the development of new approaches and tactics for strengthening and sustaining bones and implant attachment, as well as their interactions with the biological process. Patients of various ages are increasingly choosing implants, which has increased their appeal. Numerous non-metallic biomaterials used in medical devices have superior, long-term biocompatibility and physiological functionality. Estimating biocompatibility is required before using such materials in biomedical implants or sensors.

Conformal coating on hard surfaces is a current orthopaedic research problem. The clinical prognosis of patients might be dramatically impacted if the implant covering delaminates from the implant surface. Establishing a uniform coating on the implant surface of metallic additive manufactured implants is difficult due to their peculiar topography. Hence, new coating processes are required for highly specialized topographical geometric implants and corrosion protection for increasing the load-carrying capacity of the artificial joints.

Mg metal and its alloys have adequate biocompatibility and mechanical qualities that deteriorate in a living system (Pogorielov et al., 2017). There has been no current research on Mg-based biodegradable composites that examined how they degrade in the lab or interact with cells. An investigation of how a substance breaks down in the body can lead to new research.

In vitro investigations of biodegradable Mg composites reveal that they elicit a greater immunological response, which has to be matched with in vivo studies. In addition, fresh studies should be conducted to determine if the Mg composite can be utilized to heal fractures in large and small animal models (Dutta et al., 2020). Currently, there are very few research approaches that have been published for developing biocompatible and antibacterial attributes together in the implant materials. So, further research could be done in this area. Many researchers have used laser texturing for enhancing the surface properties of the bio-implant and surgical tool operation. The current technologies for coating and modifying surfaces are insufficient for long-term durability. Laser surface texturing (LST) is the most revolutionary technique in this situation because it allows for fine control of surface topography, morphology, wettability, and chemistry, making it ideal for creating biocompatible, antimicrobial, and early bone-healing surfaces.

In future, we should expect to see innovative composite biomaterials that improve patient satisfaction. Thus, detailed investigations are required to identify the behaviour of these innovative materials prior to clinical application, as well as a technique to increase biocompatibility (i.e. immediate biological responses). However, strong collaboration between biologists, surgeons, and engineers is required to meet the challenges of biomedical applications.

REFERENCES

Alvarado, J., Maldonado, R., Marxuach, J., & Otero, R. (2006). Biomechanics of Hip and Knee Prostheses 1. https://www.semanticscholar.org/paper/ Biomechanics-of-Hip-and-Knee-Prostheses-1-Alvarado-Maldonado/03e4118 75fa8570732dfcf1a02b97027d60470ea#extracted

Amukarimi, S., Ramakrishna, S., & Mozafari, M. (2021). Smart biomaterials—A proposed definition and overview of the field. *Current Opinion in Biomedical Engineering, 19*, 100311. https://doi.org/10.1016/J.COBME.2021.100311.

Arsiwala, A., Desai, P., & Patravale, V. (2014). Recent advances in micro/nanoscale biomedical implants. *Journal of Controlled Release, 189*, 25–45. https://doi. org/10.1016/J.JCONREL.2014.06.021.

Arunkumar, S., Subramani Sundaram, M., Suketh Kanna, K. M., & Vigneshwara, S. (2020). A review on aluminium matrix composite with various reinforcement particles and their behaviour. *Materials Today: Proceedings, 33*, 484– 490. https://doi.org/10.1016/J.MATPR.2020.05.053.

Bandopadhyay, S., Bandyopadhyay, N., Ahmed, S., Yadav, V., & Tekade, R. K. (2019). Current research perspectives of orthopedic implant materials. *Biomaterials and Bionanotechnology*, 337–374. https://doi.org/10.1016/ B978-0-12-814427-5.00010-X.

Benli, S., Aksoy, S., Havitcioğlu, H., & Kucuk, M. (2008). Evaluation of bone plate with low-stiffness material in terms of stress distribution. *Journal of Biomechanics*, *41*(15), 3229–3235. https://doi.org/10.1016/J. JBIOMECH.2008.08.003.

Bianchi, M., Urquia Edreira, E. R., Wolke, J. G. C., Birgani, Z. T., Habibovic, P., Jansen, J. A., Tampieri, A., Marcacci, M., Leeuwenburgh, S. C. G., & Van Den Beucken, J. J. J. P. (2014). Substrate geometry directs the in vitro mineralization of calcium phosphate ceramics. *Acta Biomaterialia*, *10*(2), 661–669. https://doi.org/10.1016/J.ACTBIO.2013.10.026.

Boutrand, J. P. (2012). Biocompatibility and performance of medical devices. In *Biocompatibility and Performance of Medical Devices*. https://doi. org/10.1533/9780857096456.

Chuang, A. T., Margo, C. E., & Greenberg, P. B. (2014). Retinal implants: A systematic review. *British Journal of Ophthalmology*, *98*(7), 852–856. https:// doi.org/10.1136/BJOPHTHALMOL-2013-303708.

Dimitriadis, K., Tulyaganov, D. U., & Agathopoulos, S. (2021). Development of novel alumina-containing bioactive glass-ceramics in the CaO-MgO-SiO$_2$ system as candidates for dental implant applications. *Journal of the European Ceramic Society*, *41*(1), 929–940. https://doi.org/10.1016/J. JEURCERAMSOC.2020.08.005.

Dutta, S., Gupta, S., & Roy, M. (2020). Recent developments in magnesium metal–matrix composites for biomedical applications: A review. *ACS Biomaterials Science & Engineering*, *6*(9), 4748–4773. https://doi.org/10.1021/ ACSBIOMATERIALS.0C00678.

Eliaz, N. (2019). Corrosion of metallic biomaterials: A review. *Materials*, *12*(3). https://doi.org/10.3390/MA12030407.

Fekete, Z., & Pongrácz, A. (2017). Multifunctional soft implants to monitor and control neural activity in the central and peripheral nervous system: A review. *Sensors and Actuators B: Chemical*, *243*, 1214–1223. https://doi. org/10.1016/J.SNB.2016.12.096.

Gamble, D., Jaiswal, P. K., Lutz, I., & Johnston, K. D. (2017). The use of ceramics in total hip arthroplasty. *Review Article*, *4*. https://doi.org/10.19080/ OROAJ.2017.04.555636.

Gangwar, A. K. S., Rao, P. S., Kumar, A., & Patil, P.P. (2019). Design and analysis of femur bone: BioMechanical aspects. *Journal of Critical Reviews*, *6*(4), 133–139.

Gangwar, A. K. S., Rao, P. S., & Kumar, A. (2021). Bio-mechanical design and analysis of femur bone. *Materials Today: Proceedings*, *44*(Part 1), 2179–2187. https://doi.org/10.1016/j.matpr.2020.12.282.

Gaviria, L., Salcido, J. P., Guda, T., & Ong, J. L. (2014). Current trends in dental implants. *Journal of the Korean Association of Oral and Maxillofacial Surgeons*, *40*(2), 50–60. https://doi.org/10.5125/JKAOMS.2014.40.2.50.

Geetha, M., Singh, A. K., Asokamani, R., & Gogia, A. K. (2009). Ti based biomaterials, the ultimate choice for orthopaedic implants – A review. *Progress in Materials Science*, *54*(3), 397–425. https://doi.org/10.1016/J. PMATSCI.2008.06.004.

Goldhagen, P. R., O Connor, D. R., Schwarze, D., & Schwartz, E. (1994). A prospective comparative study of the compression hip screw and the gamma nail. *Journal of Orthopaedic Trauma*, *8*(5), 367–372. https://doi. org/10.1097/00005131-199410000-00001.

Goodman, S. B., Yao, Z., Keeney, M., & Yang, F. (2013). The future of biologic coatings for orthopaedic implants. *Biomaterials, 34*(13), 3174–3183. https://doi.org/10.1016/J.BIOMATERIALS.2013.01.074.

Greco, F., & Mattoli, V. (2012). *Introduction to Active Smart Materials for Biomedical Applications,* pp. 1–27. https://doi.org/10.1007/978-3-642-28044-3_1.

Hee, A. C., Zhao, Y., Jamali, S. S., Bendavid, A., Martin, P. J., & Guo, H. (2019). Characterization of tantalum and tantalum nitride films on Ti6Al4V substrate prepared by filtered cathodic vacuum arc deposition for biomedical applications. *Surface and Coatings Technology, 365,* 24–32. https://doi.org/10.1016/J.SURFCOAT.2018.05.007.

Hin, T. S. (2004). *Engineering Materials for Biomedical Applications,* Vol. 1. https://doi.org/10.1142/5673.

House, W. F., Berliner, K., & Crary, W. (2016). Cochlear implants. *Annals of Otology, Rhinology & Laryngology, 85*(3_Suppl). https://doi.org/10.1177/00034894760850S303.

Ibrahim, M. Z., Sarhan, A. A. D., Yusuf, F., & Hamdi, M. (2017). Biomedical materials and techniques to improve the tribological, mechanical and biomedical properties of orthopedic implants – A review article. *Journal of Alloys and Compounds, 714,* 636–667. https://doi.org/10.1016/J.JALLCOM.2017.04.231.

Kaliaraj, G. S., Bavanilathamuthiah, M., Kirubaharan, K., Ramachandran, D., Dharini, T., Viswanathan, K., & Vishwakarma, V. (2016). Bio-inspired YSZ coated titanium by EB-PVD for biomedical applications. *Surface and Coatings Technology, 307,* 227–235. https://doi.org/10.1016/J.SURFCOAT.2016.08.039.

Kaliaraj, G. S., Thukkaram, S., Alagarsamy, K., Kirubaharan, A. M. K., Paul, L. K., Abraham, L., Vishwakarma, V., & Sagadevan, S. (2021). Silver-calcia stabilized zirconia nanocomposite coated medical grade stainless steel as potential bioimplants. *Surfaces and Interfaces, 24,* 101086. https://doi.org/10.1016/J.SURFIN.2021.101086.

Kamachi Mudali, U., Sridhar, T. M., & Baldev, R. A. J. (2003). Corrosion of bio implants. *Sadhana, 28*(3), 601–637. https://doi.org/10.1007/BF02706450.

Klee, D., & Höcker, H. (2000). Polymers for biomedical applications: Improvement of the interface compatibility. *Biomedical Applications Polymer Blends,* 1–57. https://doi.org/10.1007/3-540-48838-3_1.

Kulshrestha, A. S., & Mahapatro, A. (2008). Polymers for biomedical applications. *ACS Symposium Series, 977,* 1–7. https://doi.org/10.1021/BK-2008-0977.CH001.

Kumar, A., Behmad, S. I., & Patil, P. (2014a). Vibration characterization and static analysis of cortical bone fracture based on finite element analysis. *Engineering and Automation Problems,* No. 3, 115–119.

Kumar, A., Jaiswal, H., Garg, T., & Patil, P. (2014b). Free vibration modes analysis of femur bone fracture using varying boundary conditions based on FEA. *Procedia Materials Science, 6,* 1593–1599. https://doi.org/10.1016/j.mspro.2014.07.142.

Kumar, A., Mamgain, D.P., Jaiswal, H., & Patil, P. (2015). Modal analysis of hand arm vibration (humerus bone) for biodynamic response using varying boundary conditions based on FEA. *Advances in Intelligent Systems and Computing, 308,* 169–176. https://doi.org/10.1007/978-81-322-2012-1_18.

Kumar, A., Datta, S., & Kalyanasundaram, D. (2018). Reduction of hydraulic friction in confined flows by laser texturing: Experiments and theoretical validation. *ASME 2018 16th International Conference on Nanochannels, Microchannels, and Minichannels, ICNMM 2018.* https://doi.org/10.1115/ICNMM2018-7740.

Kumar, A., Gori, Y., Rana, S., Sharma, N. K., & Yadav, B. (2022). FEA of humerus bone fracture and healing. *Advanced Materials for Biomechanical Applications* (1st ed.) CRC Press. https://doi.org/10.1201/9781003286806.

Kumar Seth, A. (2012). Fabrication and parameter optimization of CO_2 laser machined photo mask for photolithography process. Flow over textured topographies View project. https://www.researchgate.net/publication/274513783.

Liu, Z., Chen, H., Sui, J., Yuan, Z., Chen, Z., Fu, J., & Wang, C. (2021). Failure behavior and influence of surgical tool edges in soft tissue cutting. *Journal of Manufacturing Processes, 68*, 69–78. https://doi.org/10.1016/J.JMAPRO.2021.07.025.

Munir, K., Biesiekierski, A., Wen, C., & Li, Y. (2020). Introduction to biomedical manufacturing. *Metallic Biomaterials Processing and Medical Device Manufacturing, 3–29.* https://doi.org/10.1016/B978-0-08-102965-7.00001-1.

Okazaki, Y. (2019). Selection of metals for biomedical devices. *Metals for Biomedical Devices, 31–94.* https://doi.org/10.1016/B978-0-08-102666-3.00002-X.

Okazaki, Y., & Gotoh, E. (2005). Comparison of metal release from various metallic biomaterials in vitro. *Biomaterials, 26*(1), 11–21. https://doi.org/10.1016/J.BIOMATERIALS.2004.02.005.

Pande, S., & Dhatrak, P. (2021). Recent developments and advancements in knee implants materials, manufacturing: A review. *Materials Today: Proceedings, 46*, 756–762. https://doi.org/10.1016/J.MATPR.2020.12.465.

Parihar, A., Pandita, V., Kumar, A., Parihar, D. S., Puranik, N., Bajpai, T., & Khan, R. (2021). 3D printing: Advancement in biogenerative engineering to combat shortage of organs and bioapplicable materials. *Regenerative Engineering and Translational Medicine, 1–27.* https://doi.org/10.1007/S40883-021-00219-W.

Pogorielov, M., Husak, E., Solodivnik, A., & Zhdanov, S. (2017). Magnesium-based biodegradable alloys: Degradation, application, and alloying elements. *Interventional Medicine & Applied Science, 9*(1), 27–38. https://doi.org/10.1556/1646.9.2017.1.04.

Prasadh, S., Suresh, S., Ratheesh, V., Wong, R., & Gupta, M. (2021). Biocompatibility of metal matrix composites used for biomedical applications. *Encyclopedia of Materials: Composites, 474–501.* https://doi.org/10.1016/B978-0-12-803581-8.11834-X.

Patel, N. R., & Gohil, P. P. (2012). A review on biomaterials: Scope, applications & human anatomy significance. *International Journal of Emerging Technology and Advanced Engineering, 2*(4). http://citeseerx.ist.psu.edu/viewdoc/download?doi=10.1.1.413.7368&rep=rep1&type=pdf.

Radwan, N. H., Nasr, M. S., Ishak, R. A., & Awad, G. (2020). Recent trends in the use of bioceramics for treatment of osteomyelitis. *Archives of Pharmaceutical Sciences Ain Shams University, 4*(1), 1–19. https://doi.org/10.21608/APS.2020.2001.1021.

Rajan, S. T., & Arockiarajan, A. (2021). Thin film metallic glasses for bioimplants and surgical tools: A review. *Journal of Alloys and Compounds, 876*, 159939. https://doi.org/10.1016/J.JALLCOM.2021.159939.

Renugadevi, K., Devan, P. K., Chandra Sekhara Reddy, M., Karthik, P., & Thomas, T. (2020). Optimization of surface treatment in Calotropis Gigantea (CG)-fibre yarn by simple techniques and characterization of CG fibre yarn reinforced laminate. *Journal of Materials Research and Technology, 9*(6), 12187–12200. https://doi.org/10.1016/J.JMRT.2020.08.058.

Rezaie, H. R., Bakhtiari, L., & Ochsner, A. (1998). New LC-Materials and their Applications. In *ITG-Fachbericht* (Issue 150).

Schild, H. G. (1992). Poly(N-isopropylacrylamide): Experiment, theory and application. *Progress in Polymer Science, 17*(2), 163–249. https://doi.org/10.1016/0079-6700(92)90023-R.

Shakiba, M., Rezvani Ghomi, E., Khosravi, F., Jouybar, S., Bigham, A., Zare, M., Abdouss, M., Moaref, R., & Ramakrishna, S. (2021). Nylon—A material introduction and overview for biomedical applications. *Polymers for Advanced Technologies, 32*(9), 3368–3383. https://doi.org/10.1002/PAT.5372.

Sharma, M., & Khurana, S. M. P. (2018). Biomedical engineering: The recent trends. *Omics Technologies and Bio-Engineering: Volume 2: Towards Improving Quality of Life,* pp. 323–336. https://doi.org/10.1016/B978-0-12-815870-8.00017-6.

Sivakumar, M., & Rajeswari, S. (1992). Investigation of failures in stainless steel orthopaedic implant devices: Pit-induced stress corrosion cracking. *Journal of Materials Science Letters, 11*(15), 1039–1042. https://doi.org/10.1007/BF00729754.

Sivakumar, M., Mudali, U. K., & Rajeswari, S. (1994). In vitro electrochemical investigations of advanced stainless steels for applications as orthopaedic implants. *Journal of Materials Engineering and Performance, 3*(6), 744–753. https://doi.org/10.1007/BF02818375.

Sumayli, A. (2021). Recent trends on bioimplant materials: A review. *Materials Today: Proceedings, 46*, 2726–2731. https://doi.org/10.1016/J.MATPR.2021.02.395.

Trask, R. S., Williams, H. R., & Bond, I. P. (2007). Self-healing polymer composites: Mimicking nature to enhance performance. *Bioinspiration & Biomimetics, 2*(1). https://doi.org/10.1088/1748-3182/2/1/P01.

Valiulis, A. (2007). The advanced structural materials for living beings implants. *Journal of Vibroengineering, 9*, 323.

Wegner, G., Allard, N., Al Shboul, A., Auger, M., Beaulieu, A.-M., Bélanger, D., Bénard, P., Bilem, I., Byad, M., Byette, F., Chahine, R., Claverie, J., Cloutier, M., de Bonis, C., D'Epifanio, A., Drouin, B., Durette, D., Florek, J., Fortin, M.-A., ... Vlad, M. (2014). Advanced materials for biomedical applications. *Functional Materials, 12*, 277–332. https://doi.org/10.1515/9783110307825.277/HTML.

Wu, D. Y., Meure, S., & Solomon, D. (2008). Self-healing polymeric materials: A review of recent developments. *Progress in Polymer Science, 5*(33), 479–522. https://doi.org/10.1016/J.PROGPOLYMSCI.2008.02.001.

Xu, J., Zhao, Y., Peng, S., Zhao, Y., Jiang, S., & Lu, H. (2021). Multifaceted Ag-alloyed α-Ta5Si3 nanostructured coating for high-performing bioimplants. *Surface and Coatings Technology, 427*, 127853. https://doi.org/10.1016/J.SURFCOAT.2021.127853.

Zadehnajar, P., Mirmusavi, M. H., Soleymani Eil Bakhtiari, S., Bakhsheshi-Rad, H. R., Karbasi, S., RamaKrishna, S., & Berto, F. (2021). Recent advances on akermanite calcium-silicate ceramic for biomedical applications. *International Journal of Applied Ceramic Technology*, *18*(6), 1901–1920. https://doi.org/10.1111/IJAC.13814.

Zhao, Q., Wang, T., Wang, J., Zheng, L., Jiang, T., Cheng, G., & Wang, S. (2011). Template-directed hydrothermal synthesis of hydroxyapatite as a drug delivery system for the poorly water-soluble drug carvedilol. *Applied Surface Science*, *257*(23), 10126–10133. https://doi.org/10.1016/J.APSUSC.2011.06.161.

Chapter 3

Design and fabrication of augmented glenoid implants in total shoulder arthroplasty

Chamaiporn Sukjamsri
Srinakharinwirot University Nakhon Nayok

Vamsi Krishna Pasam
National Institute of Technology Warangal

CONTENTS

DOI: 10.1201/9781003344810-3

3.1 INTRODUCTION

Total shoulder arthroplasty (TSA) is a surgical procedure performed in patients with severe osteoarthritis to restore shoulder function and relieve pain. This method generally requires polyethylene glenoid and metal humeral components to replace the damaged joint. Although TSA is considered a successful treatment with high survival rates, mechanical failure of the TSA prosthesis, particularly glenoid component loosening, is often reported. Glenoid component loosening is believed to be associated with the rocking horse effect. It can happen when the glenoid component is repeatedly subjected to eccentric loading, leading to extensive stress and deteriorated component fixation.

Osteoarthritis patients are commonly accompanied by glenoid deformity, particularly glenoid retroversion due to posterior wear. Severely retroverted glenoids are often associated with humeral head subluxation. The replacement of a standard glenoid component for a severely retroverted glenoid without correcting the humeral head position may induce rocking horse effect, causing eccentric loading and consequently resulting in glenoid component loosening. Therefore, a special procedure is required when performing TSA on glenoids with this condition. Besides eccentric reaming and bone graft filling, augmented glenoid components have been introduced to normalize the glenoid version and reposition the humeral head.

In this chapter, the concept of TSA and the materials used for glenoid and humeral components are discussed. TSA complications such as glenoid component loosening and the management of retroverted glenoid are introduced. A review of studies including different designs of the augmented glenoid component is included. The construction of a finite element model to predict the outcomes of using augmented glenoid components is described. Moreover, fabrication methods through additive manufacturing of glenoid components are presented.

3.2 CONCEPT OF TOTAL SHOULDER ARTHROPLASTY

3.2.1 Shoulder anatomy

The human shoulder comprises three bones: the scapula, the humerus, and the clavicle, as shown in Figure 3.1. Compared with other joints in the body, the shoulder has the largest mobility. Shoulder mobility is stimulated by the shoulder complex formed by four joints. These joints are the acromioclavicular (AC) joint, the sternoclavicular (SC) joint, the scapulothoracic (ST) joint, and the glenohumeral (GH) joint. The GH joint plays a vital role in connecting the arm to the trunk. It is considered a ball-socket joint where the humeral head (ball) articulates with the glenoid fossa (socket), a

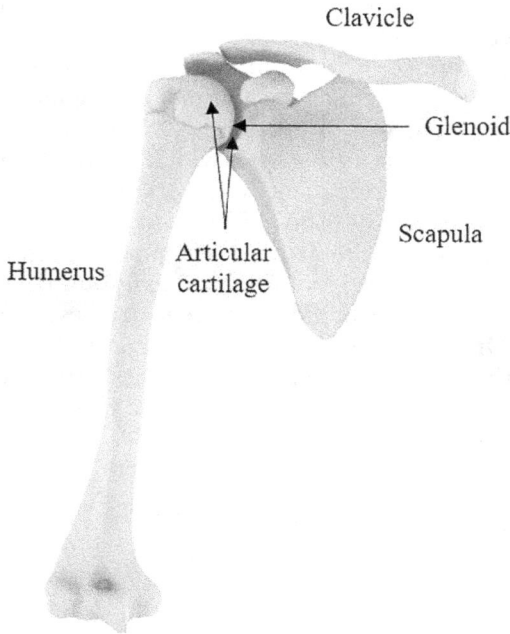

Figure 3.1 The right shoulder consisting of the scapula, the humerus, and the clavicle. (Modified from BodyParts3D, ©The Database Center for Life Science licensed under CC Attribution-ShareAlike 2.1 Japan.)

concave part of the scapula. The humeral head and glenoid fossa surface are covered with cartilage to reduce friction within the joints and provide smooth joint motion. The GH joint is enclosed entirely by the joint capsule and ligaments, which helps stabilize the joint. However, the major stabilizer of the GH joint is the rotator cuff, a group of four muscles composed of the supraspinatus, the infraspinatus, the teres minor, and the subscapularis.

3.2.2 Shoulder joint replacement

Shoulder arthroplasty is a treatment that replaces the damaged shoulder joint with prosthetic components to restore function and relieve pain. Since contact forces on the shoulder joint are smaller than those on the weight-bearing joints such as the knee and the hip, the incidence of joint replacement for the shoulder is less frequent. However, shoulder arthroplasty is still a common joint replacement procedure and has been increasing over the years (Best et al., 2021). Shoulder arthroplasty is classified into three types. The first type is hemiarthroplasty (HA), a surgical procedure in which only the damaged humeral head is replaced with a prosthetic component. The major indication for HA is proximal humerus fracture. The second type is reverse shoulder arthroplasty (RSA) or reverse polarity total shoulder replacement (RTSR). RSA is performed on both the ball and socket sides. However, the orientation of the replaced joint is opposite to the shoulder joint anatomy. The humeral is replaced with a prosthesis having a concave head, while the glenoid is replaced with a prosthesis with a convex hemispherical ball. RSA is typically indicated for patients with rotator cuff tears. The last type is total shoulder arthroplasty (TSA). TSA involves replacing the damaged humeral head and glenoid with artificial components while preserving the anatomical orientation of the joint. The National Joint Registry (NJR), the UK, reported the number of shoulder replacement cases performed between 2012 and 2019. Of these cases, 41.3%, 30.6%, and 14.9% were RSA, TSA, and HA, respectively. Although TSA has been less performed compared to RSA, it is a major treatment for patients indicated with osteoarthritis (NJR, 2020).

3.3 MATERIALS IN TOTAL SHOULDER ARTHROPLASTY APPLICATIONS

TSA prosthesis is divided into the glenoid and humeral components. The humeral components are usually modularly designed, consisting of the humeral stem and humeral head components. The glenoid and humeral components were made of metals in the early stages of development. However, because of the extensive research, the glenoid components are currently made of polyethylene and the humeral components are made of various types of materials, including metals and ceramics. The desirable properties of a material for TSA components include wear resistance, biocompatibility, and reliability in service. Although the shoulder joints are not subjected to high loads compared to the knee and hip joints, their fatigue strength must also be considered. The following sections will briefly review each material, its biomedical properties, and various pros and cons that establish its suitability for TSA applications.

3.3.1 Polyethylene

Polyethylene (PE) is the most common type of polymer used in various industrial applications. Because of its biocompatibility, PE is also suitable for bio-implant fabrication. PE can be categorized by density and chemical branching into several types, one of which is ultra-high molecular weight polyethylene (UHMWPE). The properties of UHMWPE are suitable for applications involving high loads. In TSA, UHMWPE is used for fabricating the glenoid component. However, PE glenoid components often suffer from degradation and wear under oxidation, ultimately damaging the implant. Wear debris subsequently leads to osteolysis, resulting in glenoid component loosening, which is a main problem of TSA. In modern manufacturing, vitamin E acting as an antioxidant is added to the PE components to reduce wear and improve life expectancy (Alexander et al., 2019).

3.3.2 Titanium alloys

The use of titanium (Ti) and alloys of Ti for biomedical implants has been investigated by many researchers in terms of mechanical properties, corrosion resistance, and cytocompatibility. Ti and alloys of Ti for improving their biocompatibility have also been addressed. According to the literature, pure titanium is not preferred for manufacturing implants because of its inferior bearing strength and low wear resistance, particularly in long-term applications. Hence, Ti alloys that have superior mechanical properties are used in many applications such as knee and hip prostheses and dental implants (Talib Mohammed, 2018). Ti alloys also have high fatigue strength, high hardness, and excellent biocompatible characteristics. Ti alloys are widely used in TSA for fabricating humeral stem components. It can also be used for humeral head components.

3.3.3 Cobalt alloys

Cobalt alloys are used in the fabrication of medical implants, especially the parts related to the bearing surfaces of the artificial joints. In TSA, cobalt-chromium-molybdenum (CoCrMo) alloys are mostly used to fabricate the humeral head components due to their high wear resistance, hardness, and superior fatigue strength even under corrosive atmosphere. However, the high fabrication cost and the incidence of wear in the PE glenoid component, which is the contact counterpart, are limitations of using cobalt alloys (Ibrahim et al., 2017).

3.3.4 Stainless steel

The use of stainless steel in shoulder prosthesis fabrication is less frequent than that of Ti and CoCrMo alloys. However, it is still found in the manufacture of humeral head prostheses. The corrosion resistance of stainless steel makes it a suitable material for biomedical fabrication. Stainless steel also has the advantages of biocompatibility, low cost, and good mechanical properties. The formation of chromium oxide as a film inhibits oxidation. Adding nickel (Ni) and reducing carbon content improves the corrosion resistance of stainless steel (Ibrahim et al., 2017). Despite the aforementioned properties, stainless steel is limited to short-term implants and medical devices. This is due to the release of Ni ions, which affect human health. However, this led to the development of Ni-free stainless steel that has excellent cytocompatibility, high fatigue strength, and enhanced corrosion resistance.

3.3.5 Bioceramics

Bioceramic materials are another class of biocompatible materials gaining popularity nowadays. These materials are bioinert and non-toxic. They offer high resistance to wear and corrosion (Kang & Fang, 2018). They also exhibit better tribological properties and have high hardness. The most common biomedical applications are scaffolds, dental implants, and artificial joints. In TSA applications, ceramic materials, particularly alumina and zirconia, have been used to manufacture the humeral head components. Using ceramic humeral head components is reported to help reduce the PE wear of glenoid components compared to using metal humeral head components (Mueller et al., 2017).

3.4 COMPLICATIONS OF TOTAL SHOULDER ARTHROPLASTY

3.4.1 Glenoid component loosening

Compared with RSA and HA, TSA exhibits superior postoperative outcomes, with the survival rate reported to range between 96% and 99% (Jensen et al., 2021; Rasmussen et al., 2018). However, the most common complications were reported to be glenoid component loosening, glenoid wear, and component instability, accounting for 37.7%, 22.6%, and 10.1%, respectively (Bohsali et al., 2017). Glenoid component loosening was also reported to be the most common reason for revision surgery in TSA (Parada et al., 2021). The cause of glenoid component loosening is multifactorial, but is believed to be associated with the rocking horse phenomenon. The rocking proceeds when a glenoid component is eccentrically loaded on one side, causing the other side to be distracted, leading to high stress at the bone-component interface and deteriorating the component fixation. The eccentric load often occurs posteriorly, associated with posterior glenoid wear in osteoarthritis patients (Walch et al., 1999).

3.4.2 Glenoid with osteoarthritis

Osteoarthritis (OA) is a pathologic condition classified into primary and secondary OA. Primary OA occurs due to aging, while secondary OA is a consequence of other causes, such as previous diseases or injuries that are found in young patients. OA can occur in almost any joint in the body, including the shoulder. Glenohumeral osteoarthritis (GHOA) involves the wear and tear of articular cartilage and abnormal remodeling of the subchondral bone, which is the bony component lying just below the articular cartilage. GHOA is also associated with bone erosion, bone spur formation, and narrowing of the GH joint (Li et al., 2013). The disease may damage and weaken soft tissues surrounding the shoulder joint, including the joint capsule, ligaments, and muscles (Donell, 2019; Ibounig et al., 2020). The prevalence of GHOA rises with an increased aging population. Symptoms associated with GHOA include pain, stiffness, and limited range of motion, causing difficulty in performing occupation tasks and daily-life activities. GHOA can be initially managed by non-operative treatments such as oral medications, injections, and physical therapy. However, shoulder replacement may be indicated in cases with end-stage GHOA (Pandya et al., 2018).

3.4.3 Glenoid morphology

It is recognized that GHOA is the most common cause leading to TSA. GHOA alters bony structure resulting in glenoid morphology changes, leading to decreased or insufficient bone stock for glenoid implantation (Lo et al., 2021). Most importantly, erosion and deformity of the glenoid can cause subluxation, tilt, or dislocation of the humeral head. This condition can induce eccentric load, which may alter the biomechanical characteristics of the GH joint due to the rocking horse effect. All these consequences increase the complexity of TSA procedure and the risk of glenoid component loosening, which is the most common problem in shoulders treated by TSA (Bohsali et al., 2017). For these reasons, a preoperative assessment of glenoid morphology pattern or bone loss due to GHOA is essential for surgical planning to increase the success of TSA.

Walch et al. classified the erosion patterns of the glenoid with primary GHOA into five subtypes, namely A1, A2, B1, B2, and C, as shown in Figure 3.2 (Walch et al., 1999). Type A refers to a glenoid with a centralized humeral head. Subtypes A1 and A2 demonstrate minor and extensive symmetrical erosion, respectively. Type B classifies a glenoid with posterior humeral head subluxation. Subtype B1 exhibits narrowing articular joint space with no signs of posterior erosion, whereas Subtype B2 shows posterior biconcave erosion. Finally, type C refers to a dysplastic glenoid with a retroversion angle greater than 25, regardless of erosion. The classification system proposed by Walch is the most commonly used in shoulder surgery practice. However, it has been extended to cover more glenoid wear patterns to accommodate surgical planning and increase treatment success. Additional types of glenoid morphology patterns proposed by Bercik et al. are B3 and D (Bercik et al., 2016). Type B3 defines a glenoid with retroversion and/or humeral head subluxation, combined with posterior monoconcave wear. Type D defines an antroverted glenoid or anterior humeral head subluxation. According to a study by Walch et al., most glenoids with GHOA were in type A, accounting for 59%, followed by type B, which accounted for 32% (Walch et al., 1999). However, it is generally accepted that managing glenoids with posterior wear, categorized in types B2, B3, and C, is incredibly challenging as they are often associated with high revision rates. Additionally, type B2 is the most common type of glenoid in OA shoulders undergoing TSA (Gates et al., 2019; Grey et al., 2020).

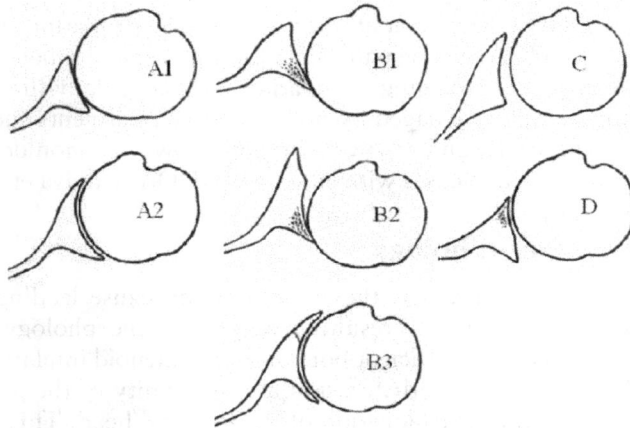

Figure 3.2 Walch classification of glenoid morphology in primary glenohumeral osteoarthritis (A1, A2, B1, B2, and C). Two more types (B3 and D) have been added to the original Walch classification system by Bercik et al. (2016). (Reprinted from Bercik, M. J., Kruse, K., 2nd, Yalizis, M., Gauci, M. O., Chaoui, J., & Walch, G. (2016). A modification to the Walch classification of the glenoid in primary glenohumeral osteoarthritis using three-dimensional imaging. *J Shoulder Elbow Surg*, 25(10), 1601–1606, with permission from Elsevier.)

3.4.4 Management of glenoid erosion

There are different surgical approaches to performing TSA in osteoarthritis patients with posteriorly eroded glenoids. The least complex approach is eccentric reaming, which involves cutting the high side of the glenoid rim to correct the glenoid version angle and then placing a standard glenoid component on the prepared surface. Eccentric reaming has not been suggested in glenoids with retroversion angle greater than 15° to avoid adverse effects such as insufficient bone stock for implant seating, glenoid component subsidence due to the removal of subchondral bone, and cortical wall perforation due to glenoid component misalignment (Borque et al., 2017; Kyriacou et al., 2019).

Bone grafting is another technique used to reconstruct the version angle of the glenoid with posterior wear. The graft can be obtained autologously from the cut humeral head while undergoing TSA surgery. Bone grafting overcomes the limit of eccentric reaming in that it can build up the posterior volume of the glenoid while retaining the anterior volume. As a result, it increases bone stock for implant seating, reduces the risk of cortical wall perforation, and restores joint kinematics. Although bone graft has been reported with successful clinical and radiographic outcomes in early and mid-term follow-up, long-term studies remain limited (Nicholson et al., 2017). Moreover, complications such as graft dissolution, nonunion, resorption, subsidence, technical demanding, and fixation failure are of concern and remain controversial (Gates et al., 2019).

Augmented glenoid component has been considered an alternative approach for correcting glenoid version without worrying about graft incorporation. Conceptually, this approach can prevent eccentric loading, lowering the risk of implant loosening and enhancing TSA success (Friedman & Garrigues, 2019; Sabesan et al., 2014).

3.5 AUGMENTED GLENOID COMPONENT DESIGNS

Augmented glenoid components have been manufactured in various designs such as wedge and step. Each design has a figure to compensate for the lost volume of the glenoid bone caused by varying degrees of posterior wear. The type of anchor is typically either keel or peg with cemented fixation. In general, augmented glenoid components available for TSA surgery are monoblock made from polyethylene.

The step-augmented glenoid component with multi-peg fixation, shown in Figure 3.3, has been introduced and evaluated in several clinical studies (Favorito et al., 2016; Iannotti et al., 2021). The postoperative outcomes in patients with severe retroverted glenoid classified into types B2, B3, and C were focused. Positive clinical and radiographic results, including improved pain relief, increased shoulder motion and function, and excellent component seating, were reported in most studies. However, the risk of central peg osteolysis was observed in some cases with B3 glenoid. These studies were based on short-term follow-ups, so long-term studies are necessitated to assess implant survival and clinical outcomes associated with the step-augmented design.

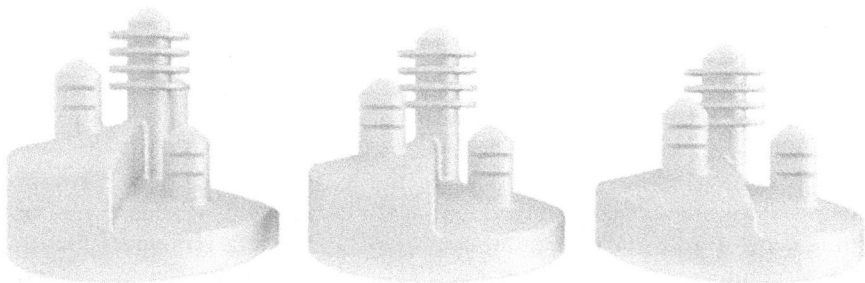

Figure 3.3 Thee different augmentation levels in the step augmented glenoid component commercialized by DePuy Orthopaedics, Inc. (Reprinted from Sabesan, V., Callanan, M., & Sharma, V. (2014). Guidelines for the selection of optimal glenoid augment size for moderate to severe glenohumeral osteoarthritis. *J Shoulder Elbow Surg*, 23(7), 974–981, with permission from Elsevier.)

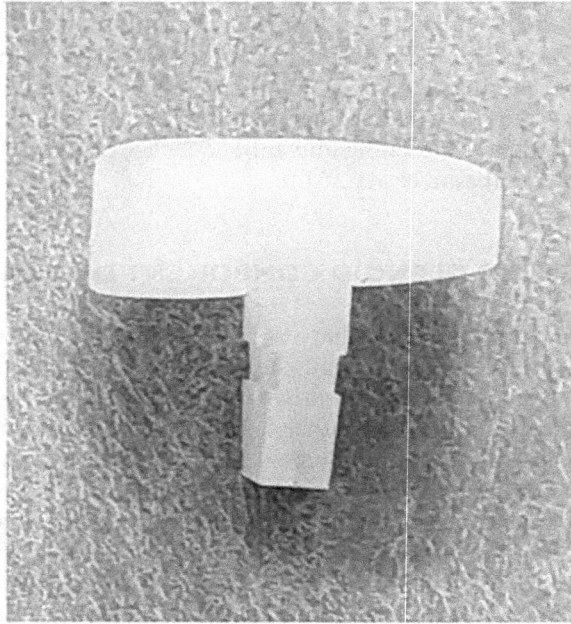

Figure 3.4 The half-wedge augmented glenoid component commercialized by Wright Medical Group, Inc. (Reprinted from Das, A. K., Wright, A. C., Singh, J., & Monga, P. (2020). Does posterior half-wedge augmented glenoid restore version and alignment in total shoulder arthroplasty for the B2 glenoid? *J Clin Orthop Trauma*, 11(Suppl 2), S275–S279, with permission from Elsevier.)

The design of the glenoid component with wedge augmentation can be classified into two types, full-wedge and half-wedge. A clinical study reported by Das et al. showed that the half-wedge all-polyethylene augmented component with keel fixation, shown in Figure 3.4, was a promising option for treating patients with B2 glenoid. Postoperative results showed that the humeral head was well repositioned, and no complications associated with surgery were found (Das et al., 2020).

Hybrid fixation has been applied to the half-wedge augmented component, shown in Figure 3.5, meaning that the component is secured via both bone cement and porous-coated central peg, inducing biological fixation via osseointegration (Marigi et al., 2021). Conceptually, the hybrid fixation can prevent component loosening and enhance component longevity. However, further studies are required to provide long-term results.

The full-wedge augmented glenoid component has been designed with multi-peg fixation, with or without ingrowth central cage, shown in Figure 3.6. A postoperative study in patients mostly with B2 and B3 glenoid deformity implanted with this component was reported by Priddy et al.

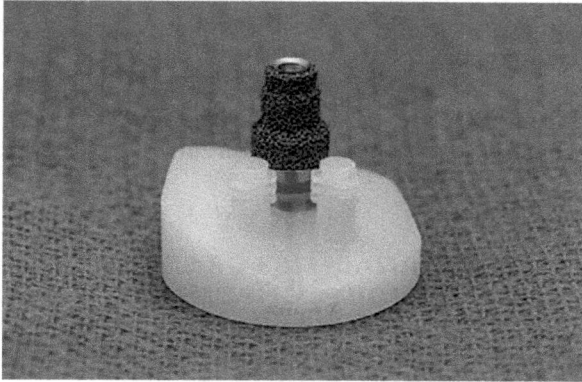

Figure 3.5 The half-wedge augmented glenoid component with a porous-coated central peg and three peripheral pegs commercialized by Zimmer Biomet. (Reprinted from Marigi, E. M., Duquin, T. R., Throckmorton, T. Q., & Sperling, J. W. (2021). Hybrid fixation in anatomic shoulder arthroplasty: surgical technique and review of the literature. *JSES Rev, Reports, Tech*, 1(2), 113–117, with permission from Elsevier.)

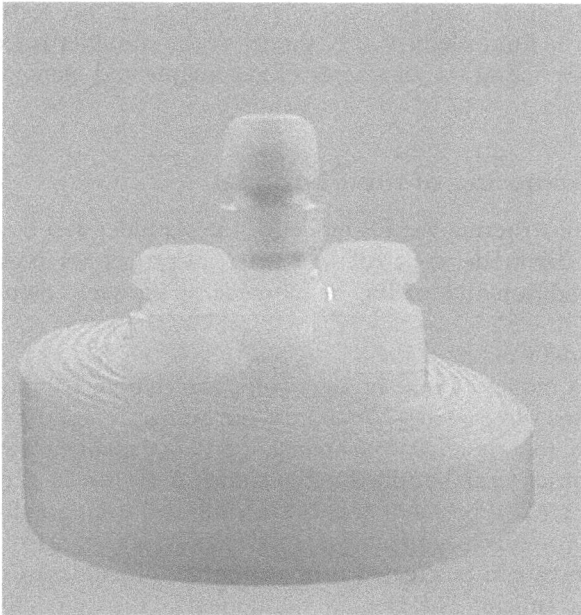

Figure 3.6 The full-wedge augmented glenoid component with multi-peg fixation commercialized by Exactech, Inc. (Reprinted from Priddy, M., Zarezadeh, A., Farmer, K. W., Struk, A. M., King, J. J., 3rd, Wright, T. W., & Schoch, B. S. (2019). Early results of augmented anatomic glenoid components. *J Shoulder Elbow Surg*, 28(6S), S138–S145, with permission from Elsevier).

A minimum of 2-year follow-up showed that the full-wedge augmented component exhibited improved clinical outcomes in shoulder mobility and pain relief. Radiographic results and revision rates were comparable with TSA using the standard glenoid component. However, cases of using the glenoid component with a higher level of wedge augmentation were associated with higher clinical and radiographic failure rates (Priddy et al., 2019).

3.6 FINITE ELEMENT ANALYSIS FOR STUDYING AUGMENTED GLENOID COMPONENT

The implementation of augmented glenoid components has intensively been studied to prevent glenoid component loosening and enhance TSA survival rate. The results from clinical studies, particularly in long-term follow-ups, are a valid measure of TSA success. However, clinical studies are complicated and require a large number of patients and clinical and ethical approvals. Finite element analysis (FEA) is a well-known computational technique that can simulate and analyze clinical problems. In addition, FEA provides insight into the mechanical state so that stress and deformation of the bone and implant can be accessibly evaluated. In this section, the construction of the finite element (FE) model of the shoulder is explained. FE studies for predicting the outcomes of the augmented glenoid component are discussed.

3.6.1 Construction of the FE model

In general, constructing the FE model of the shoulder can be divided into three stages: 3D model construction, material properties assignment, and boundary condition and loading assignment, as shown in Figure 3.7.

I. *3D Model Construction*

A 3D model of the shoulder joint for glenoid component studies comprises three parts: the scapula, the humeral, and the glenoid components. In a more complex study, the joint capsule, rotator cuff, and other muscles can be added to the model. A 3D model of the scapula is usually created based on a clinical computed tomography (CT) dataset using image segmentation software. A 3D model of the glenoid component can be created using computer-aided design (CAD) tools or 3D scanners. The glenoid component is then virtually implanted into the glenoid vault. At this point, the glenoid component should be aligned and positioned with reference to the scapula axis, and experienced surgeons should assist or approve the virtual implantation. The volume of the scapula overlaid with the glenoid component is then Boolean-subtracted to simulate reaming and drilling procedures

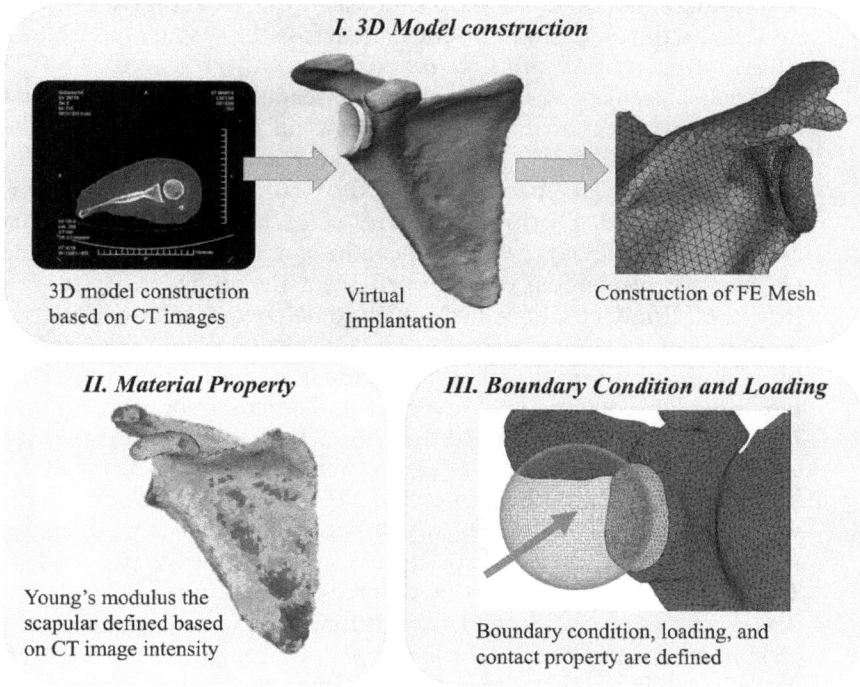

Figure 3.7 Overview of the process of constructing the FE model for shoulder analysis.

consistent with actual surgery. The FE mesh of the implanted scapula and glenoid models is then constructed. The mesh convergence test should be carried out to obtain optimal mesh size. The humeral head component can be modeled as a rigid body sphere. The FE mesh of the humeral component is, therefore, unnecessary.

II. *Material Property*

Material assignment with homogeneous and isotropic properties is usually applied to orthopedic implants. Young's modulus and poison's ratio of the glenoid component are defined according to the type of implant material. Homogeneous material properties can also be applied to the scapula. However, it is recommended that the bone should be divided into cancellous and cortical parts. Each has its own property. Many studies assign the scapula properties under the assumption of being non-homogeneous with different isotropic properties across individual elements. In this case, Young's modulus of each element can be defined based on the grayscale value in Hounsfield unit (HU) of the CT dataset at the same coordinate position. The relationship between grayscale value and bone density, as well as bone density and Young's modulus, has been proposed in several studies. Poison's ratio is usually assumed to be constant across the scapula model.

III. *Boundary Condition and Loading*

The displacement at some parts of the scapula, such as the scapula border, must be constrained to prevent rigid body motion, and the constrained parts should not affect the FE results. Since the shoulder consists of two contact counterparts, the Coulomb's contact model is usually employed. Friction coefficients of each contact pair must be assigned. Loading of the GH joint can be assigned in any form, static or dynamic, depending on the purpose of the study. Many studies load the FE model with a force magnitude comparable to GH contact forces during daily activities. These forces have been investigated by many experimental and computational studies. Bergmann et al. measured GH contact forces in a patient undergoing shoulder replacement using an implant embedded with a force sensor. Their results showed that GH contact forces ranged between 14% and 151% of the body weight (BW) (Bergmann et al., 2007). This finding is consistent with a study by Klemt et al., which was performed using a combination of motion capture experiments and musculoskeletal models. They reported that the GH contact forces ranged from 24% to 164% BW (Klemt et al., 2018). GH contact force and contact point on the glenoid vary depending on the arm position. Applying load in the FE model should take this into account. FE results in terms of the stress in the glenoid vault, cement mantle, and glenoid component are the main focus. Stress magnitude that is close to the damage limit shows an increased risk of material failure.

3.6.2 FE studies of augmented glenoid component

The FE study of augmented glenoid components conducted by Hermida et al. was reported earlier in the literature (Hermida et al., 2014). Hermida et al. constructed FE models representing both normal and arthritic retroverted scapula. Each was implanted with a standard and a wedge augmented component. The implantation alignments were set to be retroversion and neutral. In this study, a GH force of 85% BW was applied to the rigid humeral sphere. Stresses on bone structure, cement mantle, and glenoid component were measured and used to calculate fatigue life. Their results suggested that correcting posterior eroded glenoids with the wedge augmented component significantly decreased stress and improved fatigue life.

In a study by Allred et al., FEA was used to compare the performance of two augmented glenoid components, wedged and stepped design, with a standard glenoid design (Allred et al., 2016). The FEA was based on a static load of 85% BW. The fatigue life of the bone structure and cement mantle was determined. Moreover, this study measured the removal of bone volume and the area of the cortical bone that supported the glenoid component. According to their results, the wedged design demonstrated excellent performance by requiring less bone removal and providing greater cortical bone support. In addition, the wedged design also generated lower stresses, resulting in longer bone and cement fatigue life.

A more recent study by Sabesan et al. performed an FEA to compare biomechanical outcomes between wedged and stepped glenoid components (Sabesan et al., 2019). The study created an integrated model comprising the scapula with 20° retroversion, humeral head, joint capsule, and rotator cuff to simulate shoulder joint behavior under dynamic physiological load during 0°–90° abduction. GH contact forces, relative micromotion, and stress distribution in the glenoid, cement mantle, and implant were measured. Overall results suggested that the wedged component provided better outcomes than the stepped component.

3.7 FABRICATION METHODS ASSISTING SHOULDER ARTHROPLASTY

Patients with glenoid bone loss have been treated with several surgical techniques depending on the morphology of their glenoid vault. Augmented glenoid components have shown promising results in treating mild to moderate glenoid deformity. However, the available augmented components may not successfully address some types of glenoid deformity, such as those with severe erosion in any plane. Also, it has been accepted that positioning the glenoid component in a severely eroded glenoid is technically challenging, and malpositioning can cause early component loosening. Thus, preoperative and intraoperative procedures must be well prepared.

Additive manufacturing is one of the best established and studied manufacturing methods in various applications. It is also called 3D printing. Its application is mainly related to printing polymers. However, metal additive manufacturing has evolved in recent times. Printing in biomedical applications has acquired greater importance and has a variety of printing techniques available. 3D printing can potentially improve TSA success in many ways. It has been used to fabricate a custom-made glenoid implant with porous titanium structure for reconstructing a severely eroded glenoid (Stoffelen et al., 2015). In preoperative planning, a 3D printed model of glenoid morphology, especially in severe cases, prior to undergoing TSA is beneficial. A clear morphologic perspective allows surgeons to decide on surgical planning and select appropriate surgical techniques (Wang et al., 2019). In addition, 3D printing of polymer, usually polyamide, has been used to produce a patient-specific instrument (PSI), which is a surgical guide that fits individual glenoid morphology. The printed guide intraoperatively helps the surgeon correctly position the glenoid component in place (Cabarcas et al., 2019).

In the 3D printing process, the product will be modeled in a CAD package, followed by slicing the model. Then the model is fed to a 3D printing machine, which deposits the material layer by layer in a stepwise manner (Prakash et al., 2018). The 3D printer consists of a heat source for melting the raw material. The material is either fused by heating in the given shape or melted and deposited into the required shape. The choice depends on factors such as properties needed, heat source availability, and the material used. Additive manufacturing is classified based on the feed mechanism and the energy source (Herzog et al., 2016): powder feed, wire feed, and powder bed systems according to the former, and laser beam and electron beam as per the latter. Although the nature of material plays a major role, manufacturing the chosen material into a biomedical product is also crucial. Some of the processes are discussed here in the following sections.

3.7.1 Laser beam melting

The process is also called selective laser melting (SLM), direct metal laser sintering (DMLS), and laser metal fusion (LMF). The schematic representation of the process is shown in Figure 3.8. The polymer is fed by a hopper. The scan speed and laser power are adjusted to suit the material being fused. A coater blade deposits a layer equal to the thickness of one layer. Then the laser is directed onto it in a predefined pattern. The powder exposed to the heat gets melted and fused in the scanned shape. Then the build platform is lowered by a distance equal to the layer thickness. The recoater blade again deposits the material (Dumas et al., 2018). The process is thus repeated

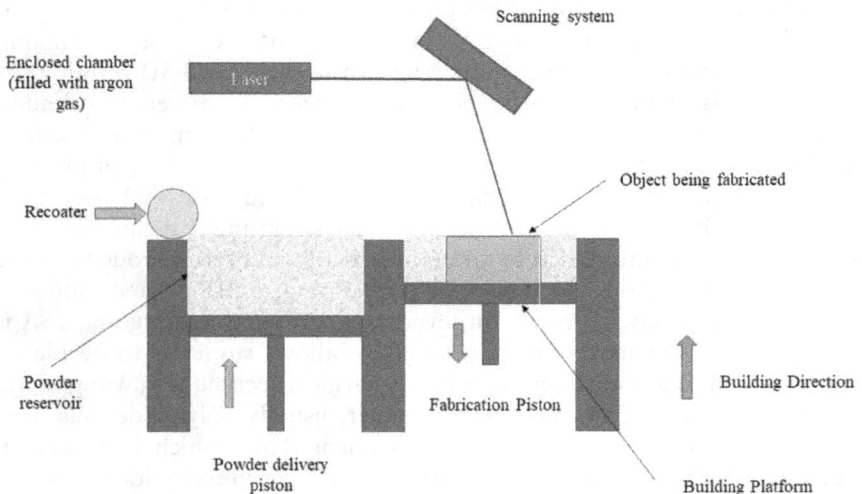

Figure 3.8 Schematic of laser beam melting (SLM) process.

until the entire component is produced. Titanium alloys and synthetic polymers such as hydroxyapatite, high-density polyethylene (HDPE), and polypropylene (PP) are widely used materials in this 3D printing technique.

3.7.2 Fused deposition modeling

The schematic of fused deposition modeling (FDM) is shown in Figure 3.9. In this method, the polymer is fed through a nozzle, generally in the form of wire. The polymer wire is heated and then extruded through a nozzle. The nozzle is mechanically manipulated. The molten polymer is deposited onto the build plate, and further layers are deposited one over the other, forming the entire component (Prakash et al., 2018). This is a simple and reliable method of printing thermoplastic materials, commonly used for building scaffolds with HDPE and polycaprolactone (PCL). However, its application to PE often suffers from a shrinkage effect. Also, the adhesion of PE to the build plate posed difficulties (Paxton et al., 2019).

In addition to the above, other techniques such as stereolithography (SLA) (Prakash et al., 2018) and direct wire electrospinning are also used to print polymer components in many biomedical applications. A comprehensive study of different additive manufacturing techniques revealed that each process has its own merits and demerits. Also, not all the materials are compatible with a particular technique. For example, 3D printing of

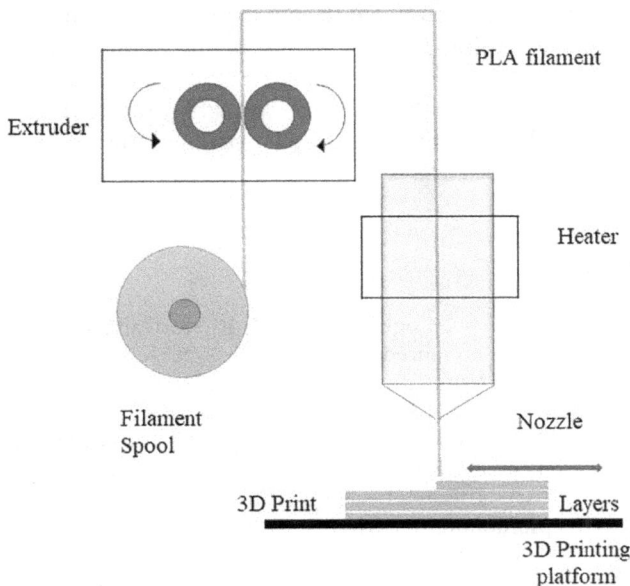

Figure 3.9 Schematic of fused deposition modeling (FDM).

UHMWPE for producing the glenoid component is not compatible with certain 3D printing techniques such as melt electrowriting (MEW). This is because the high melting temperature of UHMWPE requires a high-energy heat source. In addition, as UHMWPE is non-reactive to many solvents, it requires harmful solvents to increase its flow characteristics by reducing the viscosity (Paxton et al., 2019). Hence, further research is being done in this area to determine a suitable technique for UHMWPE printing. However, UHMWPE, like other polymers of PE family, may be printed with SLM and FDM techniques.

3.8 SUMMARY

In this chapter, basic shoulder anatomy, TSA concept, and implant materials were discussed. TSA complications in OA patients were reviewed. It was found that OA patients often have retroverted glenoid and implantation of the retroverted glenoid is challenging. An augmented glenoid component was designed to restore a neutral version of the glenoid and re-center the humeral head to prevent the glenoid component from loosening. According to recent clinical studies, the use of augmented glenoid components was promising. However, the studies were based on short-term follow-up. Finite element analysis can provide insight into the mechanical state, such as stress distribution in the bone and implant. Therefore, it can help improve the implant design and forecast surgical outcomes. However, a glenoid with extreme bone loss may not be successfully treated by using an augmented implant. Fabricating a custom-made 3D printed implant is a potential approach to address this problem. Moreover, 3D printing techniques are possibly adopted to fabricate a surgical guide and bone model that assist surgical planning. All of these can enhance the success of TSA.

REFERENCES

Alexander, J. J., Bell, S. N., Coghlan, J., Lerf, R., & Dallmann, F. (2019). The effect of vitamin E-enhanced cross-linked polyethylene on wear in shoulder arthroplasty-a wear simulator study. *J Shoulder Elbow Surg, 28*(9), 1771–1778. https://doi.org/10.1016/j.jse.2019.01.014.

Allred, J. J., Flores-Hernandez, C., Hoenecke, H. R., Jr., & D'Lima, D. D. (2016). Posterior augmented glenoid implants require less bone removal and generate lower stresses: a finite element analysis. *J Shoulder Elbow Surg, 25*(5), 823–830. https://doi.org/10.1016/j.jse.2015.10.003.

Bercik, M. J., Kruse, K., 2nd, Yalizis, M., Gauci, M. O., Chaoui, J., & Walch, G. (2016). A modification to the Walch classification of the glenoid in primary glenohumeral osteoarthritis using three-dimensional imaging. *J Shoulder Elbow Surg, 25*(10), 1601–1606. https://doi.org/10.1016/j.jse.2016.03.010.

Bergmann, G., Graichen, F., Bender, A., Kaab, M., Rohlmann, A., & Westerhoff, P. (2007). In vivo glenohumeral contact forces--measurements in the first patient 7 months postoperatively. *J Biomech*, 40(10), 2139–2149. https://doi.org/10.1016/j.jbiomech.2006.10.037.

Best, M. J., Aziz, K. T., Wilckens, J. H., McFarland, E. G., & Srikumaran, U. (2021). Increasing incidence of primary reverse and anatomic total shoulder arthroplasty in the United States. *J Shoulder Elbow Surg*, 30(5), 1159–1166. https://doi.org/10.1016/j.jse.2020.08.010.

Bohsali, K. I., Bois, A. J., & Wirth, M. A. (2017). Complications of shoulder arthroplasty. *J Bone Joint Surg Am*, 99(3), 256–269. https://doi.org/10.2106/JBJS.16.00935.

Borque, K. A., Chang, M. J., Welp, K., Wagner, E. R., Woodmass, J. M., & Warner, J. J. P. (2017). Managing glenoid bone loss in total shoulder arthroplasty: role of augmented patient-specific implants. *Semin Arthroplasty*, 28(3), 134–139. https://doi.org/10.1053/j.sart.2017.12.004.

Cabarcas, B. C., Cvetanovich, G. L., Gowd, A. K., Liu, J. N., Manderle, B. J., & Verma, N. N. (2019). Accuracy of patient-specific instrumentation in shoulder arthroplasty: a systematic review and meta-analysis. *JSES Open Access*, 3(3), 117–129. https://doi.org/10.1016/j.jses.2019.07.002.

Das, A. K., Wright, A. C., Singh, J., & Monga, P. (2020). Does posterior half-wedge augmented glenoid restore version and alignment in total shoulder arthroplasty for the B2 glenoid? *J Clin Orthop Trauma*, 11(Suppl 2), S275–S279. https://doi.org/10.1016/j.jcot.2020.02.005.

Donell, S. (2019). Subchondral bone remodelling in osteoarthritis. *EFORT Open Rev*, 4(6), 221–229. https://doi.org/10.1302/2058-5241.4.180102.

Dumas, M., Cabanettes, F., Kaminski, R., Valiorgue, F., Picot, E., Lefebvre, F., . . . Rech, J. (2018). Influence of the finish cutting operations on the fatigue performance of Ti-6Al-4V parts produced by selective laser melting. *Procedia CIRP*, 71, 429–434. https://doi.org/10.1016/j.procir.2018.05.054.

Favorito, P. J., Freed, R. J., Passanise, A. M., & Brown, M. J. (2016). Total shoulder arthroplasty for glenohumeral arthritis associated with posterior glenoid bone loss: results of an all-polyethylene, posteriorly augmented glenoid component. *J Shoulder Elbow Surg*, 25(10), 1681–1689. https://doi.org/10.1016/j.jse.2016.02.020.

Friedman, L. G. M., & Garrigues, G. E. (2019). Anatomic augmented glenoid implants for the management of the B2 glenoid. *J Shoulder Elbow Arthroplasty*, 3, 2471549219870350. https://doi.org/10.1177/2471549219870350.

Gates, S., Cutler, H., & Khazzam, M. (2019). Outcomes of posterior glenoid bone-grafting in anatomical total shoulder arthroplasty: a systematic review. *JBJS Rev*, 7(9), e6. https://doi.org/10.2106/JBJS.RVW.19.00005.

Grey, S. G., Wright, T. W., Flurin, P. H., Zuckerman, J. D., Roche, C. P., & Friedman, R. J. (2020). Clinical and radiographic outcomes with a posteriorly augmented glenoid for Walch B glenoids in anatomic total shoulder arthroplasty. *J Shoulder Elbow Surg*, 29(5), e185–e195. https://doi.org/10.1016/j.jse.2019.10.008.

Hermida, J. C., Flores-Hernandez, C., Hoenecke, H. R., & D'Lima, D. D. (2014). Augmented wedge-shaped glenoid component for the correction of glenoid retroversion: a finite element analysis. *J Shoulder Elbow Surg*, 23(3), 347–354. https://doi.org/10.1016/j.jse.2013.06.008.

Herzog, D., Seyda, V., Wycisk, E., & Emmelmann, C. (2016). Additive manufacturing of metals. *Acta Materialia*, *117*, 371–392. https://doi.org/10.1016/j.actamat.2016.07.019.

Iannotti, J. P., Jun, B. J., Derwin, K. A., & Ricchetti, E. T. (2021). Stepped augmented glenoid component in anatomic total shoulder arthroplasty for B2 and B3 glenoid pathology: a study of early outcomes. *J Bone Joint Surg Am.* https://doi.org/10.2106/JBJS.20.01420.

Ibounig, T., Simons, T., Launonen, A., & Paavola, M. (2020). Glenohumeral osteoarthritis: an overview of etiology and diagnostics. *Scand J Surg*, 1457496920935018. https://doi.org/10.1177/1457496920935018.

Ibrahim, M. Z., Sarhan, A. A. D., Yusuf, F., & Hamdi, M. (2017). Biomedical materials and techniques to improve the tribological, mechanical and biomedical properties of orthopedic implants – A review article. *J Alloys Compd*, *714*, 636–667. https://doi.org/10.1016/j.jallcom.2017.04.231.

Jensen, A. R., Tangtiphaiboontana, J., Marigi, E., Mallett, K. E., Sperling, J. W., & Sanchez-Sotelo, J. (2021). Anatomic total shoulder arthroplasty for primary glenohumeral osteoarthritis is associated with excellent outcomes and low revision rates in the elderly. *J Shoulder Elbow Surg*, *30*(7S), S131–S139. https://doi.org/10.1016/j.jse.2020.11.030.

Kang, C.-W., & Fang, F.-Z. (2018). State of the art of bioimplants manufacturing: part I. *Adv Manuf*, *6*(1), 20–40. https://doi.org/10.1007/s40436-017-0207-4.

Klemt, C., Prinold, J. A., Morgans, S., Smith, S. H. L., Nolte, D., Reilly, P., & Bull, A. M. J. (2018). Analysis of shoulder compressive and shear forces during functional activities of daily life. *Clin Biomech (Bristol, Avon)*, *54*, 34–41. https://doi.org/10.1016/j.clinbiomech.2018.03.006.

Kyriacou, S., Khan, S., & Falworth, M. (2019). The management of glenoid bone loss in shoulder arthroplasty. *J Arthrosc Jt Surg*, *6*(1), 21–30.

Li, G., Yin, J., Gao, J., Cheng, T. S., Pavlos, N. J., Zhang, C., & Zheng, M. H. (2013). Subchondral bone in osteoarthritis: insight into risk factors and microstructural changes. *Arthritis Res Ther*, *15*(6), 223. https://doi.org/10.1186/ar4405.

Lo, L., Koenig, S., Leong, N. L., Shiu, B. B., Hasan, S. A., Gilotra, M. N., & Wang, K. C. (2021). Glenoid bony morphology of osteoarthritis prior to shoulder arthroplasty: what the surgeon wants to know and why. *Skeletal Radiol*, *50*(5), 881–894. https://doi.org/10.1007/s00256-020-03647-x.

Marigi, E. M., Duquin, T. R., Throckmorton, T. Q., & Sperling, J. W. (2021). Hybrid fixation in anatomic shoulder arthroplasty: surgical technique and review of the literature. *JSES Rev, Reports, Tech*, *1*(2), 113–117. https://doi.org/10.1016/j.xrrt.2021.01.005.

Mueller, U., Braun, S., Schroeder, S., Schroeder, M., Sonntag, R., Jaeger, S., & Kretzer, J. P. (2017). Influence of humeral head material on wear performance in anatomic shoulder joint arthroplasty. *J Shoulder Elbow Surg*, *26*(10), 1756–1764. https://doi.org/10.1016/j.jse.2017.05.008.

Nicholson, G. P., Cvetanovich, G. L., Rao, A. J., & O'Donnell, P. (2017). Posterior glenoid bone grafting in total shoulder arthroplasty for osteoarthritis with severe posterior glenoid wear. *J Shoulder Elbow Surg*, *26*(10), 1844–1853. https://doi.org/10.1016/j.jse.2017.03.016.

NJR. (2020). National Joint Registry 17th Annual Report 2020 (17). https://reports.njrcentre.org.uk/.

Pandya, J., Johnson, T., & Low, A. K. (2018). Shoulder replacement for osteoarthritis: a review of surgical management. *Maturitas, 108,* 71–76. https://doi.org/10.1016/j.maturitas.2017.11.013.

Parada, S. A., Flurin, P. H., Wright, T. W., Zuckerman, J. D., Elwell, J. A., Roche, C. P., & Friedman, R. J. (2021). Comparison of complication types and rates associated with anatomic and reverse total shoulder arthroplasty. *J Shoulder Elbow Surg, 30*(4), 811–818. https://doi.org/10.1016/j.jse.2020.07.028

Paxton, N. C., Allenby, M. C., Lewis, P. M., & Woodruff, M. A. (2019). Biomedical applications of polyethylene. *Eur Polym J, 118,* 412–428. https://doi.org/10.1016/j.eurpolymj.2019.05.037.

Prakash, K. S., Nancharaih, T., & Rao, V. V. S. (2018). Additive manufacturing techniques in manufacturing -An overview. *Mater Today: Proc, 5*(2), 3873–3882. https://doi.org/10.1016/j.matpr.2017.11.642.

Priddy, M., Zarezadeh, A., Farmer, K. W., Struk, A. M., King, J. J., 3rd, Wright, T. W., & Schoch, B. S. (2019). Early results of augmented anatomic glenoid components. *J Shoulder Elbow Surg, 28*(6S), S138–S145. https://doi.org/10.1016/j.jse.2019.04.014.

Rasmussen, J. V., Hole, R., Metlie, T., Brorson, S., Aarimaa, V., Demir, Y., . . . Jensen, S. L. (2018). Anatomical total shoulder arthroplasty used for glenohumeral osteoarthritis has higher survival rates than hemiarthroplasty: a Nordic registry-based study. *Osteoarthr Cartil, 26*(5), 659–665. https://doi.org/10.1016/j.joca.2018.02.896.

Sabesan, V., Callanan, M., & Sharma, V. (2014). Guidelines for the selection of optimal glenoid augment size for moderate to severe glenohumeral osteoarthritis. *J Shoulder Elbow Surg, 23*(7), 974–981. https://doi.org/10.1016/j.jse.2013.09.022.

Sabesan, V. J., Lima, D. J. L., Whaley, J. D., Pathak, V., & Zhang, L. (2019). Biomechanical comparison of 2 augmented glenoid designs: an integrated kinematic finite element analysis. *J Shoulder Elbow Surg, 28*(6), 1166–1174. https://doi.org/https://doi.org/10.1016/j.jse.2018.11.055.

Stoffelen, D. V., Eraly, K., & Debeer, P. (2015). The use of 3D printing technology in reconstruction of a severe glenoid defect: a case report with 2.5 years of follow-up. *J Shoulder Elbow Surg, 24*(8), e218–222. https://doi.org/10.1016/j.jse.2015.04.006.

Talib Mohammed, M. (2018). Mechanical properties of SLM-titanium materials for biomedical applications: a review. *Mater Today: Proc, 5*(9), 17906–17913. https://doi.org/10.1016/j.matpr.2018.06.119.

Walch, G., Badet, R., Boulahia, A., & Khoury, A. (1999). Morphologic study of the glenoid in primary glenohumeral osteoarthritis. *J Arthroplasty, 14*(6), 756–760. https://doi.org/10.1016/s0883-5403(99)90232-2.

Wang, K. C., Jones, A., Kambhampati, S., Gilotra, M. N., Liacouras, P. C., Stuelke, S., . . . Siegel, E. L. (2019). CT-based 3D printing of the glenoid prior to shoulder arthroplasty: bony morphology and model evaluation. *J Digit Imaging, 32*(5), 816–826. https://doi.org/10.1007/s10278-019-00177-4.

Chapter 4

Fabrication and cost optimization of 3D printed mandible for applications in dentistry

Anil Kumar Birru
National Institute of Technology Manipur

Amandeep Kaur
RIMS Imphal Manipur

Khundrakpam Nimo Singh
National Institute of Technology Manipur

CONTENTS

4.1 INTRODUCTION

With the advent of three-dimensional (3D) technology, fabrication of a customized 3D object from a digital image has become a reality. An abstract idea can be transformed into a physical object. It involves construction of physical objects directly from 3D computer-aided design layer by layer and hence is also known as additive manufacturing technology. It is based on the principle of stacking two-dimensional (2D) layers to form 3D objects. It has varied applications in the fields of engineering, medicine, pharmaceuticals, architecture, biotechnology, robotics, aerospace industries and research. Advantages include freedom of design, accuracy, rapid prototyping, no inventory requirement, wide material range and low cost. In dentistry, 3D printing is employed for making patterns for metal casting of dental crowns and for the fabrication of copings, drill guides for dental implants, models for restorations and dental aligners.

DOI: 10.1201/9781003344810-4

Types of technologies involved include fused deposition modelling (FDM), fused filament fabrication (FFF), electron-beam freeform fabrication (EBF), direct metal laser sintering (DMLS), electron-beam melting (EBM), selective laser melting (SLM), selective heat sintering (SHS), selective laser sintering (SLS), plaster-based 3D printing (PP), laminated object manufacturing (LOM), stereolithography (SLA), digital light processing (DLP) and continuous liquid interface production (CLIP). Various materials utilized include thermoplastic materials (PLA and nylon), rubber, modelling clay, plasticine, RTV silicone, porcelain, metal alloy, metal matrix composite (MMC), titanium alloys, cobalt–chrome alloys, stainless steel and aluminium.

The process involves printing a 3D model from a digital image with the help of a 3D printer. The software of the 3D printer converts the 3D design into slices that can be printed and produces a slicer output "gcode". This controls the positioning of the print head, extruder temperature, bed temperature and extrusion speed. The host software sends the "gcode" to the printer for execution. The steps involved are as follows: image acquisition (DICOM), segmentation: DICOM→STL format conversion, mesh correction, selection of 3D printer and materials, printing and validation.

Caligiana et al. (2017) analysed quality function deployment (QFD) and TRIZ (Russian acronym of Theory of Inventive Problem Solving) in order to validate a design method for direct open moulds: hybrid manufacturing, which can reduce production time, use of material and energy and increase waste consumption employing subtractive and additive techniques combined. QFD can assess the product design by choice and definition of parameters that can be qualitatively discussed. The purpose was to meet a need in new and innovative ways. Castillo-Oyague et al. (2013) evaluated the marginal misfit and microleakage of cement-retained implant-supported crown copings. Single-crown structures were constructed with: (i) laser-sintered Co–Cr (LS); (ii) vacuum-cast Co–Cr (CC); and (iii) vacuum-cast Ni–Cr–Ti (CN). Samples of each alloy group were randomly luted in standard fashion onto machined titanium abutments using: (i) GC Fuji PLUS (FP); (ii) Clearfil Esthetic Cement (CEC); (iii) RelyX Unicem 2 Automix (RXU); and (iv) DentoTemp (DT) ($n = 15$ each). The results demonstrated that regardless of the cement type, LS samples exhibited the best fit, while CC and CN performed equally well. It was concluded that DMLS of Co–Cr may be a reliable alternative to the casting of base metal alloys to obtain well-fitted implant-supported crowns, although all the groups tested were within the clinically acceptable range of vertical discrepancy. Chang et al. (2019) evaluated the marginal gaps of dental restorations manufactured using conventional loss wax and casting, computer-aided design/computer-aided manufacturing (CAD/CAM) and 3D printing methods. A total of 10 Co–Cr–Mo metal crowns were individually obtained using the conventional loss wax and casting method (Group A), selective laser sintering (Group B) and CAD/CAM (Group C), respectively. Statistical analyses revealed significant differences in the marginal gaps in Group A with Groups B and C ($p < 0.05$). The mean marginal gaps between dental crowns with die models were 76 ± 61 μm, 116 ± 92 μm and 121 ± 98 μm for Groups A, B, and C, respectively.

Dawood et al. (2015) reviewed the types of 3D printing technologies available and their various applications in dentistry and in maxillofacial surgery. The technology has a particular resonance with dentistry, and with advances in 3D imaging and modelling technologies such as cone-beam computed tomography and intraoral scanning, and with the relatively long history of the use of CAD CAM technologies in dentistry, it has become of increasing importance. The uses of 3D printing include the production of drill guides for dental implants; the production of physical models for prosthodontics, orthodontics and surgery; the manufacture of dental, craniomaxillofacial and orthopaedic implants; and the fabrication of copings and frameworks for implant and dental restorations.

Erdil and Arani (2019) developed a framework for the implementation of QFD as a quality improvement tool. A case study approach was used to test this framework, and quality issues were analysed using the framework in a ceramic tile manufacturing company. The results showed considerable improvements in the critical quality characteristics identified and sales rates, demonstrating the potential of QFD to be used in assessing and prioritizing areas of improvement, and converting them into measurable process or product requirements. Joerg et al. (2006) reviewed the existing CAD/CAM systems, describing the components of CAD/CAM technologies and addressing the limitations of current systems, and suggesting possibilities for future systems. It was concluded that the existing dental CAD/CAM systems vary dramatically in their capabilities; each has distinct advantages and limitations. None can yet acquire data directly in the mouth and produce the full spectrum of restoration types (with the breadth of material choices) that can be created by traditional techniques. Konstantoulakis et al. (1998) evaluated the marginal fit and surface roughness of complete crowns made with a conventional and an accelerated casting technique. A conventional technique was compared with an accelerated technique that used 13- to 17-minute bench set time and 15-minute wax elimination cycle in a 815°C (1500°F) preheated furnace. For the marginal discrepancy and surface roughness, crowns fabricated with the accelerated casting technique were not significantly ($P > 0.05$) different from those fabricated with the conventional technique. However, the accelerated casting technique could be a vital alternative to the time-consuming conventional techniques.

In the study of Lei et al. (2018), investment casting (IC) using 3D stereolithography (SLA)-printed patterns was proposed to fabricate 3D metal heat transfer devices designed by topology optimization (TO). It highlighted that SLA-assisted IC is a cost-effective technology with high accuracy for fabricating TO metal parts. A natural convection experimental set-up was used to experimentally study the performance of the fabricated heat sinks. The results showed that the tested TO heat sinks performed better when compared to pin-fin heat sinks, operating under the conditions used for the optimization. Lim et al. (2020) evaluated the mechanical properties and bone regeneration ability of 3D printed pure hydroxyapatite (HA)/tricalcium phosphate (TCP) pure ceramic scaffolds with variable pore architectures. The findings showed that various pore architectures of HA/TCP scaffolds can be achieved using DLP 3D printing, which can be a valuable tool for optimizing bone scaffold properties for specific clinical treatments.

Low and Mori (1999) established a statistical model between thermal expansion values of investments and dimensional accuracy of cast titanium full crowns. A high correlation coefficient ($R = 0.87$) was found between dimensional accuracy (Y) and thermal expansion value (X). It was concluded that the dimensional accuracy expressed as the discrepancy between wax pattern and casting is easy to understand and less confusing than the traditional percentage value. The crown accuracy was highly predictable ($R = 0.87$) from the thermal expansion value of investments determined under controlled laboratory measuring conditions. Morey and Earnshaw (1995) investigated the effects of mould expansion and hot strength on the relative inaccuracy of full-crown castings. The likelihood that a strong investment could cause distortion of the casting by non-uniform restriction of casting shrinkage was also considered. Casting inaccuracy showed a significant linear correlation with total expansion and a highly significant linear correlation with the combination of total expansion and hot strength. The modified investment, with its low hot strength, gave less distortion of casting shape than did the much stronger unmodified material. This investigation revealed that while investment expansion is the major variable affecting casting inaccuracy, hot strength is an important modifying factor that also has to be considered when predicting casting inaccuracy from measured properties of the investment. Pradhan et al. (2021) reported the framework on metal/composite crown restoration, materials and design considerations of crown and different conventional and latest crown fabrication techniques (assisted with 3D thermoplastic and metal printing) for prosthetic dentistry in veterinary patients. The steps for the preparation of crown for canine teeth (with 3D printing by using stainless steel (SS) 316L powder and other conventional investment casting (IC) methods) were outlined. Clinical and histological advantages with respect to standard denture fixing procedures and classical denture geometry were demonstrated.

Sahu and Modi (2021) analysed Taguchi's design of experiment approach to optimize the process parameters of a 3D printer for enhancing the compressive strength (CS) of porous bone scaffolds. L9 orthogonal array (OA) was chosen to design and perform the experiments. LT: 89 µm, BO: 0o, BP: middle and DT: 200 ms were the optimum values of parameters obtained by S/N ratio analysis. LT was the most significant (48.18%), BO was slightly less significant than LT (45%), BP was little significant (6.39%), and DT was found non-significant (0.43%) as per the ANOVA. A linear regression model was developed to predict the CS of the fabricated scaffolds. The developed model was found adequate with 94.4% R-sq and 93% R-sq(adj) values. The confirmation test resulted in a maximum difference of 8.18% between experimental and predicted values of CS.

Seitz et al. (2005) reported a new process chain for custom-made three-dimensional (3D) porous ceramic scaffolds for bone replacement with fully interconnected channel network for the repair of osseous defects from trauma or disease. It was demonstrated that it is possible to manufacture parts with inner channels with a dimension down to 450 micron and wall structures with a thickness down to 330 microns. The mechanical strength of dense test parts was up to 22 MPa. Shao et al. (2017) evaluated the role of side-wall pore architecture in direct-ink-writing bioceramic scaffolds on mechanical properties and osteogenic capacity in rabbit calvarial defects. It was found that the dilute Mg doping and/or two-step sintering schedule was especially beneficial for improving the compressive strength (~25–104 MPa) and flexural strength (~6–18 MPa) of the calcium silicate scaffolds. The histological analysis for the calvarial bone specimens in vivo revealed that the SLP scaffolds had a high osteoconduction at the early stage (4 weeks), but the DLP scaffolds displayed a higher osteogenic capacity in the later stage (8–12 weeks). These findings demonstrate that the side-wall pore architecture in 3D printed bioceramic scaffolds is required to optimize for bone repair in calvarial bone defects, and particularly, the Mg doping wollastonite is promising for 3D printing thin-wall porous scaffolds for craniomaxillofacial bone defect treatment. Singh et al. (2020) evaluated the techno-economic and process capability analysis on the cast dentures made by thermoplastic- and wax-based patterns with investment casting (IC). Five different routes for making patterns (viz. wax-based patterns by conventional method, wax-based patterns with CAD/CAM support, thermoplastic-based acrylonitrile butadiene styrene (ABS)-based patterns prepared by FDM, combination of ABS+wax-based patterns and ABS-based patterns in combination with chemical vapour smoothening (CVS)) were used and further casted with NiCr(K) alloy by changing the Ni% F-(3) by wt. in different proportions. The observed values of process capability indices (C_p and C_{pk}) for all five process routes greater than 1.33 outlined that all selected routes are statistically controlled.

Singh and Dureja (2014) developed a framework of MMC-based dental implants by stir casting (SC) in silicon moulding (SM)-based investment shells. A comparative study of barrel finishing (BF) and CVS for improving the surface finish of FDM-based dentistry patterns made by using acrylonitrile butadiene styrene (ABS) filament material was highlighted (for a better understanding of intermediate steps). The effects of process parameters of hybrid FDM-BF and FDM-CVS were investigated using Taguchi L9 OA.

It was observed that the CVS method was more effective for improving the surface finish of ABS replicas without any countereffects on the dimensional accuracy as compared to BF.

In their study, Warnke et al. (2010) investigated the behaviour of human osteoblasts on HAP and TCP scaffolds. Cells seen on HAP scaffolds were more than on TCP scaffolds. Cell vitality staining and MTT, LDH, and WST tests showed superior biocompatibility of HAP scaffolds to BioOssVR, while BioOssVR was more compatible as compared to TCP. Zagidullin et al. (2021) demonstrated various versions of the kinematics of FDM 3D printers, the main units and parts, as well as their impact on the quality of 3D printing of parts. A qualimetric assessment of the quality of FDM 3D printers with various versions of kinematics design based on the QFD interconnection matrix was carried out. The aim of the study was to analyse the design and kinematics of FDM 3D printers for the manufacture of high-quality parts and assemblies for unmanned aerial vehicles without further post-processing based on the application of the QFD methodology. Based on the results of the study, recommendations and proposals for improving the design of FDM 3D printers were developed. Zhang et al. (2006) investigated the possibility of obtaining accurate titanium crown casts using wax patterns fabricated by a CAD/CAM system with a non-expanded mould. Three experimental magnesia-based investments (A, B and C) were made, and their properties were evaluated for dental use. Two types of wax patterns for full-coverage coping crowns (S-0: cement space of $0\,\mu m$; S-20: cement space of $20\,\mu m$) were fabricated using a commercial CAD/CAM system. The fit of the titanium crowns differed significantly between the TM and the CAD/CAM system. The ranges of thickness obtained from the TM, S-0 and S-20 were 20.78–$357.88\,\mu m$, 25.12–$107.46\,\mu m$ and 17.84–$58.92\,\mu m$, respectively. Hence, it was concluded that high-quality titanium crown casting was obtained using a combination of wax patterns fabricated by a CAD/CAM system and a non-expanded MgO-based investment, yet much work was made on QFD in 3D printing using PLA; hence, researchers made an attempt.

4.2 MATERIALS AND METHODS

In attaining the ability to function high knowledges, it is important not to ignore the necessity to educate the required scientific experts and to create a society capable of handling the high level of production difficulty. Recent economies are built around the so-called knowledge complex – a system of interaction between the abilities and mechanisms of a complex resolution. It is important to incorporate the concurrent design, i.e. the simultaneous creation of complementary solutions based on uniform architecture, and decentralized system of cooperation. The prerequisite for achieving these

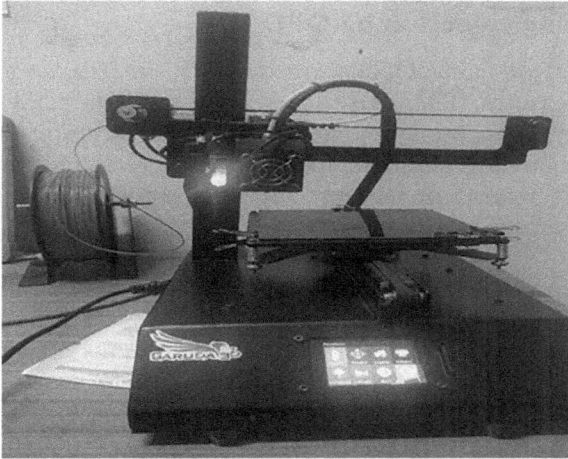

Figure 4.1 3D printing machine.

levels of ability is to break the communication barriers, to use scientific methods based on task mapping and the freedom of information exchange, and to form mutual areas of cooperation within process organization. If this fails, then it might meaningfully limit the transparency and be considerate of the dependencies and hence productive team collaboration. 3D printing might attain the solutions and may provide an easier and authentic way to achieve precise properties of the printed object with QFD.

In this research work, we used a FDM 3D printer "G3D Atom", which was manufactured by Garuda 3D. Garuda 3D is located a Hyderabad, Telangana, India. Figure 4.1 shows the image of a 3D printer. Various polymers may be used, including ABS, polycarbonate (PC), polylactic acid (PLA), high-density polyethylene (HDPE), PC/ABS, polyethylene terephthalate (PETG), polyphenylsulfone (PPSU) and high-impact polystyrene (HIPS). In this experiment, PLA filament is used to print the crown patterns. PLA is the most adopted material by most 3D printer users at domestic and industrial levels. PLA is a bio-plastic and is therefore eco-friendly, and it is not harmful to human and animal health. PLA is a green material since it is fabricated from fully renewable sources such as corn, sugarcane, wheat, or any other high carbohydrate-containing resources. PLA is preferred by most 3D printer users because it does not always need a heated bed for the adhesion to occur between the print and the platform. In its semi-crystalline form, PLA has been shown to exhibit good flexural modulus and better tensile and flexural strengths. The following are some of the important properties of the material: special property: easy to print; biodegradable uses: consumer products; strength at medium density: $1240\,kg/m^3$; filament thickness: 1.75 mm; colour: orange.

4.2.1 Processing parameters of 3D printing selection by QFD

The final goal of many QFD processes is to set the target values for the design measures. This step occurs when the data gathered throughout the process are brought together and final decisions are made to answer the following question: "What are we really going to do (with respect to this product or service)?" Setting target values should be relatively easy because:

- The team has already defined where they want their product/service to be positioned for the customer.
- The team has benchmarked the existing products/services to gain a good understanding of what level of actual performance is required in order to produce the desired level of perceived performance.
- The team has evaluated the trade-offs between design measures in order to determine what compromises may be required and how those compromises would be made.

Taking into account all of this information, the team decides upon the targets which they will shoot for. Normally, at this point, the team would not decide how they are going to achieve the target values. They are just stating, "we know that we have to achieve this level of performance if we are going to be perceived the way in which we want to be perceived". Deciding on the implementation approach will generally occur during the conceptualization process. From the survey reports, the summary of the data collected related to voice of customer, overall importance rating and current performance of the organization with respect to the concerned requirement and target values is listed in Table 4.1.

The overall importance rating could clearly be analysed by constructing a bar chart between the above-mentioned parameters, and it is represented in the following charts. After developing a voice of customer and importance

Table 4.1 Voice of customer and its importance rating in relevance to 3D printing

S. No.	Voice of customer	Overall importance rating	Current performance	Target value
1	Economic charges	8	4	8
2	Punctuality of time scheduling	10	7	10
3	Dust-free maintenance of 3D printing	7	5	7
4	Safety (including noise and vibration)	10	7	10
5	Ability to print with various materials	8	2	8
6	High print speed	10	7	10
7	Quality (accuracy and roughness) of printing	10	6	10

Table 4.2 Technical descriptors in order to realize voice of customer of 3D printing

S. No.	Technical descriptor	Relative weight
1	Weight	694
2	Dimension	243
3	Maintenance time	198
4	Material time	234
5	Type of data transfer	276

rating, a brainstorming session with a team of three members was carried out. The operational activities were identified as most important in realizing customer desires. Organization's current performance of each technical descriptor, in order to satisfy technical parameters and target values, is shown in Table 4.2.

4.2.2 Establishing relationships

Relationships between lists indicate how the two lists are related to each other. They are generally used to prioritize one list based upon the priorities of another list. Relationships can be defined by answering a particular question for each cell in a matrix. For example, the relationships between customer requirements and design measures might be defined by asking the following question: "To what degree does this measure predict the customer's satisfaction with this requirement?" By asking this same question consistently for each measure and requirement combination, a set of relationships will be defined in the matrix, which will help to determine which measures are most important to control in order to achieve a desired level of customer satisfaction. Another question that can be asked in order to define relationships is as follows: What percent of this requirement is handled by this design measure? The relationships defined using this question would result in the highest priority being assigned to the measures that control most of the functionality. These may not be the same as the measures defined in order to predict customer satisfaction. It was established that major inputs were taken for the research and are depicted in Figure 4.2. The relationship matrix of VOC & technical descriptors of the fabricated dental crown and further deployment of voice of customer of matching process parameters is shown in Figure 4.3.

Representative symbols used:
O → Represents strong relationship → 9
■ → Represents weak relationship → 1
▲ → Represents medium relationship → 3

Technical descriptors in which the following symbols were used.

O   Represents Strong Relationship   9

■   Represents Weak Relationship   1

▲   Represents Medium Relationship   3

Relation	Symbol	Rating	Importance rating.	Weight	Dimension.	Maintenance time	Material time	Type of data transfer	
Strong	o	9							
Medium	▲	3							
Weak	■	1							
Economic charges.			8					O	
Punctuality of time scheduling			10	O	▲		▲		
Maintenance of 3D Printing with dust free			7		O				
Safety (including noise and vibration)			10						
Ability to print with various materials			8	O			▲		
High print speed			10						
Quality (accuracy and roughness) of printing			10					▲	

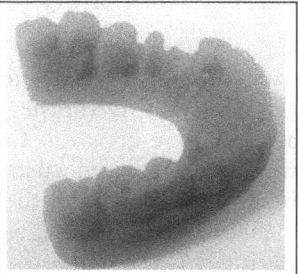

Figure 4.2 Relationship matrix of VOC & technical descriptors of fabricated dental crown.

4.3 RESULTS AND DISCUSSION OF "DEPLOYMENT OF VOC"

1. Table 4.3 depicts various technical descriptors and their corresponding relative weights obtained from the deployment of VOC.
2. The aspect of "Time scheduling activities" has a maximum relative weight, and "Ladies & P.H seating activities" has a minimum relative weight among all technical descriptors.

Relation Symbol Rating	Importance rating.	Weight	Dimension.	Maintenance time	Material time	Type of data transfer	Current performance rating.	Target rating.	Scale-up factor.	Abs. value of importance rating.
Strong o 9										
Medium ▲ 3										
Weak ■ 1										
Economic charges.	8					O	4	8	2.0	16
Punctuality of time scheduling	10	O	▲		▲		3	10	3.3	33
Maintenance of 3D Printing with dust free	7		O				3	7	2.3	16
Safety (including noise and vibration)	10						4	7	1.8	11
Ability to print with various materials	8	O			▲		4	9	2.3	21
High print speed	10						3	7	2.3	14
Quality (accuracy and roughness) of printing	10					▲	2	7	3.5	25
Absolute Weight		238	93	72	86	114				
Relative Weight		694	243	198	234	276				

Figure 4.3 Deployment of voice of customer of matching process parameters.

Table 4.3 Results of deployment of VOC of process parameters of 3D printing

S. No.	Technical descriptor	Organization's current performance
1	Weight	5
2	Dimension	3
3	Maintenance time	2
4	Material time	5
5	Type of data transfer	3

4.4 CONCLUSIONS AND FUTURE SCOPE

Conclusions:

It is a well-established fact that material time and weight of the material plays a predominant role in product design and manufacturing. The QFD method usually employs criteria weight values in their computations, which are based on the subjective judgements of the designers. In this research work, the following major conclusions were drawn:

1. The application of a QFD approach for material selection is demonstrated with 3D printing technology. As a point scale is adopted here, weights can accommodate the customers' requirements and/or technical requirements as per the standard procedure.
2. An excellent agreement is established between the rankings observed using the QFD-based approach for voice of the customer and the importance of rating for a better understanding of the conceptual design of the 3D printing products.
3. The QFD approach can be customized with parallel activities in product design to minimize the cost, improve the quality and trim down the development time of the products.

Future scope:
It also leads to a better understanding of the conceptual design of the 3D printing products during which parallel activities in product design can be performed to minimize the cost, improve the quality and trim down the development time of the products. Here, the researchers made use of only PLA. It is further directed to incorporate acrylonitrile butadiene styrene (ABS), polycarbonate (PC), high-density polyethylene (HDPE), PC/ABS, polyethylene terephthalate (PETG), polyphenylsulfone (PPSU), and high-impact polystyrene (HIPS).

Acknowledgements: We would like to thank the TEQIP-III, NPIU, Government of India and National Institute of Technology, Manipur, Imphal, India-795004, for the financial support of this research work.

REFERENCES

Caligiana, L, Francia, F, & Donnici, G. (2017). Integrating QFD and TRIZ for innovative design. *Journal of Advanced Mechanical Design, Systems, and Manufacturing*, 11(2) JAMDSM0015, Released on J-STAGE May 09, 2017, Online ISSN 1881-3054, https://doi.org/10.1299/jamdsm.2017jamdsm0015, https://www.jstage.jst.go.jp/article/jamdsm/11/2/11_2017jamdsm0015/_article/-char/en

Castillo-Oyagüe, R, Lynch, CD, Turrión, AS, et al. (2013). Misfit and microleakage of implant-supported crown copings obtained by laser sintering and casting techniques, luted with glass-ionomer, resin cements and acrylic/urethane-based agents. *Journal of Dentistry*, 41(1), 90–96.

Chang, HS, Peng, YT, Hung, WL, & Hsu, ML. (2019). Evaluation of marginal adaptation of Co-Cr-Mo metal crowns fabricated by traditional method and computer-aided technologies. *Journal of Dental Sciences*, 14, 288–294.

Dawood, A, Marti, B, Sauret-Jackson, V. et al. (2015). 3D printing in dentistry. *British Dental Journal*, 219, 521–529. Doi: 10.1038/sj.bdj.2015.914

Erdil, NO & Arani, OM. (2019). Quality function deployment: More than a design tool. *International Journal of Quality and Service Sciences*, 11, 142–166.

Joerg, R, Strub, E, Rekow, D, & Witkowski, S. (2006). Computer-aided design and fabrication of dental restorations: Current systems and future possibilities. *The Journal of the American Dental Association*, 137(9), 1289–1296.

Konstantoulakis, E, Nakajima, H, Woody, RD, & Miller, AW. (1998). Marginal fit and surface roughness of crowns made with an accelerated casting technique. *Journal of Prosthetic Dentistry*, 80(3), 337–345.

Lei, T, Alexandersen, J, Lazarov, BS, Wang, F, Haertel, JHK, Sanna, S, et al. (2018). Investment casting and experimental testing of heat sinks designed by topology optimization. *International Journal of Heat and Mass Transfer*, 127, Part B, 396–341. ISSN 0017-9310, DOI: 10.1016/j.ijheatmasstransfer.2018.07.060

Lim, HK, Hong, SJ, Byeon, SJ, Chung, SM, On, SW, Yang, BE, Lee, JH, & Byun, SH. (2020). 3D-printed ceramic bone scaffolds with variable pore architectures. *International Journal of Molecular Sciences*, 21(18), 6942.

Low, D & Mori, T. (1999). Titanium full crown casting: Thermal expansion of investments and crown accuracy. *Dental Materials*, 15(3), 185–190.

Morey, EF & Earnshaw, R. (1995). The effect of potential investment expansion and hot strength on the fit of full-crown castings made with a gypsum-bonded investment. *Dental Materials*, 11(5), 311–316.

Pradhan, SR, Singh, R, & Banwait, SS. (2021). On crown fabrication in prosthetic dentistry of veterinary patients: A review. *Advances in Materials and Processing Technologies*, 1–20. DOI: 10.1080/2374068X.2021.1970991

Sahu, KK & Modi, YK. (2021). Investigation on dimensional accuracy, compressive strength and measured porosity of additively manufactured calcium sulphate porous bone scaffolds. *Materials Technology*, 36(8), 492–503, DOI: 10.1080/10667857.2020.1774728

Seitz, H, Rieder, W, Irsen, S, Leukers, B, & Tille, C. (2005). Three-dimensional printing of porous ceramic scaffolds for bone tissue engineering. *Journal of Biomedical Materials Research. Part B, Applied Biomaterials*, 74, 782–788.

Shao, H, Ke, X, Liu, A, Sun, M, He, Y, Yang, X, Fu, J, Liu, Y, Zhang, L, Yang, G, Xu, S, & Gou, Z. (2017). Bone regeneration in 3D printing bioactive ceramic scaffolds with improved tissue/material interface pore architecture in thin-wall bone defect. *Biofabrication*, 9(2), 025003.

Singh, G, Singh, R, Singh, S, & Bhardwaj, A. (2020). Comparison of Thermoplastic and Wax Based Patterns for Investment Casting of Partial Dentures: Techno-Economic and Process Capability Analysis. *Encyclopedia of Materials: Plastics and Polymers*, 1, 94–115.

Singh, R & Dureja, JS. (2014). Development of Metal Matrix Composite-Based Dental Implants by Stir Casting in Silicon Molding-Based Investment Shells. *Materials Science and Materials Engineering*. ISBN 9780128035818. Doi: 10.1016/B978-0-12-803581-8.04154-0

Warnke, P, Seitz, H, Warnke, F, Becker, S, Sivananthan, S, Sherry, E, Wiltfang, J, & Douglas, T. (2010). Ceramic scaffolds produced by computer-assisted 3D printing and sintering: Characterization and biocompatibility investigations. *Journal of biomedical materials research. Part B, Applied biomaterials*, 93, 212–217.

Zagidullin, R, Mitroshkina T, and Dmitriev A. Quality Function Deployment and Design Risk Analysis for the Selection and Improvement of FDM 3D Printer, Published under licence by IOP Publishing Ltd. *IOP Conference Series: Earth Environmental Science*, 666, 062123. International science and technology conference "Earth science" 8 - 10 December 2020, Vladivostok, Russian Federation.

Zhang, Z, Tamaki, Y, Hotta, Y, & Miyazaki, T. (2006). Novel method for titanium crown casting using a combination of wax patterns fabricated by a CAD/CAM system and a non-expanded investment. *Dental Materials*, 22(7), 681–617.

Chapter 5

Synthesis, properties, and applications of PEEK-based biomaterials

S. Sathishkumar, P. Jawahar, and Prasun Chakraborti

National Institute of Technology Agartala

CONTENTS

DOI: 10.1201/9781003344810-5

5.1 INTRODUCTION

Recent days, the world is facing several problems in the medical field, revealing the prominent requirement of biomaterials. In this emerging world, accidents involving humans are inevitable. Due to this type of accidents, humans may severely be affected from bone fracture, bone loss, and hormone loss. In some cases, even diseases may cause these issues. To overcome these types of issues, scientists have discovered bone implants. Earlier, researchers focused on bone implant materials based on metals such as stainless steel, titanium (Ti), and cobalt-chromium (Co-Cr). These metal-based implants have some drawbacks such as toxic effects, high elastic modulus, and stress shielding. To overcome these problems, researchers moved from metal implants to polymer implants.

These days, polymer-based biomaterials have inherent spectacular properties for clinical applications. Several types of natural and synthetic polymers are substantially used in various medical applications. This chapter primarily illustrates the synthetic polymer PEEK (Polyether ether ketone). Generally, the PEEK-based polymers represent the largest and versatile class of biomaterials being extensively applied in various clinical applications. The PEEK-based materials should be satisfying some basic requirements, namely biocompatibility, bio-acceptability, and biodegradability. Particularly, PEEK-based biomaterials possess numerous favourable properties such as less weight, greater tensile strength, high toughness, flashing, low friction rate, excellent dimensional stability, exceptional insulation properties, good sterilization resistance, biocompatibility, abrasion resistance, inherent purity, excellent creep resistance, high flexural modulus, excellent corrosion resistance, high wear and fatigue resistance, low toxic gas emission, chemical resistance, and X-ray radiolucency. These PEEK-based biomaterials are highly used in many applications in the medical industry, e.g. facial and cranial implants, spinal implants, orthopaedic implants, dental and cardiac implants [1,2].

5.2 HISTORICAL BACKGROUND OF PEEK MATERIALS

PEEK is a high-performance semi-crystalline thermoplastic candidate. It is a member of the PAEK family. PEEK is the most extensively used member of aromatic polyketones, and it is originally invented by Victrex plc in the year 1980. The PEEK-based polymeric materials were manufactured by nucleophilic aromatic substitution reaction of the potassium salt of hydroquinone and 4,4'-difluorobenzophenone, such as step-growth polymerization method.

Generally, the pure PEEK polymer (Figure 5.1) possesses extraordinary, balanced physical and chemical properties because of its semi-crystalline

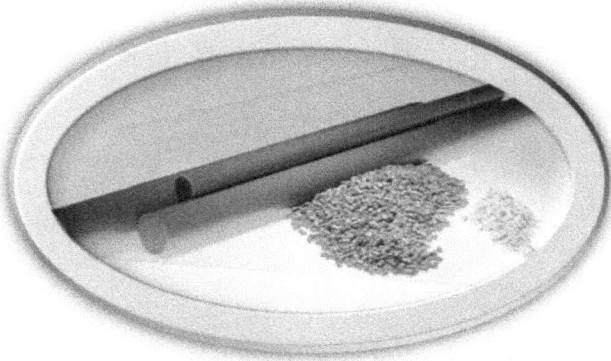

Figure 5.1 Powder, pellets, extruded rods, and film of unfilled "virgin" PEEK. (Copyright (2021) with permission from Elsevier [4].)

nature. So the PEEK has developed good bonding with the reinforced constituent. For example, pure PEEK does not have adequate wear resistance, but with the addition of carbon fibres, the property gets enhanced. In the initial stage of PEEK composites, only the carbon fibre (CF) and glass fibre (GF) were used, but nowadays, numerous filler materials are utilized depending upon the application, such as automotive, aerospace, structural, electrical, and biomedical applications [3,4].

5.3 STRUCTURE OF PAEK (PEK, PEKK, AND PEEK)

Polyetherketone (PEK) and polyetherketoneketone (PEKK) also belong to the ketone polymer group, and they are similar to the PEEK aromatic polymer.

5.3.1 Polyetherketone (PEK)

PEK is also a part of the PAEK family. It is an odourless, semi-crystalline, high-performance, engineering thermoplastic and was initially discovered by K. Dahl of Raychem in the year 1970. Its chemical structure is shown in Figure 5.2a. This type of aromatic polymer is synthesized through the nucleophilic route and electrophilic process (reaction of 4, 4'-difluorobenzophenone with 4,4'-dihydroxybenzophenone) with the help of Friedel-Crafts catalyst. This type of PAEK polymer holds a unique combination of thermal stability, chemical resistance to many organic and inorganic chemicals, and ultimate mechanical properties and has the potential as a matrix material for high-performance composites [5].

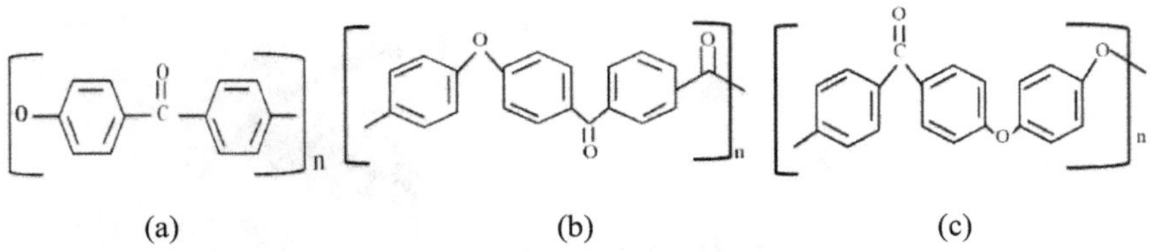

Figure 5.2 Chemical structures of (a) PEK, (b) PEKK, and (c) PEEK.

5.3.2 Polyetherketoneketone (PEKK)

PEKK is a new, evolving polymeric material, and it also belongs to the high-temperature-resistant PAEK polymer group. Its chemical structure is shown in Figure 5.2b. The benzene rings associated with ketone groups establish high modulus and long-term thermal oxidative stability. At the same time, the ether linkages grant toughness and ductility and facilitate ease of processing. This type of polymeric material possesses outstanding thermal stability, good thermal resistance, and attractive mechanical properties [6].

5.3.3 Polyether ether ketone (PEEK)

The PEEK comprises an aromatic backbone molecular chain interconnected by ether and ketone functional groups [4]. Figure 5.2c represents the chemical structures of PAEK polymers.

5.4 MATERIAL PROPERTIES OF PEEK

The material properties are the most essential aspect while selecting a material for specific applications. Initially, properties only imply a clear idea about the material to the researcher. There are numerous properties of the material that need to be considered, such as mechanical, chemical, electrical, and thermal properties. The PEEK is extremely tough and retains its excellent mechanical properties close to its melting temperature. Besides that, it has the low tendency of creep and superior sliding and wear characteristics. It is highly resistant to thermal degradation and to attacks in both aqueous and organic environments.

From a research perspective, various properties of virgin PEEK, 30 wt.% CF-infused PEEK composites, and 30 wt.% GF-infused PEEK composites are provided in this section (Figure 5.3).

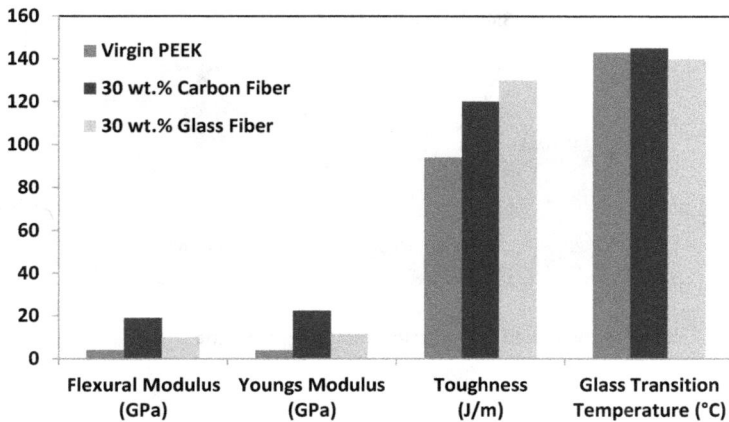

Figure 5.3 Properties of PEEK and PEEK-based composites [5–7].

5.5 SYNTHESIS OF PEEK COMPOSITES

PEEK-based composite materials are made in general by the following techniques:

1. Injection moulding
2. Compression moulding
3. Additive manufacturing.

5.5.1 Injection moulding

Injection moulding is an extensively used polymer fabrication method in which the plastic parts are made by forcing liquefied polymer into the cavity followed by solidification. The schematic diagram of injection moulding machine is shown in Figure 5.4. Currently, the injection moulding process receives interest because of short processing time, net shape moulding, and complex 3D parts that can be produced economically. Generally, the selection of injection moulding settings is most crucial because during shaping, the behaviour of the polymeric material is deeply influenced by various parameters. The standard of moulded product can be determined by following prescribed process parameters such as mould temperature, melt temperature, injection pressure, injection time, injection speed, filling time, ejection time, holding pressure, holding time, the mould geometry shape, material properties of melt, melt speed, heat transfer rate, and cooling time [8,9].

Arevalo et al. manufactured CF-reinforced PEEK composites by an injection moulding technique. To remove the residual moisture, the granules

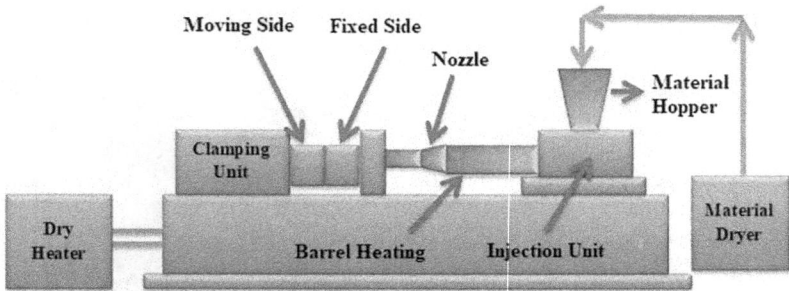

Figure 5.4 Constructional view of injection moulding machine.

were initially preheated at 70°C and then PEEK composite was fabricated at a nozzle temperature of 400°C and mould temperature of 250°C. The nanomechanical properties were investigated on injection-moulded clinical-grade PEEK and CF-reinforced PEEK composites [10].

Puertolas et al. fabricated a graphene nanoplatelet (GNP)-infused PEEK composite by injection moulding method and evaluated its tribological and mechanical properties. The processing temperature, injection time, compaction pressure, and cooling time followed were 360°C, 0.36 seconds, 1000 bar, and 3 seconds [11].

The injection-moulded multiwalled carbon nanotubes (MWCNT)-blended PEEK composite provides outstanding material properties. Toshio et al. used the injection moulding technique for composite preparation and evaluated the stress-strain characteristics of the MWCNT-PEEK composite. The processing temperature of the composite was 380°C, and the mould temperature was kept at 180°C. Here, the CNT distribution was aligned with the injection moulding direction [12].

5.5.2 Compression moulding

Compression moulding method is the most popular and common processing method to produce PEEK-based polymer composite products. The schematic diagram of compression moulding system is shown in Figure 5.5. Generally, the compression moulding is overshadowed by injection moulding techniques. The compression moulding is a high-pressure and high-volume method. It is most suited for manufacturing parts with superior strength and durability, and it is one of the first industrial techniques for metal replacement applications. To enhance the production rate and part quality, various types of parameters are considered for the compression moulding process. Typically, the principal parameters are grouped into three categories [13,14].

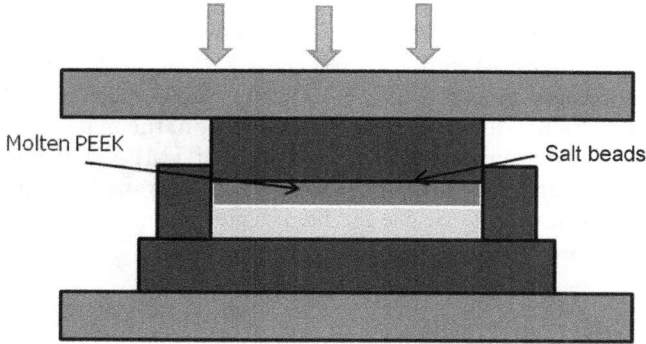

Figure 5.5 Compression moulding. (Copyright (2021) with permission from Elsevier [26].)

1. Material parameters
2. Process parameters
3. Tooling parameters.

Material parameters: Material parameters purely depend upon the type of raw material used in the compression moulding process, for example pellets and sheets (sheet thickness, pellet diameter, temperature, etc.).

Process parameters: The mainly considered process parameters are pre-charging specifications, mould temperature, mould pressure, and mould closing speed.

Tooling parameters: These parameters are strongly associated with part design, shear edge, parting line, air vent, tool material, draft angle, surface finish, and ejection system.

The PEEK-based polymer material is located into a heated metal mould and then is softened with the help of heat and forced to conform to the shape of the mould as the mould closes. Once moulding is complete, the excess amount of flash should be removed.

Compression moulding provides excellent real-time monitoring and accurate temperature control during the compaction and consolidation of PEEK composites. Ruaa et al. studied the influence of process parameters on crystal morphology and mechanical properties of compression-moulded high-performance PEEK composites. Generally, the compression mould-ing process will improve the material properties of PEEK-based polymer composites; besides that, the compression moulding also provides various supportive advantages such as cost reduction, prevention of quenches, and gasket size reduction [15].

Ahmad et al. prepared an ionic liquid-modified MWCNT-reinforced PEEK composite by the compression moulding method. The compression moulding was executed at 350°C for 10 minutes, and the PEEK composites' morphological and thermo-mechanical properties are evaluated. The compression-moulded PEEK composite possesses outstanding material properties and hence the most suitable replacement material for bone implants [16]. A compression-moulded CF-PEEK composite's crystallinity behaviour was examined by Batista et al. In this investigation, the material was heated up to 390°C for 30 minutes under the pressure of 5 MPa [17]. The compression moulding infiltration process produces a broad range of pore sizes and enhances the connectivity of the medical devices, aimed at enhanced bone growth and improved mechanical performance [18].

5.5.3 Additive manufacturing

Additive manufacturing is also called "3D printing" or "rapid prototyping". The schematic diagram is shown in Figure 5.6. The rapid prototyping is a layer-by-layer manufacturing technique, which is used to quickly fabricate complex geometries with the use of three-dimensional CAD data. In additive manufacturing, it is possible to manufacture intricate parts, which may not be possible with conventional technique, and a 3D model can be produced at a low cost without the requirement of any special tooling.

Fused deposition modelling (FDM) is a versatile tool used in additive manufacturing technique. A polymer thread is heated with a print head (nozzle) and placed over a fixtureless platform layer by layer. The principle of FDM is purely based on surface chemistry, thermal energy, and layer manufacturing technology. The material in the filament (spool) form is melted in a specially designed head, which extrudes on the model and is followed by cooling. The various parameters that disturb the performance and functionalities of the system such as material flexural modulus, material column strength, road width, deposition speed, positioning accuracy, material viscosity, envelope temperature, volumetric flow rate, tip diameter, and part geometry [19].

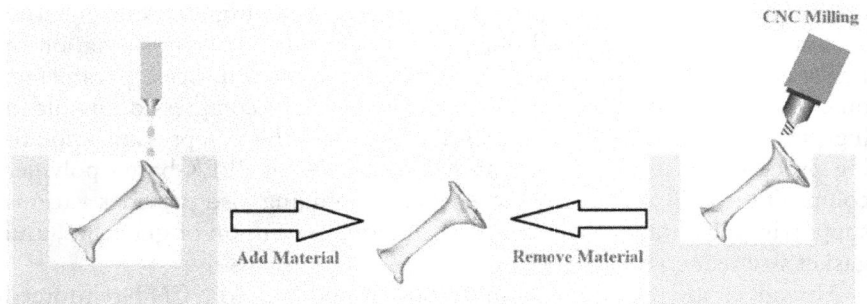

Figure 5.6 Process of rapid prototyping.

Arif et al. studied the multifunctional performance of CNT- and GNP-fortified PEEK composites by FDM. The additive manufactured PEEK-based polymer nanocomposite reveals interfacial voids between the beads and intra-bead pores and thus indicates the density level of the PEEK composite. This rapid prototyped PEEK composite's tensile properties, dynamic mechanical properties, friction, wear, and hardness characteristics are investigated, and these FDM AM PEEK-GNP and PEEK-CNT nanocomposites are potential materials for load-bearing and functional applications in orthopaedics and automotives [20].

Wang et al. manufactured a short CF-GF-reinforced PEEK composite via FDM and evaluated its comprehensive properties. The density and melting temperature were 1.3 g/cm^3 and 343°C, respectively. Generally, various types of 3D printing process parameters are widely used for the manufacture of fibre-fortified PEEK nanocomposites, such as nozzle diameter, nozzle temperature, platform temperature, printing speed, infill density, layer thickness, wall thickness, infill pattern, raster angle, and overlap interval [21]. Berretta et al. investigated the layer bonding, tensile strength, and microstructure of a CNT-loaded PEEK composite with the help of the FDM method. The short beam test was used to measure the layer-to-layer bonding of FDM components [22].

5.6 COMPOSITION OF PEEK

The PEEK composition is generally classified into two different segments based on the material participation on the composite as follows:

1. Binary composition
2. Ternary composition.

5.6.1 Binary composition

When a PEEK-based system possesses two components as major constituents, then it is said to have binary composition. In this section, some PEEK-based compositions are discussed in detail.

5.6.1.1 Hydroxyapatite (HA)-PEEK composites

PEEK-based polymer composites are widely used in versatile applications. In particular, hydroxyapatite (HA)-infused PEEK composites possess outstanding performance. HA is the most significant inorganic mineral component and has the chemical composition of $Ca_{10}(PO_4)_6(OH)_2$. It can establish harmless ions to the body and contribute to the body metabolism. Synthetic HA is a bioactive, biocompatible, and clinically used material for bone substitution [23]. HA possesses remarkable osteoconductive abilities, so it can be easily bound with the bones. While deploying the HA-PEEK composite for clinical purposes, its bioactivity characteristics occupy the most essential place. In general, the bioactivity of the composite is validated through proliferation, spreading, and ACP activity of osteoblast precursor cell (MC3T3-E1), cell attachment, apatite formation after impression in simulated body fluid (SBF), and osseointegration [24].

Nowadays, PEEK composites with different concentrations of HA are widely used in clinical industries. Ma et al. [24] developed PEEK composites with different concentrations (10, 20, 30, and 40 wt.%) and evaluated their elastic and tensile modulus. The PEEK composite infused with 30 wt.% HA possessed good tensile strength, which is better than that of the natural cortical bone (50 MPa). Hence, the PEEK composite with 30 wt.% HA seems optimal for orthopaedic implants. This HA-PEEK composite, when immersed in SBF, had enhanced osseointegration effectiveness compared to UHMWP (ultra-high molecular weight polyethylene) and virgin PEEK.

The mechanical performance of the HA-PEEK composite is most significant for orthopaedic implants. The mechanical characteristics of the HA-based PEEK composite are mainly evaluated based on their impact strength, tensile strength, compressive strength, bending strength, and hardness. In general, PEEK composites with nano-HA (nHA) reinforcement in the range of 10–30 wt.% possess better mechanical properties. The nHA delays the microcrack expansion and arrests its growth by stress distribution. Agglomerates need to be avoided as they don't hinder crack propagation and growth in the PEEK composites significantly. Meanwhile, the addition of inorganic nHA improves the density and crystallinity of the polymer material, which is beneficial for enhancing the hardness of the composite. The bio-interfacial affinity is mainly based on the thickness of muscle encapsulation by the addition of nHA, which obviously improves the bio-interfacial affinity. Hence, the adjustment of nHA with PEEK/nHA composite improves the mechanical performance. The PEEK-nHA composite is the most suitable for extensive applications such as hard tissue repair and orthopaedic surgery [25].

5.6.1.2 Carbon fibre-PEEK composites

Carbon fibre (CF) is considered as the most important constituent in PEEK-based polymer composites. The CF reinforcement has established outstanding enhancement in the mechanical strength of PEEK, and hence, it can be provide accurate matching of elasticity modulus between CF-PEEK composite and human cortical bone. The elastic modulus of CF-based PEEK composite is comparatively greater than that of the virgin PEEK and lower than that of metallic materials (7.8–18 GPa).

The mechanical characteristics of CF-PEEK composites are most similar to those of bone tissue. The strain variable is consistent, which can issue better mechanical compatibility. These CF-based PEEK composites enhance the bending power of the interface; reduce fretting, shear stress (σ_s), and vertical displacement; and further assure that bone tissue develops into the prosthesis to attain biological fixation. Due to their superior mechanical properties, CF-fortified PEEK composites have attained widespread attention in the industrial as well as in academic domain.

The property of bioactivity for polymer composite is more significant for clinical applications, but pure PEEK has not shown any capacity for providing sufficient bioactivity. The bioactivity improvement is achieved by the dispersion of CF reinforcement in PEEK [26]. High mechanical strength and bioactivity improvement in CF-PEEK composites makes them most suitable for spinal reconstruction. Wear handling is one of the essential requirements for biomedical applications. It purely depends upon the type of material used. The CF-infused PEEK composite provides outstanding wear resistance compared with UHMWPE. Generally, the mechanical performance of medical-grade PEEK composites is characterized by the nano-indentation technique. The nano-indentation is a potential tool for finding the fibre-matrix interaction and computing the mechanical behaviour of CF-reinforced PEEK composites and is also used to optimize biomaterial properties in structural applications [26].

The stiffness and strength of the PEEK composite have been enhanced due to the incorporation of short CF with ductility reduction [27]. The CF-reinforced PEEK composite has high compressive strength, bending strength, and hardness compared with virgin PEEK material, but its impact strength has been reduced. The CF-PEEK composite has demonstrated excellent nano-tribological and nanomechanical performances; hence, it is a potential candidate for clinical applications [28,29]. Earlier, the CF-induced PEEK composite was mostly used in cardiac implants, neurological leads, spinal cages, and bone fixation screws. Recently, CF-PEEK composites have extensively been used in orthopaedic implants, dental implants, and knee replacement products because of their ability to withstand prolonged fatigue strain; meanwhile, the modulus is very similar to that of human bone [30].

5.6.2 Ternary PEEK composites

When a PEEK-based system possesses three components as major constituents, then it is said to have ternary composition. Sometimes, the binary PEEK composite does not provide sufficient mechanical and biological performances. The real biomedical material in clinical implants has a complex structure and often requires being compatible with numerous biological characteristics in order to attain the greatest biological function substitution. Hence, the researchers are focusing on developing ternary PEEK composites. In this section, some PEEK-based compositions are discussed in detail.

5.6.2.1 CNT-BG-PEEK composites

The mechanical characteristics and biocompatibility are the most important characteristics for bone repair biomaterials. Jianfei et al. investigated the thermal stability, morphology, mechanical properties, bioactivity, and preliminary cell responses of MC3T3-E1 osteoblast cells on MWCNT-filled BG (bioactive glass)-PEEK ternary composites. With this ternary PEEK, the composite scaffold was fabricated by an injection moulding process [31]. They reported that the mechanical characteristics of the ternary PEEK composite are significantly better than the binary PEEK (BG-PEEK) composite. With the addition of MWCNT with BG-PEEK, the thermal stability has been improved. The bone-like apatite layer that was developed on the surface of the ternary composite after immersion in SBF reveals better apatite-forming ability. The cell culture experiment deeply illustrated the metabolic activity and osteogenic differentiation capability of osteoblasts. Moreover, MTT (tetrazolium-based colorimetric assay) and ACP (amorphous calcium phosphate) results emphasized the importance of MWCNT reinforcement. Therefore, the MWCNT-BG-PEEK composite is a healthy bone repair biomaterial for orthopaedic clinical applications [31].

Han et al. fabricated CNT-BG-PEEK ternary composites by the injection moulding method. Bioactivity is the most crucial property expected for bio-inert materials. The bioactive glass (BG) was mixed to the composites in order to enhance the bioactive characteristics of the ternary PEEK composite. The adsorption and co-precipitation were used to preserve the mechanical characteristics of the CNT-PEEK composite while adding bioactive glass. The addition of CNT improves the mechanical characteristics of the composite. Immersion of ternary CNT-BG-PEEK composites in SBF actually improves their bioactivity when immersed for up to 15 days [31]. They also possess good mechanical strength and excellent biological activity, hence making them most suitable for use as a bone substitute material [32].

5.6.2.2 CF-HA-PEEK composites

Hydroxyapatite and CF are effective reinforcement materials for improving the mechanical properties of PEEK-based bio-nanocomposites. In particular, HA possesses superior biological activity and osteoinductivity; besides that, it can potentially encourage bone growth and biological tissue adhesion.

Deng et al. prepared a PEEK ternary composite (PEEK-CF-HA) and evaluated active bone repairing materials by estimation of growth and assessment of osseointegration in vivo. HA is mainly associated with bone regeneration, and CF provides outstanding mechanical properties and non-toxicity to the PEEK ternary composite. The modulus of elasticity and tensile strength his most identical to the human cortical bone. The cell experiment outcome showed that the ternary composite (CF-HA-PEEK) promoted cell attachment proliferation and enhanced calcium nodule formation. In vivo evaluation emphasized newly formed bone. The volume of ternary PEEK composite is higher than that of virgin PEEK. Therefore, the PEEK-based ternary composite is the most appropriate bone repair material and it will be advisable for many challenging dental and orthopaedic applications [33].

Xu et al. developed a novel nHA-CF-PEEK ternary composite with the improvement of osteogenesis as an efficient bioactive material for bone grafting and bone tissue engineering (BTE) application. The combined modification of oxygen plasma and sandblasting could enhance the hydrophily and create nano-micro topographical structure on the surface of PEEK ternary composites. Hence, this type of biocomposites issued excellent ability to promote the proliferation and increase the osseointegration between the bone and implant [34].

PEEK is used to fabricate high-porosity bio-nanocomposite foam materials for new bone formation. The HA-, CF-, and CNT-infused PEEK foam materials were prepared via melt casting and salt porogen leaching methods. The porosity plays an important role in the composite preparation because cell implantation and growth mainly depend upon the pore size. CF and HA were used to enhance the cell attachment and interaction with the porous PEEK, and uniformly distributed CNT can increase the mechanical properties of scaffold materials.

The addition of HA, CF, and CNT with PEEK foam in general increases the yield strength and elastic modulus. Even $0.5\,\mathrm{wt.\%}$ CNT incorporation in PEEK has provided excellent mechanical properties. The yield strength and compression modulus of the prepared biocomposite are much greater than those of the virgin PEEK material. As the concentration of CF increases, the mechanical properties decrease due to the agglomeration of the carbon particles, which increases the local stress. Hence, PEEK composite foams containing HA, CF, and CNT have potential for being deployed in various biomedical applications [35].

5.7 CHARACTERIZATION OF PEEK COMPOSITES

Characterization is the most predominant tool to evaluate the properties of PEEK composites. Numerous types of techniques have been employed to characterize the intrinsic properties of PEEK-based polymer composites. To name a few, particle size, surface area, surface topography, and surface composition may be identified by characterization techniques such as electron microscopy (SEM and TEM), X-ray diffraction, magnetic measurements, dynamic light scattering, X-ray photo-electron spectroscopy, and Auger electron spectroscopy. Some crucial and regularly used characterization techniques are described below.

5.7.1 X-ray diffraction

X-ray diffraction is a widely used non-destructive technique for characterizing crystalline and semi-crystalline materials. It is widely used to find and evaluate the crystal structure, chemical composition, and physical properties of the material. The X-ray diffracted by a set of crystallographic planes interfaces constructively depending upon the path differences. Generally, the XRD peaks issued by the constructive interface of monochromatic beam X-rays scattered at an approximate angle from every set of lattice planes, and the atomic positions within the lattice planes are obviously determined by the peak intensities. Generally, the material's structural changes due to the blending of other constituents are easily monitored by the XRD technique. It is the most familiar characterization technique for the polymer and polymer-based nanocomposites in contrast to the single crystal method the demands the sample in the form of individual (single) and independent crystal [36–38].

Yu et al. analysed the phase and surface information of nHA-PEEK composites by XRD diffraction and FTIR. Figure 5.7 shows the XRD pattern of PEEK composites with various wt.% of nHA.

The diffraction peaks were achieved in the range of 15°–30° for PEEK, whereas it was shown that HA diffraction peaks were indexed in the range of 30°–45°. With increasing nHA content in PEEK composites, the diffraction of peaks decreased. There are no additional diffraction peaks noticed when nHA-PEEK is physically combined and without the making of new chemical bonds [25].

Miyazaki et al. characterized the crystalline structure of CF-PEEK composites by thin-film X-ray diffraction. Figure 5.8 shows the XRD pattern of the virgin PEEK and carbon (C)-fortified PEEK composites subjected to

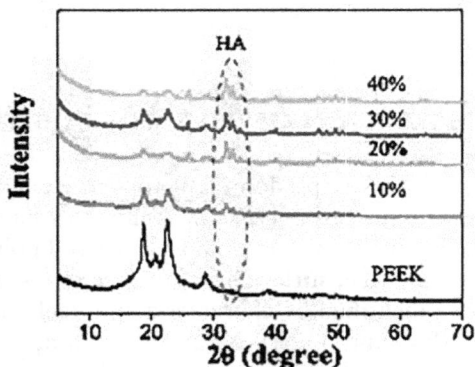

Figure 5.7 XRD patterns of PEEK/nHA composites. (Reprinted with permission from Ref. [25].)

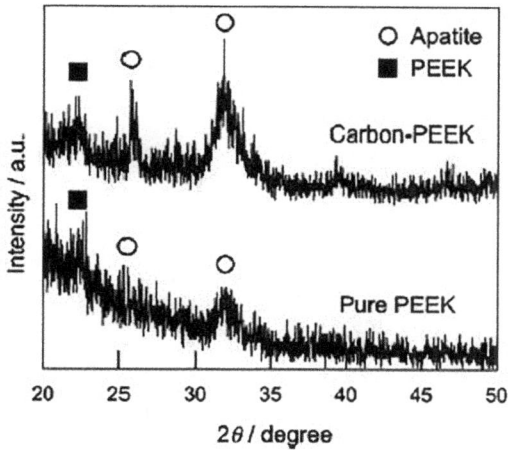

Figure 5.8 XRD patterns of virgin PEEK and carbon fibre (CF)-PEEK composites under H$_2$SO$_4$ and CaCl$_2$ treatments, which were soaked in SBF for 336 hours. (Copyright (2021) with permission from Elsevier [26].)

H$_2$SO$_4$ and CaCl$_2$ treatments, which were soaked in SBF for 336 hours. The peaks dispensed to very low crystalline apatite discovered at 26° and 32° [26].

Fedel et al. evaluated the microstructure and crystallinity behaviour of PEEK material by XRD measurements. This XRD analysis obviously indicates the plasma treatment had created non-measurable effects in PEEK's crystalline structure [39].

Li et al. handled X-ray diffraction for characterization and efficiency analysis of the virgin PEEK material. XRD was used to discover the properties of the FDM printed PEEK materials. Generally, the virgin PEEK material mainly reveals typical crystal peaks under various printing parameters and also different diffraction intensities have been achieved [40]. The scattered light from the virgin PEEK material may also be studied by XRD by analysing the crystallinity of PEEK material before and after thermocycling. Here, all diffraction peaks were calculated and divided by the total area of the pattern [41].

5.7.2 Scanning electron microscopy

Scanning electron microscopy (SEM) is a convenient and widespread technique for illustrating the surface topography and material composition of PEEK-based polymer composites. It takes a photograph of a sample by scanning with a focused beam of electrons. The electron obviously interacts with the surface region of the workpiece, produces multiple signals that

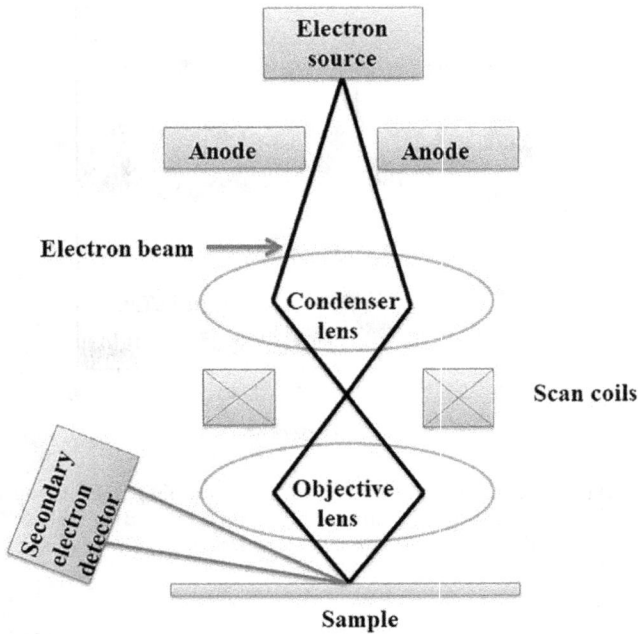

Figure 5.9 Working principle of SEM. (Copyright (2021) with permission from Elsevier [42].)

can be deflected, and contains details about the surface morphology and composition of the workpiece or sample.

SEM has been used in a broad range of polymer and polymer composite studies and applications, such as fibre distribution in a polymer matrix, adhesion between the fibre and matrix, surface roughness, phase boundaries in blends, adhesive failure, networks, and fracture surfaces.

A schematic diagram of working of a scanning electron microscopy is shown in Figure 5.9.

Ma et al. characterized the surface morphology and chemical composition of PEEK infused with 30 wt.% HA by SEM. SEM is also used to investigate cell spreading by observing cells. The surface morphology of HA-PEEK composite is shown Figure 5.10. Virgin PEEK and HA-PEEK composite surfaces after and before immersion in SBF for 168, 336, and 672 hours were analysed. SEM observations reveal that cells on HA-PEEK composites have a greater spreading efficiency and connect the neighbouring cells compared to that of virgin PEEK and UHMWPE [24].

Qin et al. observed the fracture morphology and flexural cross section of bending test sample by SEM. This SEM image reveals CF distribution in PEEK matrix and its shape [28].

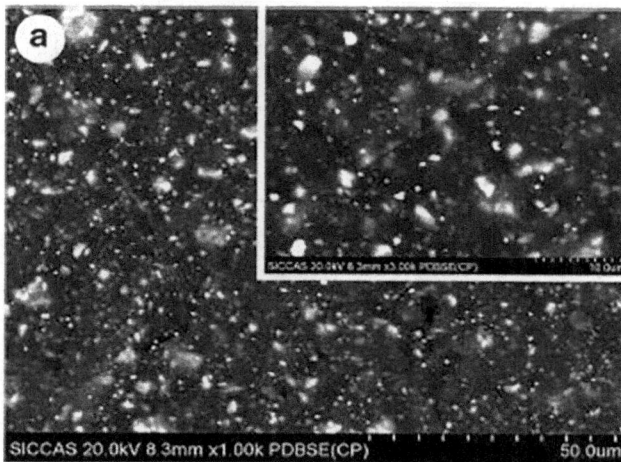

Figure 5.10 Surface morphology of HA-PEEK composite by SEM. (Reprinted with permission from Ref. [24].)

Cao et al. measured the surface morphology of a ternary PEEK (MWCNT-BG-PEEK) composite by SEM. SEM images exhibited the surface morphology of virgin PEEK and PEEK composites infused with 4% MWCNT and 10% BG (bioactive glass) after static immersion in SBF for 336 and 672 hours. The result shows that there is no apatite formation on pure PEEK material, but in the surrounding of MWCNT-BG-PEEK composite, numerous apatite particles have been formed, which confirms that it possesses better bioactivity than the virgin PEEK material [31].

Deng et al. examined the microstructure, fracture morphology, and cellular morphology of a nHA-CF-PEEK composite by FE-SEM. The surface morphology of this PEEK ternary composite was evaluated after 72 and 336 hours of static immersion in SBF. SEM reveals that the cell attachment and calcium nodule formation of ternary composite have been increased compared with pure PEEK material, and hence, it is the most appropriate material for orthopaedic clinical applications [33].

5.7.3 Raman spectroscopy

Raman spectroscopy is an extensively used spectroscopic technique. This eminent, optimal, vibrational spectroscopic technique provides details about the molecular composition and molecular structure of the required materials. This method yields excellent spatial resolution, and it is much easier to analyse smaller samples. The Raman spectroscopy is attracting growing interest from various scientific disciplines because of its outstanding characteristics such as biological imaging, chemical sensing, and material characterization.

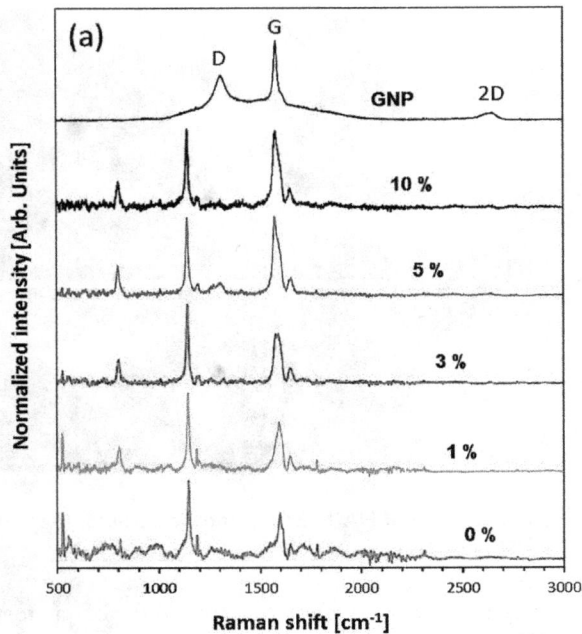

Figure 5.11 Raman signal at different wt.% GNP additions of PEEK. (Copyright (2021) with permission from Elsevier [11].)

Chai et al. used Raman spectroscopy for characterizing the chemical structure of PEEK with laser spot diameter 1 μm and spectral resolution less than 0.35 cm^{-1}; besides that, the transfer film formation was also analysed by Raman spectroscopy. The Raman spectroscopy characterization was done on irradiated PEEK transfer film at 20 MGy (dose). The result indicated that there are no changes noticed in the Raman signal of the transfer film of virgin PEEK and the degradation layer removed after 200 and 5400 laps, so the micro-tribological behaviour of the surface degradation layer is more critical and highly complex [43]. With the help of Raman Spectroscopy, the GNP-fortified PEEK composite was evaluated. The Raman signal was shown for PEEK composites with different concentrations of GNP (Figure 5.11). The Raman band emphasized that the addition of GNP progressively improves the mechanical and wear characteristics of the PEEK composites [11].

Raman spectroscopy is the most significant method for the qualitative analysis of organic molecules, biomolecules, polymers, and inorganic mixed materials as individual and as bulk particles. Besides that, it is also extensively used for quantitative and semi-quantitative analyses [11,21,23].

5.8 PROPERTIES OF PEEK COMPOSITES

Generally, material selection is purely based on the properties of materials. There are several types of insightful material properties deeply associated with the PEEK-based polymer composites for various biomedical applications. In recent days, the PEEK and PEEK-based polymer composites have been highly demanded biomaterials due to their outstanding biological properties. The biological properties of PEEK-based polymer composites are mainly concerned with the following aspects [44]:

1. Biocompatibility
2. Bioactivity
3. Bio-tribology
4. Biomechanics.

5.8.1 Biocompatibility

Biocompatibility is the most predominant requirement for biomaterials. The PEEK composite has attracted noticeable attention by its efficient application in hard tissue repair due to its excellent biocompatibility. Among the various inorganic fillers, HA is a potential candidate for improving the biocompatibility feature of PEEK-based polymer composites.

Yu et al. evaluated the biocompatibility of nHA-PEEK composites through in vitro analysis by measuring the hydrophobicity and biomimetic formation of HA on the surface of the PEEK composite. Based on in vitro evaluation, the PEEK composite obtains excellent biocompatibility features with the incorporation of HA. Hence, this type of composite is the most appropriate implant material for orthopaedic surgery [25]. Xu et al. developed a nHA-CF-PEEK ternary composite and modified it by the combined treatments of sandblasting and oxygen plasma to obtain enhanced biocompatibility and osseointegration nano-microtopographical surface, which promises for orthopaedic and dental repair applications [34].

In recent years, the PEEK-based polymer composites have widely been used in various biomedical applications such as orthopaedic, spinal implants, and bone plates due to their outstanding biocompatibility. Generally, the HA produces excellent biocompatibility. The biocompatibility and biodegradability of PEEK composites together can form potential bone bonding with bone tissue. Furthermore, HA addition also produces biological properties in HA-PEEK bio-nanocomposite scaffolds for bio-tissue engineering field [35].

5.8.2 Bioactivity

Bioactivity is a key property that promotes osseointegration for bonding and superior stability of clinical implants. The biocompatibility and bioactivity of implants are influenced by the chemistry and topography of the implant surfaces. The bioactivity improvement of orthopaedic implants is significantly developed for the short- and long-term stability of the implant in contact interfaces with the bone tissues [44,45].

Typically, the PEEK composite bioactivity properties are improved by two different strategies. One approach mainly deals with impregnating bioactive ceramics with the PEEK material. In recent days, various types of bioactive ceramics possessing significant properties are available, such as HA, calcium phosphate (CP), bioactive glass (BG), and calcium silicate (CS). The addition of bioactive ceramics to PEEK has resulted in a trade-off between mechanical and bioactivity properties. Another approach is dealing with surface treatment or surface coating of PEEK and its reinforcements. By this approach, the bioactivity of PEEK is greatly enhanced [46].

Ma et al. evaluated the bioactivity of a HA-incorporated PEEK composite. The bioactivity of the HA-PEEK composite is measured and compared to that of pure PEEK and UHMWPE. The apatite formation and osseointegration were evaluated in vitro and in vivo; besides that, the osteoblast interaction was also investigated. SBF immersion test is widely used to evaluate the in vitro bioactivity of PEEK materials. The HA blended with the pure PEEK material in different concentrations such as 10, 20, 30, and 40 wt.% and the results of various investigations purely indicate that the bioactivity of HA-PEEK composite enhanced with an increase in HA content in the composite. Therefore, the HA-PEEK composite has achieved excellent bioactivity with the addition of HA and osteogenesis of PEEK also enhanced substantially after the incorporation of HA [24].

Miyazaki et al. prepared a carbon-based PEEK composite by chemical surface treatment method and also evaluated its bioactivity. The surface chemical modification plays an important role in enhancing the bioactivity of the carbon PEEK composite. H_2SO_4 and $CaCl_2$ solutions are used for chemical modification. The result indicates that the bioactivity of carbon PEEK composite is significantly improved compared to pure PEEK material. Therefore, the carbon PEEK has become the most important novel biomaterial for spinal reconstruction application due to its higher mechanical strength and bioactivity [26].

The in vitro analysis was used to evaluate the bioactivity and biocompatibility of MWCNT-BG-PEEK ternary composite, and the ternary composite was immersed in SBF for enhancing its bioactivity. After 672 hours of immersion in SBF, many clustered globular apatite molecules appeared and it nearly covers the entire surface of the composite. Hence, the MWCNT-BG-PEEK composite provides an outstanding bioactivity compared with virgin PEEK material [31].

5.8.3 Bio-tribology

Bio-tribology is the study of tribology in biological systems, especially the human body. It is mainly concerned with friction, wear, and lubrication at biological interfaces. Bio-tribology is one of the emerging and most exciting disciplines of tribology and tribological issues, which plays a significant role in determining the performance and service life. In recent days, PEEK-based biomaterials have successfully been used to replace metal components in various clinical applications such as spinal cages, dental implant systems, a femoral component of total hip replacements, and fracture fixation. The PEEK-based biomaterials occupy an essential place in the biomedical field due to their excellent strength and outstanding wear-resisting characteristics.

Schroeder et al. studied and evaluated the wear characteristics of CF-reinforced PEEK composites for flexion bushings of rotating hinged knee joints. Total knee replacement (TKR) provides patients with end-stage arthritis a possibility to restore the function of the knee joint as well as reduce pain. Researchers have investigated four different types of materials such as CF-PEEK pitch fibres, CF-PEEK PAN fibres, pure PEEK, and UHMWPE. Results indicated that the CF-PEEK composite provides a higher wear resistance compared to virgin PEEK material. So the pure PEEK is considered an alternative material to UHMWPE and it is the most appropriate material for flexion bushing in hinged knee joint applications [47].

The bio-tribological performance of PEEK and PEEK-based polymer composites was also systematically investigated under bovine serum lubrication. Three different types of PEEK composites were successfully evaluated, such as CF-fortified PEEK, CF-graphene-PTFE (polytetrafluoroethylene)-fortified PEEK, and GF-fortified PEEK. The wear test incorporated by pin-on-disc tribometer and experimental result emphasized CF-reinforced PEEK composite produced low wear rate under the condition of bovine serum lubrication [48].

The biocompatibility and tribological characteristics of PEEK composites were modified by the interface of CF, potassium titanate whisker (PTW), and HA [49]. The CF (30%)-, PTW (15%)-, and HA (5%)-infused PEEK composites exhibited superior wear resistance than single-phase reinforcement; particularly, PTW can defend the wear degree of the PEEK matrix and enhance the wear characteristics of PEEK composites. Hence, the CF-PTW-HA-PEEK composite satisfies the requirement of replacing the conventional Ti (titanium) alloy to make the potential internal fixation implants.

Song et al. studied nanomechanical and nano-tribological behaviours of PEEK and CF-PEEK composites. The CF reinforcement effectively improves the nanohardness and elastic modulus; besides that, it reduces friction coefficient and wear rate of PEEK composites. The wear rate of CF-PEEK composites is lower than that of the pure PEEK, and hence, it is a potential candidate for biomedical applications [29].

5.8.4 Biomechanics

Biomechanics is the science of mechanical laws applied to living organisms. This study is mainly concerned with the material structure, function, and motion of the biological system. Biomechanics is also associated with the design of prostheses, artificial organs, anthropomorphic test devices, and bio-instrumentation as well as with the macro- and microscale analysis of biological systems, such as cellular mechanics. The PEEK-based biomaterial confers an excellent modulus and high strength compared with conventional implants. These PEEK-based biomaterials potentially reduce stress shielding due to a match in elastic modulus and stiffness between the bone and implant.

Xu et al. investigated the mechanical properties (tensile, bending, and shear strength) of a unidirectional continuous carbon fibre (UDCCF)-fortified PEEK composite by wrapped yarn method. The mechanical properties of PEEK composites are enhanced with the increase in moulding temperature and hold time. Beyond the mould temperature of 430°C and mould time of 90 minutes, the mechanical characteristics of the PEEK composite began to decrease due to the degradation of the matrix. Moreover, the slow cooling rate creates slight impact on the mechanical properties of PEEK composites [50]. The addition of 3D braided CF significantly enhanced the mechanical strength of the PEEK composite [51]. The filler material surface treatment also helps in improving the adhesion between PEEK and inorganic content, leading to improved mechanical strength of the PEEK composite. Hence, this composite seems more compactible for orthopaedic applications.

The CF-fortified PEEK composite is a potential aspirant to replace the metals for load-bearing applications, such as knee replacement, artificial hip joint, fracture fixation plates, and nails. Wang et al. evaluated the mechanical properties of the CNT-fortified PEEK composite by molecular dynamic simulation. CNT improves the interfacial strength of the PEEK composite. The ultra-fine molecular design of the CNT processing and molecular chain modification of PEEK enhances the mechanical performance of PEEK nanocomposites. Hence, these composites are the most appropriate material for lightweight structural components in clinical industries [52].

The bioactive ceramics (HA) improve the bioactivity and mechanical performance of the PEEK composite system, especially modulus of elasticity, compression strength, and micro-indentation hardness, whereas the tensile strength and strain to failure reduced with an increasing amount of HA. HA-reinforced PEEK composites exhibited mechanical compatibility more or less equivalent to the natural bone. These injection moulded HA-infused PEEK biocomposites have promising mechanical properties, which makes them an efficient material for load-bearing orthopaedic applications [53].

5.9 APPLICATIONS

PEEK-based biomaterials received much attraction due to their special characteristics stated above. In medical industries, the PEEK is the most predominant replacement material for metallic implants. The PEEK and

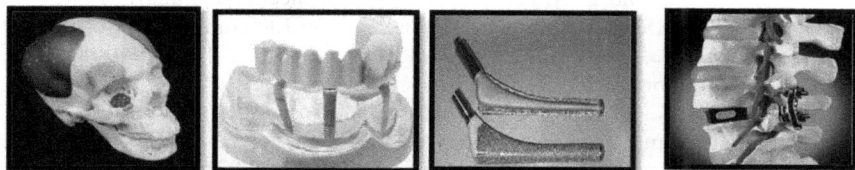

Figure 5.12 Medical applications of PEEK. (Copyright (2021) with permission from Elsevier [17,54–56].)

PEEK-based biomaterials are majorly associated with several biomedical applications such as bone replacement (facial and cranial implants), spine surgery (spinal cages), orthopaedic surgery (bone and hip replacement, articulation implants), tooth replacement from CFR (dental prosthesis, infra-radicular post), and cardiac surgery (infra-cardiac pump, heart valves) (Figure 5.12).

REFERENCES

1. Kulshrestha, A. S., and A. Mahapatro. (2008). Polymers for biomedical applications. American Chemical Society, *ACS Symposium Series*, Washington, DC, pp. 1–5.
2. Gila, M. H., J. F. J. Coelho, P. Ferreira, and P. Alves. (2011). Polymers for biomedical applications: Chemical modification and bio functionalization. Edited by Trindade T., Silva. A., *Nano Composite Particles for Bio Applications*, Jenny Stanford Publishing, Singapore, pp. 1–32.
3. Peters, E. N., and R. K. Arisman. (2000). *Engineering Thermo Plastics*. Elsevier, NewYork, pp. 177–196.
4. Kurtz, S. M. (2000). *An Overview of PEEK Biomaterials*. Elsevier Inc., pp. 1–7. DOI: 10.1016/B978-1-4377-4463-7.10001-6.
5. Omnexus. (2021) Poly Ether Ether Ketone (PEEK): A complete guide on high-heat engineering plastic. Special Chem. Selection Guide.
6. Wypych, G. (2012). PEK poly ether ketone. Edited by Wypych G., *Handbook of Polymers*. ChemTec Publishing, Ontario Canada, pp. 364–366.
7. Reitman, M., D. J. Jaekel, R. Siskey, and S. M. Kurtz. (2019). Morphology and crystalline architecture of poly aryl ether ketones. Edited by Kurtz S.M., *PEEK Biomaterials Handbook (Second Edition)*. William Andrew Publishing, Elsevier, Norwich NY, United States, pp. 53–66.
8. Lal, S. K, and H. Vasudevan. (2013). Optimization of injection moulding process parameters in the moulding of Low Density Polyethylene (LDPE). *International Journal of Engineering Research and Development*, 7(5), 35–39.
9. Bikas, A., N. Pantelelis, and A. Kanarachos. (2002). Computational tools for the optimal design of the injection moulding process. *Journal of Materials Processing Technology*, 122, 112–126.

10. Arevalo, S. E., and L. A. Pruitt. (2020). Nano mechanical analysis of medical grade PEEK and carbon fiber-reinforced PEEK composites. *Journal of the Mechanical Behaviour of Biomedical Materials*, 111, 104008. DOI: 10.1016/j.jmbbm.2020.104008.

11. Puertolas, J. A., M. Castro, J. A. Morris, R. Rios, and A. A. Casaos. (2018). Tribological and mechanical properties of Graphene Nano platelet/PEEK composites. *Carbon*. DOI: 10.1016/ j.carbon.2018.09.036.

12. Ogasawara, T., T. Tsuda, and N. Takeda. (2011). Stress–strain behaviour of multi-walled carbon nanotube/PEEK composites. *Composites Science and Technology*, 71, 73–78.

13. Park, C. H., and W. I. Lee. (2012). *Compression Moulding in Polymer Matrix Composites*. Wood head Publishing Limited, Sawston, Cambridge, pp. 47–93.

14. Tatara, R. A. (2017). Compression moulding. *Applied Plastics Engineering Handbook*. Elsevier Inc. pp. 291–320. DOI: 10.1016/ B978-0-323-39040-8.00014-6.

15. Mezrakchi, R. A., T. Creasy, H. J. Sue, and T. Bremner. (2020). Manipulation of thick-walled PEEK bushing crystallinity and modulus via instrumented compression moulding. *Journal of Applied Polymer Science*. DOI: 10.1002/ app.49930.

16. Ahmad, A., H. Mahmood, N. Mansor, T. Iqbal, and M. Moniruzzaman. (2021). Ionic liquid modified PEEK-MWCNTs nano composites with enhanced thermo mechanical properties. *Journal of Physics: Conference Series*, 1793, 012044. DOI: 10.1088/1742-6596/1793/1/012044.

17. Batista, N. L., M. C. Rezende, and E. C. Botelho. (2021). The influence of crystallinity on the weather resistance of CF/PEEK composites. *Applied Composite Materials*, 28, 235–246. DOI: 10.1007/s10443-020-09863-x.

18. Siddiq, A., and A. R. Kennedy. (2020). Compression moulding and injection over moulding of porous PEEK components. *Journal of the Mechanical Behavior of Biomedical Materials*, 111, 103996.

19. Singh, S., C. Prakash, and S. Ramakrishna. (2019). 3D printing of polyether-ether-ketone for biomedical applications. *European Polymer Journal*, 114, 234–248. DOI: 10.1016/j.eurpolymj.2019.02.035.

20. Arif, M. F., H. Alhashmi, K. M. Varadarajan, J. H. Koo, and A. J. Hart, et al. (2019). Multifunctional performance of carbon nano tubes and Graphene Nano platelets reinforced PEEK composites enabled via FFF additive manufacturing. *Composites Part B*. DOI: 10.1016/j.compositesb.2019.107625.

21. Wang, P., B. Zou, S. Ding, C. Huang, and Z. Shi, et al. (2020). Preparation of short CF/GF reinforced PEEK composite filaments and their comprehensive properties evaluation for FDM-3D printing. *Composites Part B*. DOI: 10.1016/j.compositesb.2020.108175.

22. Shahrubudin, N., T. C. Lee., and R. Ramlan. (2019). An overview on 3D printing technology: Technological, materials, and applications. *Procedia Manufacturing*, 35, 1286–1296. DOI: 10.1016/j.promfg.2019.06.089.

23. Ma, H., A. Suonan, J. Zhou, Q. Yuan, and L. Liu, et al. (2021). PEEK (Polyether-ether-ketone) and its composite materials in orthopaedic implantation. *Arabian Journal of Chemistry*, 14, 102977. DOI: 10.1016/j.arabjc.2020.102977.

24. Ma, R., and D. Guo. (2019). Evaluating the bioactivity of a hydroxyapatite-incorporated poly ether ether ketone bio composite. *Journal of Orthopaedic Surgery and Research*, 14, 32. DOI: 10.1186/s13018-019-1069-1.

25. Yu, X., S. Yao, C. Chen, J. Wang, and Y. Li, et al. (2020). Preparation of poly(ether-ether-ketone)/nano hydroxyapatite composites with improved mechanical performance and bio interfacial affinity. *ACS Omega*, 5, 29398–29406. DOI: 10.1021/acsomega.0c04257.
26. Miyazaki, T., C. Matsunami, and Y. Shirosaki. (2017). Bioactive carbon–PEEK composites prepared by chemical surface treatment. *Materials Science and Engineering C*, 70, 71–75. DOI: 10.1016/j.msec.2016.08.058.
27. Gonzalez, D., R. Millan, M. Rusinek, and A. Arias. (2015). Investigation of mechanical impact behaviour of short carbon-fiber-reinforced PEEK composites. *Composite Structures*. DOI: 10.1016/j.compstruct.2015.08.028.
28. Qin, W., J. Ma, Y. Li, Q. Liang, and B. Tang. (2018). Mechanical properties and cytotoxicity of hierarchical carbon fiber-reinforced poly (ether-ether-ketone) composites used as implant materials. *Journal of the Mechanical Behaviour of Biomedical Materials*. DOI: 10.1016/j.jmbbm.2018.09.040.
29. Song, J., H. Shi, Z. Liao, S. Wang, and Y. Liu. (2017). Study on the nano mechanical and nanotribological behaviours of PEEK and CFRPEEK for biomedical applications. *Polymers*, 10, 142. DOI: 10.3390/polym10020142.
30. Li, C. S., C. Vannabouathong, S. Sprague, and M. Bhandari. (2014). The use of carbon-fiber-reinforced (CFR) PEEK material in orthopaedic implants: A systematic review. *Clinical Medicine Insights: Arthritis and Musculoskeletal Disorders*, 8, 33–45. DOI: 10.4137/CMAMD.S20354.
31. Cao, J., Y. Lu, H. Chen, L. Zhang, and C. Xiong. (2018). Preparation, properties and in vitro cellular response of multi-walled carbon nano tubes/bioactive glass/poly(ether ether ketone) bio composite for bone tissue engineering. *International Journal of Polymeric Materials and Polymeric Biomaterials*. DOI: 10.1080/00914037.2018.1455679.
32. Han, C.T., M. Chi, Y. Y. Zheng, L. X. Jiang, and C. D. Xiong, et al. (2013). Mechanical properties and bioactivity of high-performance poly(ether ether ketone)/carbon nano tubes/bioactive glass biomaterials. *Journal of Polymer Research*, 20, 203. DOI: 10.1007/s10965-013-0203-8.
33. Deng, Y., P. Zhou, X. Liu, L. Wang, and X. Xiong, et al. (2015). Preparation, characterization, cellular response and in vivo osseointegration of poly ether ether ketone/nano hydroxyapatite carbon fiber ternary bio composite. *Colloids and Surfaces B: Biointerfaces*. DOI: 10.1016/j.colsurfb.2015.09.001.
34. Xu, A., X. Liu, X. Gao, F. Deng, and Y. Deng, et al. (2015). Enhancement of osteogenesis on micro/nano-topographical carbon fiber-reinforced poly ether ether ketone – nano hydroxyl apatite biocomposite. *Materials Science and Engineering C*, 48, 592–598. DOI: 10.1016/j.msec.2014.12.061.
35. Uddin, M. D. N., P. S. Dhanasekaran, and R. Asmatulu. (2019). Mechanical properties of highly porous PEEK bio nano composites incorporated with carbon and hydroxyapatite nano particles for scaffold applications. *Progress in Biomaterials*. DOI: 10.1007/s40204-019-00123-1.
36. Benjwal, R. S. P., and K. K. Kar. (2015). *Carbon Nanotubes: Synthesis, Properties and Applications Polymer Nano composites Based on Inorganic and Organic Nanomaterial's*. Scrivener Publishing LLC, New York, United States, pp. 89–138.
37. Rajeswari, A., E. J. S. Christy, S. Gopi, K. Jayaraj, and A. Pius. (2020). Characterization studies of polymer-based composites related to functionalized filler-matrix interface. DOI: 10.1016/B978-0-08-102665-6.00009-1.

38. Kohli, R., and K. L. Mittal. (2019). Methods for assessing surface cleanliness. *Developments*, 12. DOI: 10.1016/B978-0-12-816081-7.00003-6.

39. Fedel, M., V. Micheli, M. Thaler, and F. Awaja. (2019). Effect of nitrogen plasma treatment on the crystallinity and self-bonding of poly ether ether ketone (PEEK) for biomedical applications. *Polymer Advanced Technology*, 1–8. DOI: 10.1002/pat.4764.

40. Li, Y., and Y. Lou. (2020). Tensile and bending strength improvements in PEEK parts using fused deposition modelling 3D printing considering multifactor coupling. *Polymers*, 12, 2497. DOI: 10.3390/polym12112497.

41. Valente, M., et al. (2021). An in vitro analysis of the physical and mechanical behaviour a poly ether ether ketone(PEEK) component for an implant supported and retained removable dental prosthesis. *International Journal of Prosthodontics*. DOI: 10.11607/ijp.6819. Epub ahead of print. PMID: 33662066.

42. Titus, D., E. J. J. Samuel, and S. M. Roopan. (2019). *Nanoparticle Characterization Techniques*. Elsevier Inc., pp. 303–319. DOI: 10.1016/ B978-0-08-102579-6.00012-5.

43. Chai, L., B. Zhang, L. Qiao, P. Wang, and L. Weng. (2021). Influence of gamma irradiation-induced surface oxidation on tribological property of poly ether ether ketone (PEEK). *Polymer Bulletin*. DOI: 10.1007/s00289-021-03825-4.

44. Song, P. Y., W. Jing, and P. C. Ling. (2013). Research on biological properties of PEEK based composites. *Applied Mechanics and Materials*, 325–326, 3–7. DOI:10.4028/www.scientific.net/AMM.325-326.3.

45. Geetha, K. R., R. Prabhu, and S. N. Sundar. (2020). Modified bioactive PEEK material for dental implants: A review. *International Journal of Innovative Science and Research Technology*, 5(10), 2456–2165.

46. Ma, R., and T. Tang. (2014). Current strategies to improve the bioactivity of PEEK. *International Journal of Molecular Science*, 15, 5426–5445. DOI: 10.3390/ijms15045426.

47. Schroeder, S., S. Braun, U. Mueller, M. Vogel, and R. Sonntag, et al. (2020). Carbon-fibre-reinforced PEEK: An alternative material for flexion bushings of rotating hinged knee joints. *Journal of the Mechanical Behaviour of Biomedical Materials*, 101, 103434. DOI: 10.1016/j.jmbbm.2019.103434.

48. Xin, H., R. Liu, L. Zhang, J. H. Jia, and N. He, et al. (2021). A comparative biotribological study of self-mated PEEK and its composites under bovine serum lubrication. *Biotribology*, 26, 100171. DOI: 10.1016/j.biotri.2021.100171.

49. Ning, L., C. Deqiang, G. Xiyan, L. Lirong, and C. Weizeng. (2020). Biological tribology properties of the modified polyether ether ketone composite materials. *Reviews on Advanced Materials Science*, 59, 399–405. DOI: 10.1515/ rams-2020-0034.

50. Xu, Z., M. Zhang, S. H. Gao, G. Wang, and S. Zhang, et al. (2017). Study on mechanical properties of unidirectional continuous carbon fiber-reinforced PEEK composites fabricated by the wrapped yarn method. *Polymer Composite*. DOI: 10.1002/pc.24600.

51. Monich, P. R., B. Henriques, A. P. N., Oliveira, and J. C. M. Souza, et al. (2016). Mechanical and biological behaviour of biomedical PEEK matrix composites: A focused review. *Materials Letters*, 185, 593–597. DOI: 10.1016/j. matlet.2016.09.005.

52. Wang, B., K. Zhang, C. Zhou, M. Ren, and Y. Gu, et al. (2019). Engineering the mechanical properties of CNT/ PEEK nano composites. *RSC Advances*, 9, 12836. DOI: 10.1039/c9ra01212e.

53. Bakar, M. S. A., P. Cheang, and K. A. Khor. (2003). Mechanical properties of injection moulded hydroxyapatite poly ether ether ketone biocomposites. *Composites Science and Technology*, 63, 421–425.

54. Day, J., S. M. Kurtz, and K. Ong. (2019). Isoelastic PEEK implants for total joint replacement. *PEEK Biomaterials Handbook*. Elsevier Inc. DOI: 10.1016/B978-0-12-812524-3.00021-1.

55. Siewert, B. M. D., M. P. Castro, N. Serenoand, and M. J. Smith. (2019). Applications of PEEK in the dental field. *PEEK Biomaterials Handbook*. Elsevier Inc. DOI: 10..1016/B978-0-12-812524-3.00020-X.

56. Kurtz, S. M. (2019). Development and clinical performance of PEEK intervertebral cages. *PEEK Biomaterials Handbook*. Elsevier Inc. DOI: 10.1016/B978-0-12-812524-3.00015-6.

Chapter 6

Morphology and Dielectric Characteristics of OPMF/KGG biocomposites

V. Srikanth, K. Raja Narender Reddy, and R. Sai Kumar

Kakatiya Institute of Technology and Science Warangal

CONTENTS

6.1 INTRODUCTION

Increased environmental awareness and societal interest, as well as new environmental restrictions and unsustainable petroleum consumption, have prompted the consideration of environmentally friendly materials. Global concern for the protection of environment has driven the scientists and engineers to find suitable alternatives to synthetic fibre polymer composite products [1]. Natural fibres are exceptionally alluring for composite materials since they are less expensive, eco-friendly, accessible in high amounts, inexhaustible and biodegradable, as well as having excellent mechanical qualities and a low density [2,3]. Subsequently, the need for natural fibre-built composites has radically expanded in the course of recent years for different business applications in the modern sector [4,5]. On the other hand, natural fibres in composite materials have some disadvantages, such as excessive moisture absorption, poor dimensional soundness, low heat resistance, structural fluctuation, and incompatibility with polymeric matrix [6,7]. Fibre surface treatment or polymer framework adjustment procedures can be used to address these concerns. Fibre surface alterations have been studied using a variety of physical and synthetic treatment approaches aimed at enhancing the resemblance between natural fibres and polymer lattices. Crown release, cold plasma, X-ray and UV bombardment, mercerization (alkali), joining, acetylation and treatment with permanganate, silane, peroxide and anhydride are only a few of the techniques used in the previous literature [8,9]. These modifications allow composite materials to improve their mechanical characteristics as well as their moisture absorption. Preparation of new composite, oil palm mesocarp fibre is natural fibre to support natural resin to build laminates. Biocomposites are made of low-cost plant fibres and biodegradable resins. Some of the resins are made from plant proteins, and some of the natural gums such as Kondagogu gum (*Cochlospermum gossypium*), karaya gum (*Sterculia urens* Roxb.), soy protein and wheat protein isolates are some examples of biocomposites [10,11]. Kondagogu gum (KGG) belongs to Bixaceae family. It is an aqueous solution from the plant that will solidify with time and temperature. The usage of green composite materials is anticipated to have huge market potential as a result of the increased focus on natural issues such as biodegradation, sustainable assets, and lower CO_2 emissions through entire development [12]. Researchers are becoming increasingly interested in the use of regular fibres such as coir, palm kernel and Palmyra with synthetic and bio-resins as matrix materials [13]. Examination of dielectric properties of OPMF supported with KGG uncovered that it has acceptable conductivity. The unprocessed gum is more effective as a binder in food and pharmaceutical endeavours than local gum [14]. The KGG has better properties than the karaya gum and other plant gum leaves [15]. Coming to the biocomposites, they are a blend of at least two distinct sorts of materials with a variety of physical and chemical properties. In today's engineering design and development activity, these are gradually gaining more relevance as structural materials. Composites are constructed from several fibres used as the reinforcement and matrix. Regardless, one section of any kind is required. The framework materials are circled and support the impacts of their extraordinary mechanical properties to ensure those grid properties. When several broken periods of different quality of composites (natural assets) occur, a composite material often consists of more than one intermittent stage that is circulated in a continuous stage [16–19]. The intermittent stage is typically harder, and that sort of stage with mechanical properties is better than ceaseless stages. The persistent stage is known as the matrix. The irregular stage is known as the reinforcement. The reinforcement stage may comprise any material in fibre or total structure. The matrix phase must be able to flow around the reinforcement and then harden [20–22]. The parameter of a dielectric that determines its ability to form a capacitance is called permittivity. Let us take a capacitor of any shape and dimension with vacuum in the space between the electrodes and denote its capacitance by Co. The value is obtained using a strength criterion test configuration [23,24]. The dissemination factor is the cotangent of the point between the applied voltage and current and is for the most part obtained from a prompt examination of the dial on a capacitance interface. This misfortune is a protection structure and is related to the wavering of polar particles attempting to situate themselves with the exchanging electric field [25]. Natural fibres have a major role in many engineering applications, including aerospace, automobiles and sporting goods, according to a review of the literature and studies conducted around the world.

The current study is to fabricate composites using short OPMF laminates reinforced with KGG. The fibres of the composite are arranged in a random pattern. The dielectric characteristics and surface morphology are investigated in depth and presented. The effects of fibre length and fibre weight percent on the dielectric characteristics and surface morphology of broken specimen samples are also looked at.

6.2 MATERIALS AND METHODS

6.2.1 Raw materials

Extricated oil palm mesocarp fibres (OPMF) were received from viswak fibre industries, Tenali, Guntur. KGG powder (grade I) is purchased from Nutriroma, Hyderabad. Glycerol, ammonia (NH_3), glutaraldehyde, hydrochloric acid (HCl) and sodium hydroxide (NaOH) pellets were purchased from International Drugs & Chemicals Suppliers, Warangal.

6.2.1.1 Alkali treatment

The alkali treatment is to improve the collateral bonding between the fibre surface and matrix. This treatment also removes a portion of the lignin, wax and oils that coat the outside of the fibre cell, as well as depolymerizes cellulose and reveals the short-length crystallites. This method consequently increases surface hardness. OPM fibre by soaking in distilled water for a span of 24 hours in 2% of NaOH solution after washed thoroughly and dried up again for 24 hours. In order to accomplish so, we must pay attention to the mechanical characteristics of composites. The alkali treated composites are represented as TM and untreated composites: UM; 04 is represents length of fibre.

6.2.1.2 Resin preparation

The process of preparing resin from KGG powder is illustrated in Figure 6.1. A weighed amount of KGG powder is taken in a clean glass beaker, and

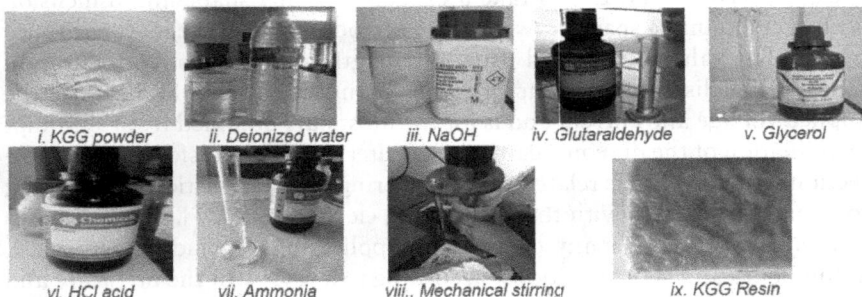

| i. KGG powder | ii. Deionized water | iii. NaOH | iv. Glutaraldehyde | v. Glycerol |

| vi. HCl acid | vii. Ammonia | viii.. Mechanical stirring | ix. KGG Resin |

Figure 6.1 Preparation of KGG resin.

deionized water of 2.5 times the weight of the gum powder is added to the glass beaker. For 20–30 minutes, the contents are agitated using a magnetic stirrer at room temperature. To neutralize the gum solution, add the necessary amount of 1M NaOH and 1M HCl to make the matrix. Glycerol and glutaraldehyde, each 25%–30% by weight of KGG powder, are weighed separately after a continuous incubation of 20 minutes and mixed with the earlier gum solution to obtain a pH of 7–8. Glycerol is the plasticizer and glutaraldehyde is the cross-linking agent and their quantity is varied to study their effect on the tensile strength and thermal stability.

6.2.1.3 Preparation of composites

Bioresin KGG was used to fabricate Palmyra fibre composites of volume $280 \times 280 \times 3$ mm with basic treated and untreated fibres of 4 mm and varying fibre weight proportions of 5%, 10% and 15%. These are fabricated in an approach to beat the shrinkage volume using the hand lay-up method.

6.2.2 Methods

6.2.2.1 Dielectric measurements

The dielectric properties of a test specimen were measured as per ASTM Standards D150, and here, we can use circular/square test samples/specimens of 20 mm diameter or $20 \times 20 \times 4$ ($L \times B \times T$). As electrodes, test samples were sandwiched between two parallel gold plates. In the frequency range of 100 Hz to 1 MHz, the dielectric constant, dielectric loss, and tan values of these samples were all evaluated at room temperature.

6.2.2.2 Scanning Electron Microscopy

The morphology of dielectric breaking non-conductive samples was examined using SEM, TESCAN, VEGA3 LMU. Before recording the micrographs, the cracked surfaces were electroplated with gold to provide electrical conduction. The collages were photographed using a digital camera in this case. With the use of a focused beam of high-energy electrons, the SEM reveals information about texture, crystalline structure and orientation of materials to produce a wide range of signals on the surface of a solid specimen. Data are collected across a specific area of the sample in most applications, and two-dimensional pictures are created to identify the sample and their properties and to analyse crystalline structure.

6.3 RESULTS AND DISCUSSION

6.3.1 Dielectric properties

Here, Figure 6.2a shows the variation of dielectric constant with the two different composites treated with 4 mm length and 5% weight of the fibre. Here, we can set the frequency between 0 and 50 Hz. From the test, we can find that the dielectric constant values of the two composites vary from 9.68 to 3.52. It was found that increasing the fibre weight percentages caused to decrease dielectric constant (Ds) and the dielectric values at different fibre ratios. According to Figure 6.2a, the dielectric constant of the untreated 4 mm length, 5% weight ratio composite was higher than that of the treated 4 mm length, 5% weight ratio composite. The polarizability of the composite will be reduced at increased fibre content and, as a result, lower fibre length, resulting in lower dielectric values. As the thickness of the sample

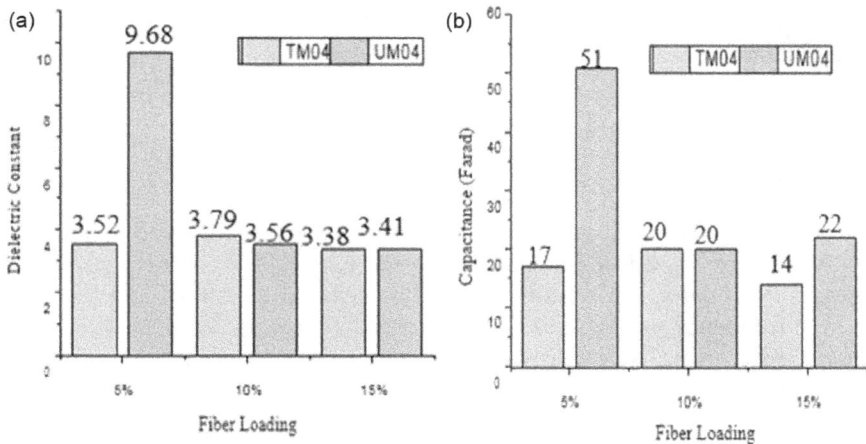

Figure 6.2 Dielectric properties of OPMF/KGG biocomposites: (a) capacitance; (b) dielectric constant. Note: UM0405; TM0405: UM – untreated mesocarp; TM – treated mesocarp; 04 – length of fibre; 05 – fibre's wt. %.

grows, so does the dielectric constant. Coming to the test reports from Figure 6.2, untreated and treated OPMF/KGG biocomposite samples are shown with different fibre loadings. We can compare treated 4 mm 5% composites in this case with untreated 4 mm 5% composites. Finally, the treated 4 mm 5% composite material with a 3.52 Ds value, the optimum insulating material, was obtained. The lesser value of dielectric constant represents the best insulating material. The untreated mesocarp fibre (UM0405) composite increased more than the treated mesocarp fibre (TM0405) composite. Increasing the thickness of a material improved the dielectric constant at a specific composition. It is well understood that as the thickness of a material increases, the dielectric value should increase proportionally. The composites created, on the other hand, do not show a proportional rise in dielectric value with thickness.

This study was undertaken due to the inhomogeneity of the samples in terms of distribution of fibre and KGG and consequently porosity of the samples. If it is possible to obtain materials with variable dielectric values simply by changing the composition or thickness, it will be easier to produce dielectrics for specific purposes. Microelectronics and ceramic capacitors both benefit from materials with a low dielectric constant, as well as strong thermal and mechanical durability. For low dielectric applications, previous research on biocomposites revealed dielectric values ranging from 3.78 to 170. The methods used in this work can be used to make composites with necessary dielectric constants. Above the frequency of 30 Hz, dielectric constants continued to decline and showed only a little change up to 50 Hz. Note that the area of the capacitor is always restricted with the help of the guard and thus remains constant. This is noted as C_x in power factor. Now measure the thickness "t" of the composite specimen (in cm) with the help of a screw gauge/micrometer. Then, use the following formula to calculate the dielectric of the solid/non-polymer specimen (Ds).

$$Ds = 0.57521 \times C_x \times t.$$

6.3.2 Dielectric strength

As per ASTM D149, a step-by-step process is used for finding or determining the Ds of a solid or polymer insulating material at commercial power frequency under specified condition. The exchanging voltage at a business power frequency of 50 Hz is applied to test (Figure 6.3a). The voltage is increased starting from zero and continues until the dielectric fails. The greater part of the regular test voltage is applied to utilize basic test cathodes on inverse appearances of the example. The test voltage is obtained from an arrangement transformer that is supplied by a variable sinusoidal low-voltage source. See Figure 6.3a; the break down voltage decreases when increasing the fibre content in biocomposites. From 5% to 10% of the fibre content, the voltage value is raised, and at 15% of the fibre content, it is

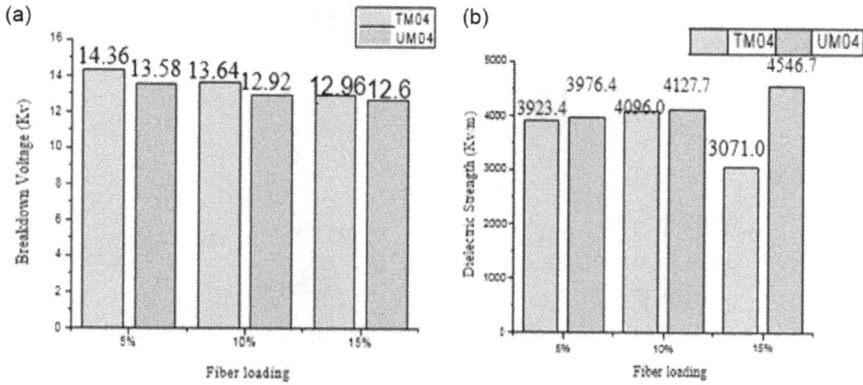

Figure 6.3 OPMF/KGG biocomposites' (a) breakdown voltage and (b) dielectric strength.

partially dropped. Here, we can observe from Figure 6.3 that untreated and treated OPMF/KGG biocomposite samples have different fibre loadings. Now, we are going to compare the dielectric strength of the treated and untreated composites. From Figure 6.3b, it can be observed that as the fibre content increases, the strength ratio also increases. In comparison to treated fibre, the untreated 15% fibre content yields the highest strength. The, at treated 5% fibre content, is 3923.479 (kV/m), and the highest is 4546.7 (kV/m), with untreated 15% fibre content. The specifications of machine: input: 120 VAC, 50 Hz, 20 A; output: 50 kV at 2 kVA, 5% below distortion value; duty: 2 kVA at 1 hour, 1.2 kVA continuous; 23" W × 72" H × 24" deep HV.

6.3.3 Dielectric losses

Here, the variations of dielectric loss and dissipation factor with respect to fibre content of the composite are shown in Figure 6.4. The dissipation factor, such as the dielectric constant, increases with fibre percentage and frequency for all composites. The reduction in the dissipation factor corresponds to a reduction in the quantity of electric current dissipated by the material. As the amount of fibre grows, electrons tend to move faster and have a higher risk of interacting with one another, resulting in energy loss. As a result of the energy loss, the dissipation factor decreases. However, lowering the fibre content in composites lowers the dissipation factor since the treated fibre can help with charge transport. The dielectric loss $P = (v)2 \times$ Frequency × Capacitance × tan D. The unit of P is watts. The force factor estimates are independent of the protected area and only rise with an increase in contamination from moisture and other foreign substances. An increase in the dielectric misfortune may speed up protection

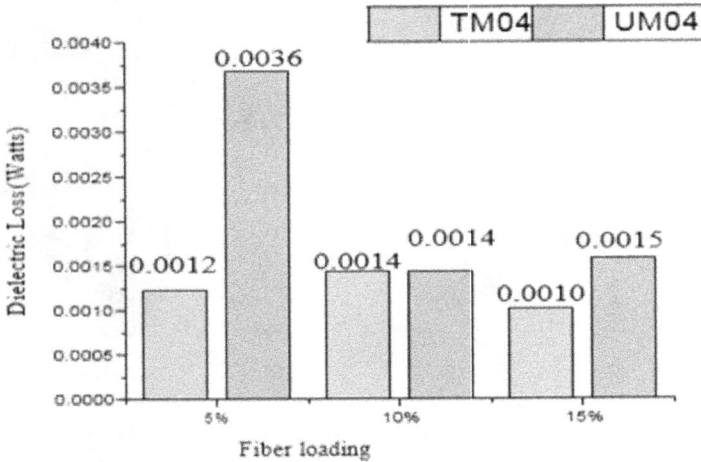

Figure 6.4 Dielectric loss values of different samples with diff. loadings.

Table 6.1 OPMF/KGG biocomposites. UM – untreated mesocarp fibre, TM – treated mesocarp fibre, with 04 mm fibre length and 5%, 10% and 15% weight of the fibre

Sample type	C_x	Q	tan D
UM0405	51	11,730	0.00434
UM0410	20	4600	0.004347
UM0415	22	5060	0.004348
TM0405	17	3910	0.004336
TM0410	20	4600	0.004329
TM0415	14	3220	0.004347

weakening due to heating. Regarding the reports, Table 6.1 and Figure 6.4 display different fibre loadings for untreated and treated OPMF/KGG bio-composite sample. Here, we can compare treated 4 mm 5% and untreated 4 mm 5%. Therefore, we got the lowest dielectric loss (P) and tan D having sample is treated 4 mm length with 5% of weight of the fibre those values are $P = 0.001230$ watts & tan $D = 0.004336$. The lesser value of dielectric loss represents the best insulating material. Here, the best insulating material we obtained is the treated 4 mm 5%. A non-destructive test, 10 kV rating bridge equipment is considered for measuring the dissipation factor. A test voltage of up to 1.5 times the nominal voltage rating of the equipment is applied for 1 minute. The tan D meter has the following specifications: 1 MHz test frequency, range of tan D 0.001 to 0.200 absolute, voltage 230 V and frequency 50 Hz.

6.3.4 SEM

The interfacial characteristics of the composites were studied using scanning electron microscopy (SEM). Failure dielectric samples surface SEM micrographs of composites of both untreated and chemically altered surfaces (treated) OPMF with 4 mm length with 5%, 10% and 15%, respectively, are shown. Figure 6.5c shows a matrix that reveals fibre debonding. Because of the low fibre–matrix similarity in untreated composites, the interaction between the fibre and the matrix was often poor. Figure 6.5c shows that untreated OPM fibres were discovered in multi-fibre bundles rather than being equally disseminated. The tested dielectric specimen is subjected to SEM examination. Figure 6.5a shows the SEM analysis of treated 4 mm length 5% wt. dielectric sample. At this weight percentage of fibre concentration, the dielectric tested high, indicating that the bonding is robust and that fibre pull-out is minimal. Due to the higher dielectric strength value, the effective stress transfer between the fibre and matrix is good at 5% composite. This composite has the largest fibre percentage, which results in the least amount of fibre pull-out. Figure 6.5b shows the SEM analysis of fragmented specimens with a 5 weight percent dielectric. Figure 6.5a–c shows the SEM investigation of a 5 wt. % dielectric specimen with a fibre loading of 4 mm length. Due to insufficient distribution matrix material, fibre pull-out and other factors, microscopic holes and voids emerge on the surface in these images. The matrix accumulation is greater with 5 wt. % fibre loading, and thus, the strength seen is lower. The dielectric research on the cross section of a fractured dielectric sample of untreated 5 wt. % with a fibre length of 4 mm is shown in Figure 6.5c. The results show that this percentage produces the most tensile stress. This is owing to the fibre–matrix adhesion being sufficient and superior to the other percentages studied. The active load transfer observed is suitable for specimens of 5 wt. %. Additionally, the results show that due to good bonding, crack onset and fibre pull-out are negligible. Misalignment and bundling of fibres are thought to have happened during the process. In SEM images of untreated 4 mm length and 5% weight content, non-uniform

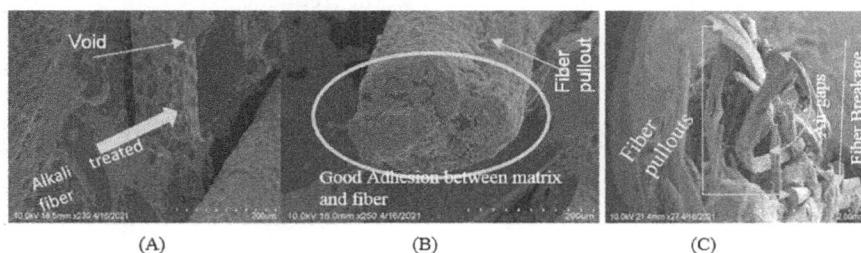

(A)   (B)   (C)

Figure 6.5 Scanning electron microscopy: (a and b) treated; (c) untreated.

voids may also be found, as depicted in Figure 6.5c. Numerous fibre pull-outs are seen, and the fibre surfaces are clean, suggesting poor matrix–fibre adhesion. Untreated composites' dielectric properties deteriorated, but as fibre % increased, the composite strength increased as well, irrespective of treated or untreated composite. This is because as the fibre % increased, the load-carrying capacity of the composites also increased. Here, the SEM micrographs of a fracture surface of the composites with untreated and chemically modified composites were investigated.

The treated and untreated fibres of 5% weight content composites are shown in Figure 6.5. In the case of NaOH-treated fibres, the study of SEM images shows that alkaline treatment increases surface roughness and contributes to the emergence of matrix reaction products on their surface. OPMF pre-treatment adds to the production of a rough surface on the fibres, resulting in thinner fibres. As a result, the alkali-treated OPMF has a larger contact area and a stronger binding to the KGG matrix. Figure 6.5 depicts the damage to the fibre–matrix interaction, which supports this finding (a & b). Untreated fibre composites (Figure 6.5c) were discovered, making it difficult for the KGG matrix binder to permeate the spaces between the fibres and lowering the material's homogeneity. Biocomposites with untreated OPMF have noticeable gaps between the shives and the KGG matrix, indicating poor interfacial adhesion and delamination, as seen in the images above. Because of the high concentration of wax, hemicelluloses and lignin on the surface, the fibre–matrix interface is deteriorating. Such morphological characteristics have been linked to poor adhesion contact at the fibre–matrix interface, according to the researchers.

6.4 CONCLUSIONS AND FUTURE SCOPE

Complete biocomposites with a range of dielectric values can be obtained using OPMF/KGG composites. Such dielectric materials are promising alternatives for conventional dielectric materials used in a variety of electronic applications such as high-speed circuits, high-performance capacitor, electrical cable insulation and printed circuit boards. Considerable variations in dielectric constant were observed at frequencies below 10 Hz, but the dielectric values decreased marginally or were nearly constant at higher frequencies. In the frequency range of 100 Hz to 1 MHz, the loss factor, dielectric constant, capacitance, and dielectric strength of KGG matrix and composites with various amounts of OPMF-reinforced biocomposites have been examined. The experimental results show that the untreated 5% weight fibre composites have better dielectric properties than all other composites, and similar observations show that the dielectric constant and loss factor decrease with increasing frequency. The untreated composites have better dielectric properties compared to treated ones. The maximum dielectric strength is observed for 15% weight content fibre untreated composites.

REFERENCES

1. Thyavihalli Girijappa, Y. G., Mavinkere Rangappa, S., Parameswaranpillai, J. and Siengchin, S. (2019), Natural Fibers as sustainable and renewable resource for development of eco-friendly composites: A comprehensive review, *Frontiers in Materials*, 6, 226.

2. Mathur, V. K. (2006), Composite materials from local resources, *Construction and Building Materials*, 20, 470–477.

3. Satyanarayana, K.G., Arizaga, G. G. and Wypych, F. (2009), Biodegradable composites based on lignocellulosic fibers—An overview, *Progress in Polymer Science*, 34, 982–1021.

4. Holbert, J. and Houston, D. (2006), Natural fiber reinforced polymer composites in automotive applications, *The Journal of The Minerals, Metals & Materials Society*, 58, 80–86.

5. Pandey, J. K., Hahn, S. H., Lee, C. S., Mohanty, A. K. and Mishra, M. (2010), Recent advances in the application of natural fiber based composites, *Micromolecular Materials and Engineering*, 295, 975–989.

6. Athijayamani, A., Thiruchitrambalam, M., Natarajan, U. and Pazhanivel, B. (2009), Effect of moisture absorption on the mechanical properties of randomly oriented natural fibers/polyester hybrid composite, *Materials Science Engineering A*, 517, 344–353.

7. Torres, F. G. and Cubillos, M. L. (2005), Study of the interfacial properties of natural fiber reinforced polyethylene, *Polymer Testing*, 24, 694–698.

8. John, M. J. and Anandjiwala, R. D. (2007), Recent developments in chemical modification and characterization of natural fiber-reinforced composites, *Polymer Composites*, 29, 187–207.

9. Thakur, V. K., Singha, A. S., Kaur, I., Nagarajarao, R. P. and Liping, Y. (2010), Silane functionalization of Saccaharum cilliare fibers: Thermal, morphological, and physicochemical study, *International Journal of Polymer Analysis and Characterization*, 15, 397–414.

10. Philips, G. O. and Williams, P. A. (2001), Tree exudates gums: Natural and versatile food additives and ingredients, *Food Ingredients Analysis of International*, 23, 26–28.

11. Sashidhar, R. B., Raju, D. and Karuna, R. (2015), Tree Gum: Gum Kondagogu. In: Ramawat K, Mérillon JM. (eds) *Polysaccharides*. Springer, Cham.

12. Vinod, V. T. P., Sashidhar, R. B., Suresh, K. I., Rama Rao, B., Vijaya Saradhi, U. V. R. and Prabhakar Rao, T. (2008), Morphological, physico-chemical and structural characterization of gum kondagogu (Cochlospermum gossypium): A tree gum from India, *Food Hydrocolloids*, 22, 899–915.

13. Jagadeesh, D., Jeevan Pradsad Reddy, D., Varada Rajulu, A. and Li, R. (2011), Green composites from wheat protein isolate and Hildegardia Populifolia natural fabric, *Polymer Composites*, 32(3), 398–406.

14. Li, X., Tabil, L. G. and Panigrahi, S. (2007), Chemical treatments of natural fiber for use in natural fiber-reinforced composites: A review, *Journals of Polymers and the Environment*, 15, 25–33.

15. Vinod, V. T. P., Sashidhar, R. B., Sarma, V. U. M. and Satyanarayana Raju, S. (2010a), Comparative amino acid and fatty acid compositions of edible gum kondagogu (Cochlospermum gossypium) and karaya (Sterculia urens), *Food Chemistry*, 123, 57–62.

16. Fidelis, M. E. A., Pereira, T. V. C., Gomes, O. D. F. M., de Andrade Silva, F. and Toledo Filho, R. D. (2013), The effect of fibre morphology on the tensile strength of natural fibres, *Journal of Materials Research and Technology*, 2, 149–157.

17. Van de Velde, K. and Kirkenes, P. (2002), Thermal degradation of flax: The determination of kinetic parameters with thermogravimetric analysis, *Journal of Applied Polymer Science*, 83, 2634–2643.

18. Obiukwu, O., Opara, I. and Udeani, H. (2016), Study on the mechanical properties of palm kernel fibre reinforced epoxy and poly-vinyl alcohol (PVA) composite material, *International Journal of Engineering and Technologies*, 7, 68–77.

19. Pothan, L. A., Thomas, S. and Neelakantan, N. R. (1997), Short banana fiber reinforced polyester composites: Mechanical, failure and aging characteristics, *Journal of Reinforced Plastics and Composites*, 16, 744–765.

20. Doddi, P. R. V., Chanamala, R. and Dora, S. P. (2019), Dynamic mechanical properties of epoxy based PALF/basalt hybrid composite laminates, *Materials Research Express*, 6(10), 105343.

21. Singha, A. S. and Thakur, V. K. (2008), Mechanical properties of natural fibre reinforced polymer composites, *Bulletin of Material Science*, 31, 791.

22. Paul, V., Kanny, K. and Redhi, G. G. (2015), Mechanical, thermal and morphological properties of a bio-based composite derived from banana plant source, *Composites Part A: Applied Science and Manufacturing*, 68, 90–100.

Chapter 7

Physical Properties of Surface Modification Impact on Coir Fiber/KGG biocomposites

V. Srikanth, K. Raja Narender Reddy, and M. Keerthika

Kakatiya Institute of Technology and Science, Warangal

CONTENTS

7.1 INTRODUCTION

Current ecological principles and sociological trouble require the advancement of bio-based materials and other new techniques that can liberate the planet from its utilization of non-renewable energy sources during the most recent times [1]. These organic substances are used as substitutes for various composites because of their inherent qualities such as ease of production, fundamental control, efficacy, accessibility, less rigorous technique and lower cost (for example, metals). Composites made out of synthesized reinforcements and polymer matrices are losing favor because of major ecological concerns and colossal expenses [2]. Thus, the interest for regular fiber-supported composites for different business applications in the modern area has soared in recent years [3]. Normal fibers in composite materials, on the other hand, have a few drawbacks, including excessive dampness retention, less durability security, low heat resistance, arrangement variation and incompatibility with polymeric matrix [4]. Surface treatment of fiber

DOI: 10.1201/9781003344810-7

or interfacial bonding alteration innovations can help address these issues. Numerous physical and chemical treatment approaches for fiber surface alteration have been investigated to improve the similarity of normal fibers to polymer matrix. Natural fibers have the potential to replace conventional artificial fibers like reinforcing steel, graphite, or crystal, which are frequently used in packaging, transportation, and building [5,6]. Commercial collection of plant fibers from agricultural ranches is extremely advanced since it improves manageability and increases the practical usage of natural assets [7]. Consequently, a few examples of fibers that are the focus of this analysis are coir fibers. Coir is biodegradable, abundant, inexhaustible, enduring and savvy; it can likewise endure high temperatures and salt water without disintegrating. Coir fibers are by a long shot the most engaging materials, in spite of having lower heat conductivity and mass thickness than other normal fibers [8]. When the fibers were correctly mixed with polymer matrices, they exhibited exceptional characteristics. The majority of fiber components were composed of highly polarized hydroxyl groups, which resulted in the unwanted hydrophilic feature [9]. This element improves fiber water reactivity, coming about in a feeble cross-link thickness between polar aquaphobic fibers and non-polar aquaphobic matrices. Superficial change is one of the methodologies used in the fiber business to decrease the water-insoluble effect. Kondagogu gum (*Cochlospermum gossypium*) is a tree that grows wild in India's woods. This plant's exudate gum has the potential to be used as a low-cost biosorbent [10,11]. With the help of grinder machine, crystals of KGG were made to form a KGG powder. In this chapter, the use of coir fiber as a reinforcement and Kondagogu gum (KGG) powder as a matrix is reported. The Arecaceae family includes the coconut tree, which is a long-lived tree. It is quite likely to be found in many regions of the world. Coconut trees provide edible fruits that are widely used in international cuisines. The coir fiber's arrangements in the composite are made in a random manner. Alkali-based synthetic treatments on the composite were investigated in this study. Infrared spectroscopy was used to describe the treatment's effects on the fibers. The overall goal of this research is to modify the coir fiber surface by alkali treatment and examine the real characteristics, interfacial holding and chemical obstruction of biocomposites with these treated coir fibers. The effect of fiber stretch and fiber weight percentage on physical characteristics is investigated. Similarly, the morphology of holding between fiber and matrix was examined.

7.2 MATERIALS AND METHODS

7.2.1 Materials

Extricated coir fibers were obtained from a neighborhood supplier. KGG powder was bought from Girijan Cooperative Society, Hyderabad. Glycerol, ammonia (NH_3), glutaraldehyde, hydrochloric acid (HCl), sodium hydroxide (NaOH) pellets were bought from Rekha Chemicals, Warangal.

7.2.1.1 Alkaline treatment

The NaOH pretreatment of fiber is aimed at improving the collateral holding between the fiber's surface and the binder. Additionally, a portion of the lignin, paraffin, and grease that coat the fiber cell's exterior layer are removed during this process. Lignin is also depolymerized, revealing the decent-length crystalline phase. This method therefore increases surface hardness. Coir fibers are obtained from the local ranchers, and the fibers are pulled out of the fiber organization and treated with 2% of NaOH by absorbing water for a time period of 24 hours and washed altogether with refined water and evaporated again for 24 hours.

7.2.1.2 Resin preparation

The process of preparing resin from KGG powder is illustrated in Figure 7.1. A weighed amount of KGG powder is taken in a clean glass beaker, and deionized water of 2.5 times the weight of the gum powder is added to the glass beaker. These substances are blended with an attractive stirrer at room temperature for 20–30 minutes. 1 mole of NaOH and 1 mole of HCl are used to produce the matrix in order to neutralize the gum arrangement. After consistent stirring for 20 minutes, glycerol 25% by weight and

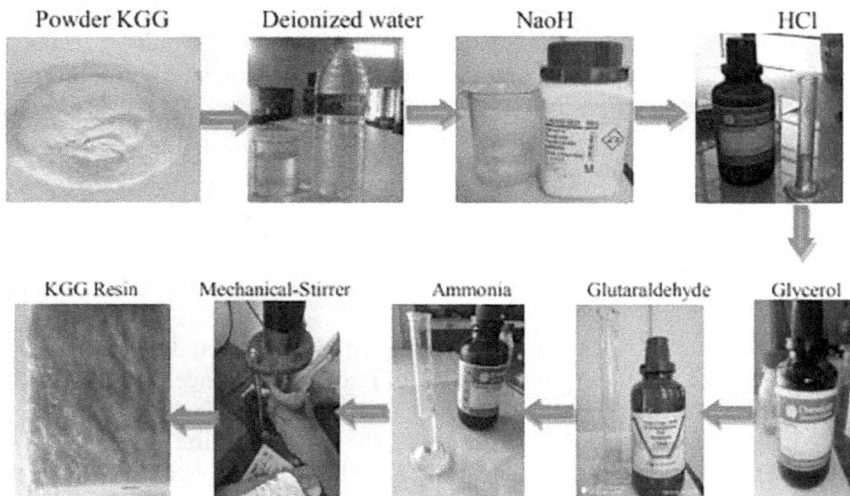

Figure 7.1 Preparation of resin (KGG).

glutaraldehyde 30% by weight of KGG granulates are weighed independently and blended in with the prior gum solution at a pH of 7–8. Glycerol is the plasticizer and glutaraldehyde is the cross-linking agent and their quantity is varied to study their effect on tensile strength and thermal stability.

7.2.1.3 Fabrication of composites

The prepared KGG resin is taken in a dish, and the fibers are separately added in different proportions, viz. 5%, 10% and 15% of the resin by weight. The substances are blended completely to guarantee uniform appropriation of fibers and resin, poured on a glass form and uniform pressing factor applied and afterward permitted to fix at room temperature for 24 hours.

7.2.2 Methods

7.2.2.1 Fourier Transform Infrared Spectroscopy (FTIR)

Fourier transform infrared (FTIR) spectroscopy was performed on unprocessed and manufactured coir fibers using a PerkinElmer Spectrum 100 Spectrometer. The bands were all recorded with 32 outputs for each scan and a resolution of $4\,cm^{-1}$ within $4000-400\,cm^{-1}$ region.

7.2.2.2 Scanning Electron Microscopy

SEM is used to dissect the fiber samples, providing a good view of the tight interaction linking the fiber and the polymer in laminates. A high-energy electron shaft is coordinated onto the example's surface, resulting in high-resolution images of each sample's crystalline structure, surface geography and laminate composition.

7.3 RESULTS AND DISCUSSION

7.3.1 Fourier Transform Infrared Spectroscopy (FTIR)

The engineering features of polymer composites are affected by the component materials' qualities (type, amount and fiber conveyance and direction). Besides these features, the concept of interconnection and load transfer tools play an important role. Because of the poor interlinking connection between the deliquescent (regular) fiber and the aquaphobic matrix, the end products have reduced engineering properties as well as structural changes owing to water retention. There are a range of enhancement approaches available to improve the connection between the lattice and the strands

Table 7.1 FTIR spectra data table of sample treated coir of 4 mm length and 5% weight of fiber (TC0405)

Wavelength (cm⁻¹)	Range	Appearance	Bond	Functional group
3385	4000–3000	Strong, wide	O–H stretching	Alcohol
2816	3000–2500	Average	C–H stretching	Alkane
1518	1600–1300	Strong	N–O stretching	Nitro compound
1380	1600–1300	Average	O–H bending	Carboxylic acid
1044	1400–1000	Strong	C–O stretching	Primary alcohol

depending on the fiber and matrix type. One of the most important difficulties in the relevance of composite materials is the expense of interface modifier synthetic chemicals. The most essential issue to be covered in this research is improving the true properties of fiber composites. Tables 7.1–7.7 summarize the FTIR characteristics of untreated and intentionally altered coir fiber/KGG composites as a function of fiber loading, and Figures 7.2–7.5 depict the related charts. In order to investigate the appearance and shifting of transmittance peaks, the FTIR spectra of altered composite are compared with the raw composite as shown in below figures.

The presence of chemical group gatherings of polysaccharide, hemicellulose and adhesives, additionally as synthetic resin and acyclic chemical group gatherings of polymer caused the O–H stretching vibrations, while the C–H characteristic peaks are due to acyclic chemical group mixtures of polysaccharide, methyl group gatherings of hemicellulose, methoxyl gatherings of polymer and group gatherings of waxes [12–15]. The carbonyl aldehyde or ketone and the carboxylic corrosive of lignin, the carbonyl of acetyl ester, the carboxyl of carboxylic corrosive of hemicellulose, the carbonyl ester of waxes, the carboxyl ester of cellulose caused C=O characteristic peaks, while the aromatic groups caused the C=C characteristic peaks.

The spectra of the treated coir sample show the treated 4 mm length 5% content fiber absorption peak from Table 7.1 at 3385 cm⁻¹, which corresponds to O–H stretching. The assimilation band at 2816 cm⁻¹ relates to alkenes with C–H stretching as seen in Figure 7.2. A thin peak at 1518 cm⁻¹, 1380 cm⁻¹ is caused by N–O stretching nitro compound and carboxylic group O–H bending. The C–O stretching caused a prominent peak to develop at 1044 cm⁻¹ in the alcohol group. The treated 4 mm length 10% content fiber absorption peak from Table 7.2 in the spectra of sample treated coir is at 3406 cm⁻¹, correlating to O–H stretching. Two peak shifts were also detected at 2896 and 1618 cm⁻¹, indicating substantial C–H stretching and C=C stretching. Similarly, the change of groups from 1394 to 1098 cm⁻¹ arises concurrently with the bands, indicating a depletion in C–H bonding to C–O stretching from the components that generated the vibrations and deformities.

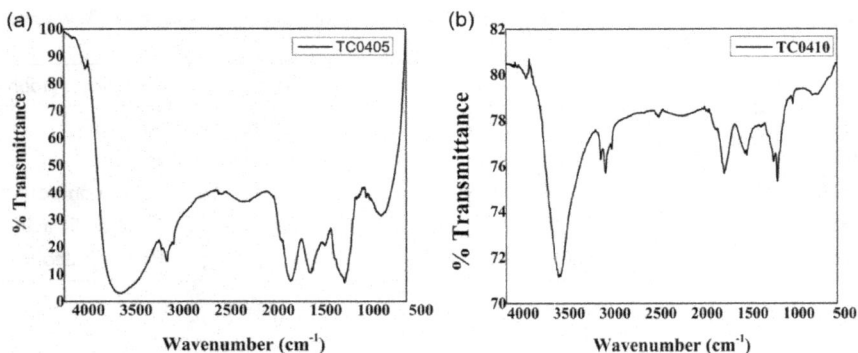

Figure 7.2 FTIR spectra of coir/KGG composites: (a) treated coir of 4mm length and 5% wt. (b) Treated coir of 4mm length and 10% wt.

Table 7.2 FTIR spectra data table of sample treated coir of 4mm length and 10% weight of fiber (TC0410)

Wavelength (cm⁻¹)	Range	Appearance	Bond	Functional group
3406	4000–3000	Strong, wide	O–H stretching	Alcohol
2896	3000–2500	Average	C–H stretching	Alkane
1618	1670–1600	Average	C=C stretching	Conjugated alkene
1394	1600–1300	Average	O–H bending	Carboxylic acid
1098	1400–1000	Strong, broad	C–O stretching	Primary alcohol

From Figure 7.3, the treated coir 4mm length 15% content fiber absorption peaks are notable from Table 7.3 in the spectra at 3426 cm⁻¹, correlating to strong O–H bond. Another two peak shifts occur in the medium C–H stretching alkane group at 2954 cm⁻¹. Furthermore, the change of intensities from 1681, 1480 to 1116 cm⁻¹ appeared concurrently with intensities, indicating solid O–H and medium O–H, along with solid C–O bending.

From Figure 7.3, the untreated coir 4mm length 5% content fiber absorption peaks are notable from Table 7.4 in the spectra of sample at 3318 cm⁻¹, correlating to strong O–H bonding. Two pinnacle shifts occur at 2782 cm⁻¹ medium C–H stretching alkane group. Furthermore, the bands shifted from 1640 to 1032 cm⁻¹ along with the band frequencies, indicating that the components that generated the vibrations and twisting were solid C=C stretching to medium O–H bending. Figure 7.4 shows an untreated coir 4mm length 10% content fiber absorption peaks, which are notable from Table 7.5. In the spectra of sample at 3386 cm⁻¹, correlating to strong and broad O–H stretching. There are two more peak shifts at 2819 cm⁻¹ in the medium C–H stretching alkane group. Furthermore, the spectrum energies shifted from 1639 to 1361 cm⁻¹, indicating that the components that generated the

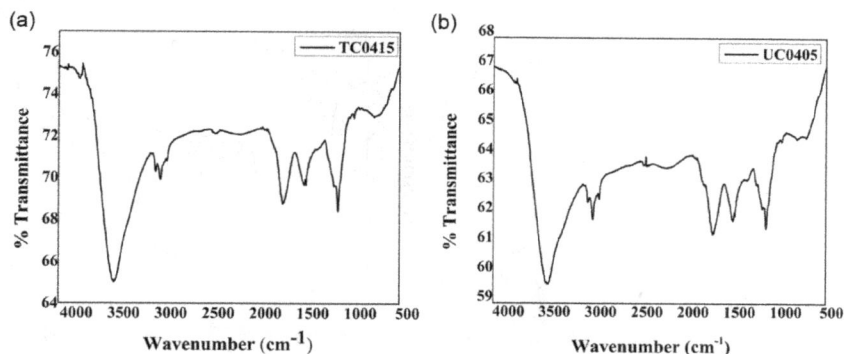

Figure 7.3 FTIR spectra of coir/KGG composites: (a) treated coir of 4 mm length and 15% wt. (b) Untreated coir of 4 mm length and 05% wt.

Table 7.3 FTIR spectra data table of sample treated coir of 4 mm length and 15% weight of fiber (TC0415)

Wavelength (cm⁻¹)	Range	Appearance	Bond	Functional group
3426	4000–3000	Strong, wide	O–H stretching	Alcohol
2954	3000–2500	Average	C–H stretching	Alkane
1681	2000–1650	Strong	C=O stretching	Conjugated ketone
1480	1600–1300	Average	O–H bending	Carboxylic acid
1116	1400–1000	Strong	C–O stretching	Primary alcohol

Table 7.4 FTIR spectra data table of sample untreated coir of 4 mm length and 5% weight of fiber (UC0405)

Wavelength (cm⁻¹)	Range	Appearance	Bond	Functional group
3318	4000–3000	Strong, wide	O–H stretching	Alcohol
2782	3000–2500	Average	C–H stretching	Alkane
1640	1670–1600	Strong	C=C stretching	Conjugated alkene
1032	1400–1000	Average	O–H bending	Alcohol

vibrations and deformations were solid C=C stretching, solid C–O stretching and medium O–H bending. Figure 7.4 shows an untreated coir 4 mm length 15% content fiber absorption peaks, which are notable from Table 7.6 in the spectra of sample at $3403\,cm^{-1}$, correlating to strong and broad O–H stretching. Another two pinnacle shifts at $2902\,cm^{-1}$ medium C–H stretching alkane bunch. Similarly, the change of bands from 1624 to $1413\,cm^{-1}$ occurred concurrently with the wave frequencies, indicating solid C=C stretching, medium O–H bending to solid C–O stretching from the

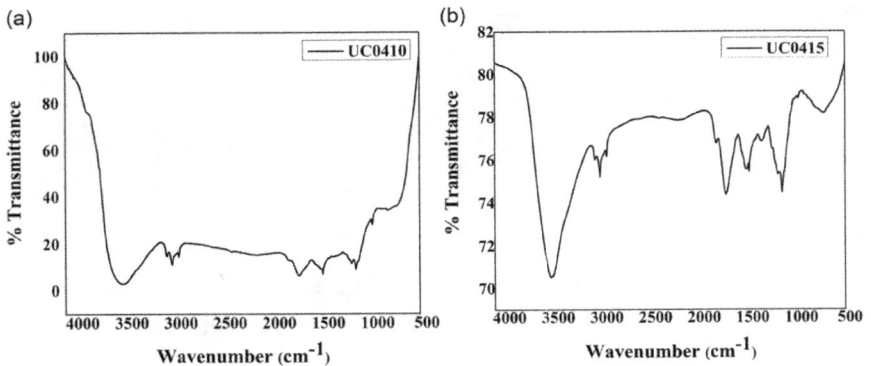

Figure 7.4 FTIR spectra of coir/KGG composites: (a) untreated coir of 4 mm length and 10% wt. (b) Untreated coir of 4 mm length and 15% wt.

Table 7.5 FTIR spectra data table of sample untreated coir of 4 mm length and 10% weight of fiber (UC0410)

Wavelength (cm⁻¹)	Range	Appearance	Bond	Functional group
3386	4000–3000	Strong, wide	O–H stretching	Alcohol
2819	3000–2500	Average	C–H stretching	Alkane
1639	1670–1600	Strong	C=C stretching	Conjugated alkene
1361	1400–1000	Average	O–H bending	Carboxylic acid
1054	1400–1000	Strong	C–O stretching	Primary alcohol

Table 7.6 FTIR spectra data table of sample untreated coir of 4 mm length and 15% weight of fiber (UC0415)

Wavelength (cm⁻¹)	Range	Appearance	Bond	Functional group
3403	4000–3000	Strong, wide	O–H stretching	Alcohol
2902	3000–2500	Average	C–H stretching	Alkane
1624	1670–1600	Strong	C=C stretching	Conjugated alkene
1413	1400–1000	Average	O–H bending	Carboxylic acid
1098	1400–1000	Strong	C–O stretching	Primary alcohol

components that generated the vibrations and deformity. Figure 7.5 shows the neat KGG resin content fiber absorption peaks notable from Table 7.7 in the spectra of sample at 3419 cm⁻¹, correlating to strong and broad O–H stretching. There are two more peak shifts at 2815 cm⁻¹ in the medium C–H stretching alkane group. Also, the spectrum frequencies shifted from 1514

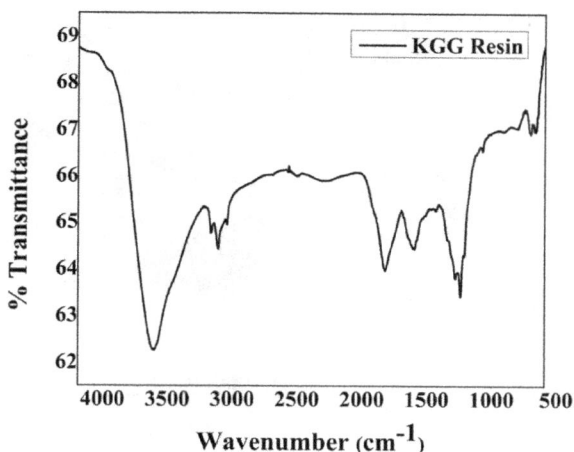

Figure 7.5 FTIR spectra of pure resin.

Table 7.7 FTIR spectra data table of sample KGG resin (neat KGG resin)

Wavelength (cm⁻¹)	Range	Appearance	Bond	Functional group
3419	4000–3000	Strong, wide	O–H stretching	Alcohol
2815	3000–2500	Average	C–H stretching	Alkane
1514	1600–1300	Strong	N–O stretching	Nitro compound
1400	1600–1300	Average	O–H bending	Carboxylic acid
1056	1400–1000	Strong	C–O stretching	Primary alcohol

to 1400 cm⁻¹, indicating that the components that generated the vibrations and mishappening were solid N–O stretching, medium O–H bending and solid C–O stretching.

FTIR spectroscopy confirmed the occurrence of dissimilarity in bonding in synthetic and raw coir fiber. As fiber material increased, the band intensities in the spectra of treated and untreated coir fibers increased as well. The primary band intensity was initially noted in the treated 15% fiber percentage range, where it is stronger compared to the resin and untreated composites. We will now look at the 15% decrease in treated band intensities from raw fibers (3403, 2902, 1624, 1413, 1098 cm⁻¹) and 3426, 2954, 1681, 1480 cm⁻¹ to pure KGG resin (3419, 2815, 1514, 1400, 1056 cm⁻¹). This may be due to a depletion in strong C=O stretching, medium C–H stretching, medium O–H bending, solid O–H stretching and solid C–O stretching. C–H, C=C, C–H and C–O bonds contributed to coir fiber components' vibrations and deformities.

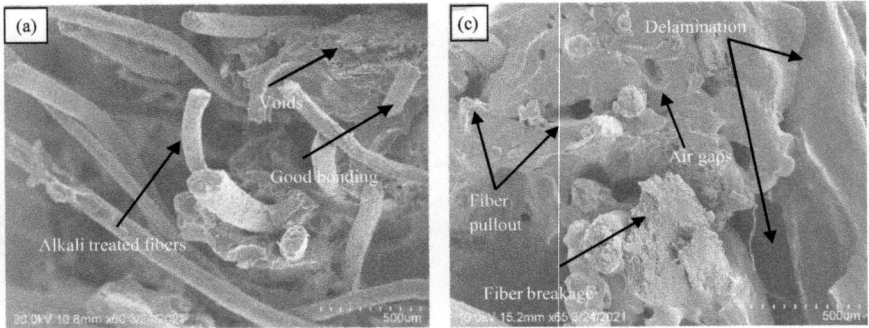

Figure 7.6 SEM images of (a) treated and (b) untreated composites.

7.3.2 Scanning Electron Microscopy

The intercellular characteristics of the prepared composites are explored using scanning electron microscopy (SEM). SEM pictures of a composite's broken surface with untreated and artificially modified composites were examined. The treated and untreated fibers of 15% weight content composites are shown in Figure 7.6. The examination of SEM pictures shown in Figure 7.6a indicates that alkaline therapy intensifies the surface harshness of the fibers and adds to the presence of results of matrix response on their surface for the situation of NaOH-treated fibers. Pretreatment of coir fiber adds to the development of a rough surface of the fibers, making them thinner. Thus, this outcome in augmentation of contact region and more grounded binding of the alkali offered coir fiber the KGG matrix. This goal is supported by the highlights of damage at the interface between the fiber and matrix illustrated in Figure 7.6b. Composites reinforced with untreated coir fiber (Figure 7.6b) were identified, making it hard to KGG matrix binder to enter the holes between the fibers and reducing the homogeneity of the material. Bio-composites with untreated coir fibers uncover noticeable holes between the shives and the KGG matrix, indicating poor interfacial attachment and delamination. With respect to composites, regions are plainly noticeable where pulling out of the fibers has occurred. The noticed morphological highlights are shown because of the weakening of the fiber–matrix attachment due to the high grouping of wax, hemicelluloses, pectin, and lignin on a superficial level. They detailed that such morphological characters are straightforwardly identified with helpless attachment contact at the fiber–matrix interface.

7.4 CONCLUSIONS

KGG composites with coir fibers were successfully built and shown. The raw and synthetic coir fiber composites had a length of 4 mm and a varying fiber substance of 5%, 10% and 15% individually. The FTIR examination of bonding in treated coir fiber of 4 mm length and 15% wt. shows that the bonding is astounding throughout the composites. This is for the most part because of better interfacial grip between the lattice and the fibers. The chemical and physical changes in untreated and treated fibers were investigated, and the following conclusions were reached. The spectra of alkali-treated composites matched those of untreated fiber. Although the peaks in the treated fiber spectra are comparable to those in the untreated fiber, there are some noticeable variations, such as weakening and sharpening at certain locations, as well as peak loss at others. The disappearance of the peak is due to the effective removal of a significant percentage of the fiber's hemicelluloses and lignin as a consequence of alkalization of the fibers. Other apparent changes in fiber spectra include a decrease in absorption intensity as well as a minor upward shift of the peak, indicating partial elimination of hemicelluloses and lignin. The treated fiber composites outperformed the untreated ones in terms of physical attributes. When compared to treated and untreated coir bio-composites, treated coir fibers demonstrated greater physical properties in the FTIR test, with a wider range of peak values. In most circumstances, as the length of the fiber in coir rises, the wavelength drops. Additionally, as the heaviness of the coir fiber develops, so does the frequency number. In SEM pictures, the surface properties binding for raw and intentionally modified fiber-reinforced composites may be easily identified. In SEM pictures, the interfacial properties adhesion for raw and chemically modified fiber-reinforced composites may be easily identified. These outcomes uncover that using coir fiber in composites with KGG resin opens up additional opportunities for the utilization of these materials in a variety of industries.

REFERENCES

1. Ronga, M. Z., Zhang, M. Q., Liu, Y., Yang, G. C., and Zeng, H. M. (2001), The effect of fiber treatment on the mechanical properties of unidirectional sisal- reinforced epoxy composites, *Composites Science and Technology*, 61, 1437–1447.
2. Ashori, A., and Nourbakhsh, A. (2010), Bio-based composites from waste agricultural residues, *Waste Management*, 30, 680–684.
3. Holbery, J., and Houston, D. (2006), Natural fiber reinforced polymer composites in automotive applications, *The Journal of The Minerals, Metals & Materials Society*, 58, 80–86.

4. Athijayamani, A., Thiruchitrambalam, M., Natarajan, U., and Pazhanivel, B. (2009), Effect of moisture absorption on the mechanical properties of randomly oriented natural fibers polyester hybrid composite, *Materials science and Engineering: A*, 517, 344–353.

5. Islam, S., Hasan, M., and Ahmad, M. B. (2014), Chemical modification and properties of cellulose-based polymer composites. In Thakur VK (ed) *Lignocellulosic polymer composites: processing, characterization, and properties*, 1st edn. Wiley, New York, pp 301–324. https://doi.org/10.1002/9781118773949.ch14

6. Yilmaz, N. D. (2015), Agro-residual fibers as potential reinforcement elements for biocomposites. In Thakur VK (ed) *Lignocellulosic polymer composites: processing, characterization, and properties*, 1st edn. Wiley, New York, pp 231–270. https://doi.org/10.1002/9781118773949.ch11

7. Khedari, J., Suttisonk, B., Pratinthong, N., and Hirunlabh, J. (2001), New lightweight composite construction materials with low thermal conductivity, *Cement and Concrete Composites*, 23, 65–70.

8. Amiandamhen, S. O., Meincken, M., and Tyhoda, L. (2020), Natural fibre modification and its influence on fibre-matrix interfacial properties in biocomposite materials. *Fibers and Polymers*, 21, 677–689.

9. Ebele, C. C., Metu Chidiebere, S., and Ojukwu Martin, C. (2016), Fourier Transform Infrared (FTIR) spectroscopy study on Coir Fiber Reinforced Polyester (CFRP) composites, *International Journal of Civil, Mechanical and Energy Science (IJCMES)*, 2, 20–28.

10. Vinod, V. T. P., Sashidhar, R. B., Suresh, K. I., Rama Rao, B., Vijaya Saradhi, U. V. R., and Prabhakar Rao, T. (2008), Morphological, physico-chemical and structural characterization of gum kondagogu (Cochlospermum gossypium): A tree gum from India, *Food Hydrocolloids*, 22, 899–915.

11. Sashidhar, R. B., Raju, D., and Karuna, R. (2015), Tree Gum: Gum Kondagogu. In: Ramawat, K., Mérillon, J. M. (eds.), *Polysaccharides*, Springer, Cham, 185–217.

12. Morán, J. I., Alvarez, V. A., Cyras, V. P., et al. (2008), Extraction of cellulose and preparation of nanocellulose from sisal fibers, *Cellulose*, 15, 149–159.

13. El Mansouri, N. E, and Salvadó, J. (2007), Analytical methods for determining functional groups in various technical lignins, *Industrial Crops and Products*, 26, 116–124.

14. Sun, S., Yuan, T., Li, M., Cao, X., Xu, F., and Liu, Q. (2012), Structural characterization of hemicelluloses from bamboo culms (*Neosinocalamus Affinis*), *Cellulose Chemistry and Technology*, 46, 165–176.

15. Heredia-Guerrero, J. A., Benítez, J. J., Domínguez, E., Bayer, I. S., Cingolani, R., Athanassiou, A., and Heredia, A. (2014), Infrared and Raman spectroscopic features of plant cuticles: A review, *Frontiers in Plant Science*, 5, 305.

Chapter 8

Thermo-Mechanical and Morphological analysis of PF/KGG bio-composites

V. Srikanth, K. Raja Narender Reddy,
P. Anil Kumar, and K. Punnam Chander
Kakatiya Institute of Technology and Science, Warangal

CONTENTS

8.1 INTRODUCTION

A composite is a mix of two unique visibly recognizable materials that are joined together to accomplish superior properties that differ from the constituent material properties. In natural fiber composites, fibers are used as a reinforcement material [1]. Bio-composites of Palmyra fiber as a reinforcement and bio-resin Kondagogu gum (Cochlospermum gossypium) as the matrix material are eco-friendly and effectively biodegradable in nature; Kondagogu gum (Cochlospermum gossypium) is an adherent of the Bixaceae family [2]. Because of their easy accessibility and low cost, distinctive gums such as Kondagogu gum (KGG), Sterculia gum, wheat protein isolate, and soy protein isolate (SPI) are getting more popular in logical exploration and industry. KGG (Cochlospermum gossypium), gum karaya and other wild gum-based trees grow abundantly in India [3]. The most fundamental perspective in characterizing the fiber/network interface is the ability to transfer loads between fiber and matrix. Natural fibers, on the other hand, have the drawback of absorbing moisture (hydrophilic), resulting in less interfacial bonding between matrix and fiber [4]. Researchers claim that surface alteration techniques increase interfacial binding between fiber surface and matrix by an accurate chemical treatment process [5]. Bio-composites are used in a variety of technological applications, including environmental protection and the production of lighter composites for vehicles, building beams, and packaging [6].

In contrast to the well-known and commercially exploited gums, an experimental work in the lab on KGG has resulted in identifying distinct features, which are similar to those of other gum plants [7]. KGG (Cochlospermum gossypium) was studied [8,9] to determine its response in watery conditions, and the corresponding properties of the gum were dictated by deacetylating gum; later, different chemical and physical properties of this gum were investigated. The removal of hemicellulose and surface contaminants (wax) from Palmyra fibers after alkali treatment resulted in an increase in the rough surface area available for matrix interaction [10]. Surface-modified fiber composites outperform untreated fiber composites in terms of mechanical properties. The effects of the therapy on the fibers were characterized by SEM [11]. According to the survey of literature and research undertaken worldwide, natural fibers play a vital role in various engineering and technological executions, including airplanes, automobiles, and recreational goods. In this work, Palmyra fibers obtained from the Palmyra tree were used to fabricate composites of varying fiber weight percentages, the fibers are accommodated in a randomly orientated way. The current work investigates and reports on the application of alkali treatment to modify the fiber surface and further improve composite qualities such as mechanical, thermal, and surface morphology. Mechanical characteristics are investigated in relation to fiber length and fiber weight percentage. In addition, the fractured tensile surfaces of composites were investigated using SEM.

8.2 MATERIALS AND METHODS

8.2.1 Materials

Palmyra fibers were procured from neighborhood farmers, and KGG powder (KGG – grade 1) was obtained from Nutriroma Pvt. Ltd. in Hyderabad, Telangana. NaOH, glycerol, glutaraldehyde, HCL, NH$_3$, and PVA were procured from Rekha Chemicals, Warangal, Telangana.

8.2.1.1 Fiber treatment

The primary goal of alkali fiber treatment is to increase interfacial binding between the surface of fiber and matrix. This treatment also depolymerizes cellulose and reveals short-length crystallites by removing a particular portion of lignin, oil and wax from fiber cell's outer surface, and it increases the surface hardness. Palmyra fiber mesh is obtained from local farmers and long fibers are extracted from the fiber network; later, they are treated with 2 percentage NaOH and soaked in water for 24 hours. Then fibers are rinsed completely with distilled water and dried for another 24 hours; later, the treated and untreated fibers are chopped according to the required length of 4 mm.

8.2.1.2 Resin preparation

To fabricate the resin, the ideal measures of powdered KGG was precisely gauged and then poured into a glass measuring utensil with 1 L of deionized water (by weight approx. 2.5 X KGG powder). The whole thing was then stirred for 20–30 minutes with the use of a mechanical stirrer, and then 1 mole of NaOH and 1 mole of HCl were added to nullify the gum solution. Separately weighed glutaraldehyde and glycerol were blended with 25–30 percentage times in a continuous incubation for 10 minutes (by wt. of KGG powder). After that, the mixture is blended with NH_3 solution to obtain a pH of 7.0–8.0 and stirred until the mixture turns pale yellow as shown in Figure 8.1, indicating the synthesis of resin and making the matrix.

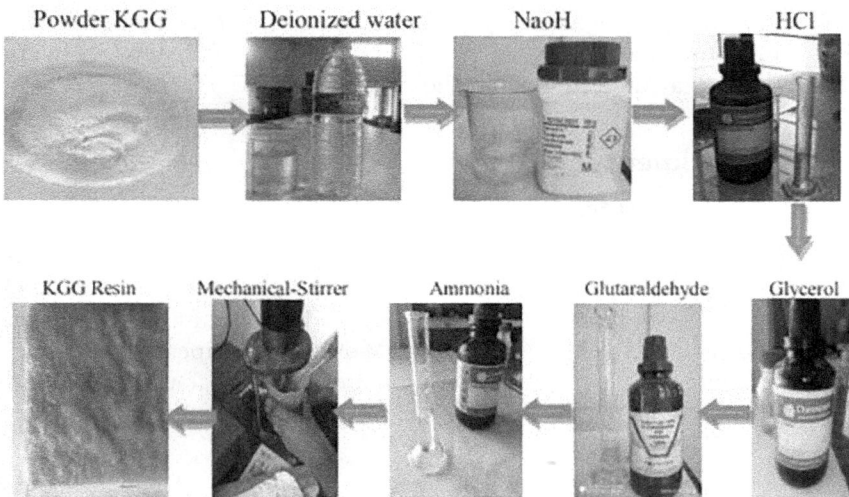

Figure 8.1 Resin preparation.

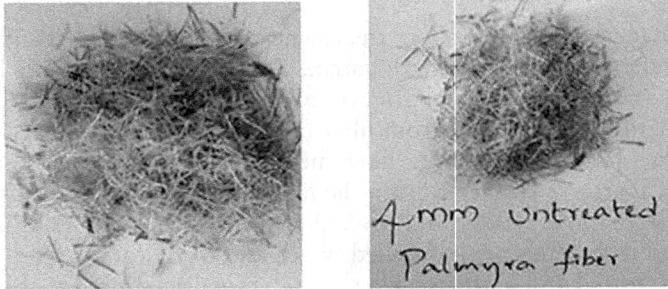

Figure 8.2 Fibers of 4 mm length treated and untreated.

Figure 8.3 PF/KGG composites.

8.2.1.3 Fabrication of composites

Bio-resin KGG was used to fabricate Palmyra fiber composites of volume (280×280×3 mm) with basic treated and untreated fibers of 4 mm length as shown in Figure 8.2 and with varying fiber weight percentages of 5, 10, and 15 using hand lay-up technique as shown in Figure 8.3.

8.2.2 Experiments

8.2.2.1 Mechanical testing

The tensile characteristics of PF/KGG bio-composites were examined utilizing a Zwick/Roell Z010 UTM with a load of 10 kN and a 40 mm check length with a cross-head speed comprising of 10 mm/min. The test standards followed are ASTM D638 of type IV dumbbell shape. Three samples were examined from each respective laminate, and the par values were utilized to evaluate the tensile strength and percentage of elongation.

8.2.2.2 Scanning Electron Microscopy

On split tensile samples, a scanning electron microscope examination is performed to assess the sample's internal structural bonding, surface topology, and composition. On a HITACHI 3700, a beam of high-energy electrons is centered on the surface of a solid specimen, generating a variety of signals that show the object's crystalline image. Prior to recording the microstructure with a 10 kV accelerating speed, the broken surfaces were glazed with gold for electrodeposition to provide electrical conductivity.

8.2.2.3 Differential Scanning Calorimetry (DSC)

A differential scanning calorimeter (DSC8000 PerkinElmer) was utilized for scrutinizing the thermal attributes of the PF/KGG laminates. Test samples of 5–10 mg were precisely measured and fixed in an aluminum dish and afterward filtered all through a temperature scope of −50°C to 450°C at a fundamental warming pace of 10°C/min. A vacant aluminum container was used as a reference pan. The glass transmission temperature (T_g) of PF/KGG was determined utilizing the articulation point of the thermographs from graph.

8.3 RESULTS AND DISCUSSION

8.3.1 Tensile test

The mechanical properties of Palmyra fiber bio-composites are determined by the component segment characteristics (type, amount, and fiber circulation and direction). Apart from these features, the concept of interfacial connections and weight transfer systems at the point of contact is also crucial. The resultant materials exhibit poor mechanical characteristics and dimensional changes owing to moisture absorption due to insufficient interfacial contact between the hydrophilic (regular) fiber and hydrophobic lattice. There are many techniques to improvise the bond between the grid and the fibers relying upon the fiber and lattice type, and the expense of surface alteration synthetics is perhaps the most basic factors in the usage of built-up composites. To address these difficulties, fibers were chemically treated using an aqueous NaOH coupling agent.

This investigation's main focus is to enhance the mechanical characteristics of fiber composites. Table 8.1 sums up the tensile properties of chemically untreated and treated PF/KGG bio-composites as an element of fiber loading, with Figures 8.4 and 8.5 as a reference. The variation of fiber weight ratio in the samples suggests that better strength is observed in the samples with higher fiber loading. It also suggests that alkaline-treated composites have more strength when contrasted with the untreated composites; this can be seen in Figures 8.4 and 8.5. This shows that treated fiber has improved strength because of strong interfacial binding between fibers and matrix.

Table 8.1 Tensile properties of PF/KGG bio-composites (neat resin, treated, and untreated)

Sample name	Tensile strength (N/mm²)	Percentage elongation
Neat resin	1.12	19.05
TP0405	1.35	15.2
TP0410	1.93	8.72
TP0415	2.81	6.73
UP0405	0.89	23.16
UP0410	1.69	18.78
UP0415	1.84	16.93

TP – treated Palmyra; UP – untreated Palmyra; 04 – the length of fiber; 05, 10, and 15 – Percentages of fiber

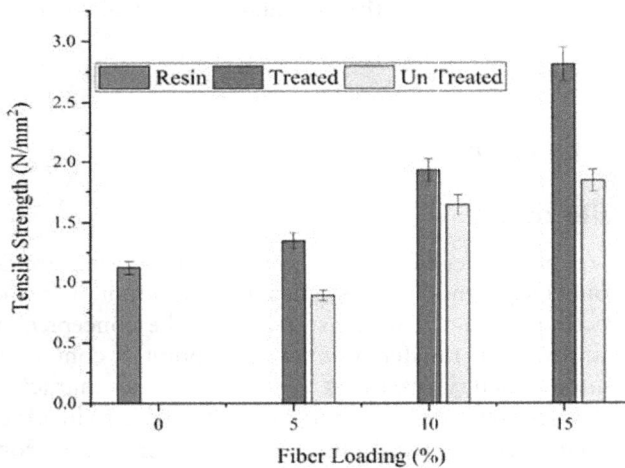

Figure 8.4 Fiber loading vs tensile strength.

The tensile characteristics of the PF/KGG bio-composites are improved with the increase in fiber content. The greatest value was found at 15 percentage weight fiber loading in both untreated and treated fiber composites when contrasted with neat resin. The improved tensile qualities of the fibers reveal their capacity to function as a load transfer agent for matrix and fiber. In every case, the treated composites' tensile characteristics were found to be superior to the matrix. Figure 8.4 shows the tensile strength of both treated and untreated fiber composites was found to be as follows for 15 percentage fiber by weight: TP0415 – 2.81 MPa and UP0415 – 1.84 MPa. The strength of treated and untreated fiber laminates has higher percentage increase over the matrix as follows: alkali-treated 94.6 – percentage and untreated – 64.2 percentage.

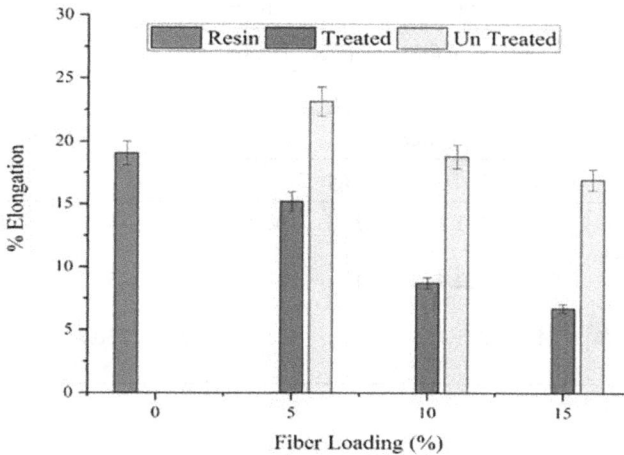

Figure 8.5 Fiber loading vs percentage elongation.

The percentage elongation (Figure 8.5) is low in fiber loading of 15 percentage weight. This is because tensile strength is more when contrasted with the other treated and untreated fiber laminates. A smaller percentage of elongation is observed in treated and untreated fibers of 15 percentage and 10 percentage weight content when compared to neat resin. This suggests that the material will perform better under tensile loading if the percentage of elongation is lower. It also implies that the fiber and matrix have high affiliate adhesion, which improves the material's tensile strength and ductility. When compared to other laminates and pure resin, the untreated fiber of 4 mm length and 5 percentage weight had a greater percent of elongation. This can be seen in Figure 8.5.

8.3.2 Melting characteristics and crystallization temperature of composites

The thermal characteristics of composites were explored using DSC. The glass transition temperature (T_g), melting temperature (T_m), crystallization enthalpy (H_c), and crystallization temperature (T_c) determined utilizing DSC are summarized in Table 8.2. The T_g and T_m of the composites varied with the addition of fiber, as shown in Table 8.2. The composite exhibits an increase in T_g with the addition of fiber. These impressions indicate that the composite's qualities have shifted from sensitive and adaptive to hard and extreme. These findings suggest that both treated and untreated PF fibers have an impact on the KGG matrix's crystallization characteristics.

When compared to the treated/untreated composites, the resin melting temperature was low, but when the fiber content increased, the melting

Table 8.2 Thermal characteristics of neat resin and PF/KGG bio-composites

Name	T_g (°C)	T_m (°C)	ΔH_c (J/g)	T_c (°C)				
Neat resin	46	220	11.06	103.2				
			Treated				Untreated	
Fibers	T_g (°C)	T_m (°C)	ΔH_c (J/g)	T_c (°C)	T_g (°C)	T_m (°C)	ΔH (J/g)	T_c (°C)
PF/KGG – 05 percentage	48	253.2	4.7	106	44	230.5	7.7	103.9
PF/KGG – 10 percentage	51	262.4	5.1	101.8	49	251.1	6.8	111.9
PF/KGG – 15 percentage	54	271.1	6.5	109.5	57	268.9	9.6	127.2

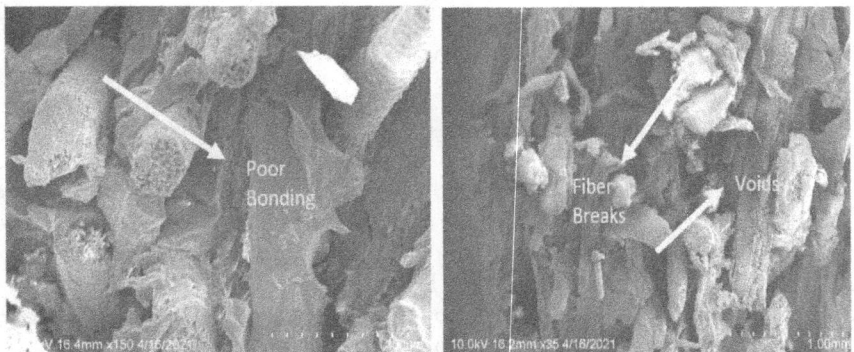

Figure 8.6 SEM micrographs of untreated PF/KGG laminates with broken surfaces.

temperature increased as well. The high melting point temperature in fiber laminates is because the fibers catch up heat quickly. Here, 15 percentage weight fiber composites have a high melting point temperature and crystallization temperature when contrasted with resin and laminates of 5 and 10 percentage fiber-loaded composites.

8.3.3 Scanning Electron Microscopy

Scanning electron microscopy was used to explore the interfacial properties of the composites. Figures 8.6–8.8 exhibit micrographs of broken tensile specimen surfaces of composites with untreated and treated composites, respectively. According to Figure 8.6, fiber debonding is indicated by the wider distance between the matrix and the untreated, 4 mm long, 5% fiber content. Because of the lack of fiber–matrix similarity, the link between the fibers and the matrix in untreated composites was typically poor. Untreated

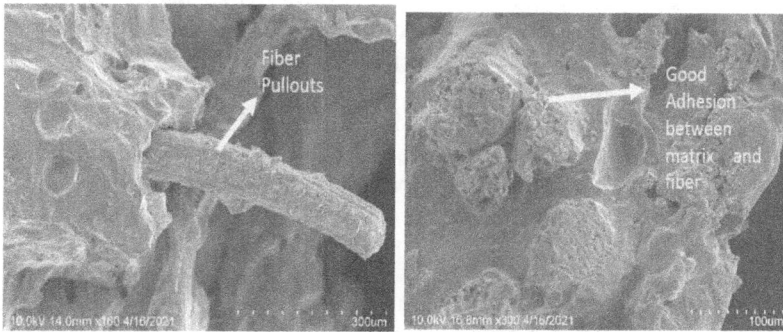

Figure 8.7 SEM micrographs of treated PF/KGG laminate with broken surfaces.

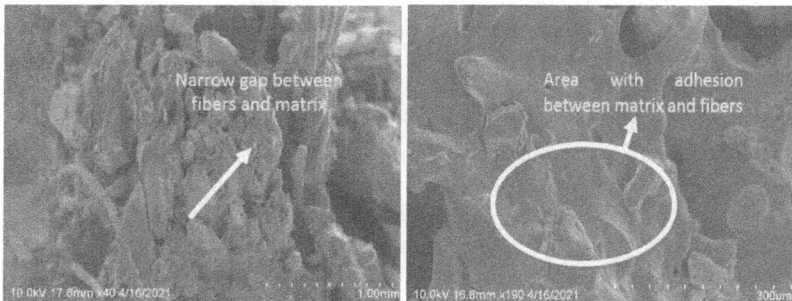

Figure 8.8 SEM micrographs of treated PF/KGG laminates showing fibers and matrix interface.

PF fibers were found in multi-fiber bundles rather than being evenly dispersed, as shown in Figure 8.6.

Misalignment and bundling of fibers are thought to have happened during processing. In SEM images of untreated 4 mm length and 10 percentage weight content, non-uniform voids may also be found, as depicted in Figure 8.6. Numerous fiber pull-outs are seen, and the fiber surfaces are clean, suggesting poor matrix–fiber adhesion. Irrespective of treated or untreated fiber composites, as the fiber percentage increased, the load-carrying capacity of the composites also increased. In untreated composites, mechanical properties deteriorated due to limited fiber–matrix compatibility; to overcome this issue, the surfaces of fibers were treated. The alkali treatment changed the surface of fibers substantially, removing surface contaminants (wax) and hemicellulose while also increasing the direct surface area accessible for matrix interaction. SEM micrographs of alkali-treated composites reveal a minor gap between the fibers of 4 mm length and 15 percentage weight and the matrix; this can be seen in Figures 8.7 and 8.8.

Even though SEM photos reveal aggregation on the surface, interfacial adhesion is influenced by surface topography because the rougher the alkali-treated fiber is, the stronger the mechanical interlocking and the better the reinforcement and matrix connection. In treated fibers of 4 mm length and fiber weight percentages of 5, 10, and 15, the maximum tensile strength is observed in 15 percentage fiber composites. These findings support that alkali treatment of Palmyra fibers increases interfacial adhesion and, as a result, the thermal and mechanical properties of composites are also improved.

8.4 CONCLUSIONS AND FUTURE SCOPE

KGG-based bio-composites with Palmyra fiber reinforcement have been successfully fabricated and characterized. The untreated and alkali-treated PF/KGG composites of randomly oriented fibers were fabricated with differing fiber weight percentages of 5, 10, and 15 with reference to the matrix. When compared to other equivalent fiber weight percentages, the composites with 15 percentage fiber weight of both treated and untreated composites exhibited better mechanical properties. Results indicate that the tensile characteristics of treated Palmyra fiber of 4 mm length and 15 percentage fiber weight, i.e., TP0415, has better strength when compared to neat resin and other composites. Regardless of treated or untreated fiber composites, as fiber weight percentage increased, the tensile strength of composites increased. According to the microscopy findings in NaOH-treated fiber composites, good adhesion between matrix and fibers increased the fiber surface roughness and a better mechanical interlocking between constituent materials. Fiber pull-outs, voids, fiber delamination, and matrix shearing were all visible in SEM images. The thermal investigations suggest composites of 15 percentage fiber weight have a high melting point temperature and crystallization temperature when contrasted with resin and composites of 5 and 10 fiber weight percentages. Overall, Palmyra fiber-reinforced bio-composites with 15 weight percentage fiber loading have superior qualities than other composites, as predicted. Because the supporting fiber material is more eco-friendly, non-harmful, affordable, and readily accessible than traditional fibers, these composites are an excellent fit for a variety of design applications. Overall, a KGG bio-resin reinforced with natural fibers might be a useful composite material.

Further, different mechanical and tribological properties of the composite can be investigated; PLA and other constituent chemicals can be added to improve the thermal and mechanical properties of the composite for better industrial applications.

REFERENCES

1. S. Santhosh, N. Bhanuprakash (2017). A review on mechanical and thermal properties of natural fiber reinforced hybrid composites. *IRJET*, 4, 3053–3057.
2. V. Srikanth, K. Rajanarender Reddy, K. Nageshwar Rao (2021). Biocomposites: A study on behavior of oil palm mesocarp fiber reinforced KGG. *IOP Conference Series: Materials Science and Engineering*, 1123, 012005.
3. T. R., Bhardwaj, Meenakshi Kanwar, Roshan Lal, Anubha Gupta (2000). Natural gums and modified natural gums as sustained-release carriers. *Drug Development and Industrial Pharmacy*, 26, 1025–1038.
4. A. Athijayamani, M. Thiruchitrambalam, U. Natarajan, B. Pazhanivel (2009). Effect of moisture absorption on the mechanical properties of randomly oriented natural fibers polyester hybrid composite. *Materials Science and Engineering: A*, 517, 344–353.
5. H. Gu, (2009). Tensile behaviors of the coir fiber and related composites after NaOH treatment. *Materials and Design*, 30, 3931–3934.
6. K. N. Bharath, S. Basavarjappa (2016). Applications of bio composite materials based on natural fibers from renewable resources: A review. *Science and Engineering of Composite Materials*, 23, 123–133.
7. V. T. P. Vinod, R. B. Sashidhar (2010). Surface morphology, chemical and structural assignment of gum Kondagogu (Cochlospermum gossypium DC): An exudate tree gum of India. *Indian Journal of Natural Products and Resources*, 1, 181–192.
8. V. T. P. Vinod, R. B. Sashidhar, K. I. Suresh, B. T. Prabhakar Rao (2008). Morphological, physico-chemical and structural characterization of gum kondagogu (Cochlospermum gossypium): A tree gum from India. *Food Hydrocolloids*, 22, 899–915.
9. V. T. P. Vinod, R. B. Sashidhar (2009). Solution and conformational properties of gum kondagogu (Cochlospermum gossypium) - A natural product with immense potential as a food additive. *Food Chemistry*, 116, 686–692.
10. M. Thiruchitrambalam, M. Logesh, D. Shanmugam, S. Muthukumar (2018). The physical, chemical properties of untreated and chemically treated palmyra palm leaf fibers. *International Journal of Engineering and Technology*, 7, 582–585.
11. C. Uma Maheswari, K. Obi Reddy, E. Muzenda, M. Shukla, A. VardaRajulu (2013). Mechanical properties and chemical resistance of short tamarind fiber/ unsaturated polyester composites: Influence of fiber modification and fiber content. *International Journal of Polymer Analysis and Characterization*, 18, 520–533.

Chapter 9

Posture analysis
Current status and future trends

Arnab Sarmah
Indian Institute of Technology Guwahati

Satoshi Ito
Gifu University Gifu

Subramani Kanagaraj
Indian Institute of Technology Guwahati

CONTENTS

9.1 INTRODUCTION

The stability of a body can be defined as the resistance of the body to a change in acceleration or its equilibrium position. It is strongly affected by both physiological and neurological factors. Balance refers to the ability to control the equilibrium (Egoyan & Moistsrapishvili, 2013). Postural stability is measured as the position of the COM and/or COP relative to the BOS, which is the area under the feet. In both static and dynamic conditions, the COM position should be within the BOS for maintaining the stability. However, in addition to its position, COM velocity also determines the stability during dynamic conditions. Postural response/reaction is the muscle activations in response to both internal and external disturbances that maintain the body alignment of the mass centers (Iqbal, 2011). Postural stabilization is maintained through visual, vestibular and somatosensory process. The somatosensory process consists of passive and active mechanisms at the muscular and the spinal level. Active torques are generated due to the contraction of muscles in response to commands from the central nervous system (CNS) from reflex loops and/or higher centers, whereas passive torques are due to the inherent viscosity and stiffness of the muscles, ligaments and tendons (Iqbal, 2011). The gait and posture of an individual changes over his/her lifetime. These changes are more common in older adults, i.e., people with more than 65 years of age, due to change in sensorimotor systems, and they are not avoidable. These changes are also caused due to chronic diseases and result in gait and posture deviation, resulting in static and dynamic instability. It increases the fall risk factor and thus is associated with increased mortality, morbidity, disability, loss of independent living and altered quality of life, leading to high healthcare expenditures. During the activities of daily life (ADL), falls are prevented by the stability. Loss of stability and falls result in injuries, which are prevalent and have been reported in many countries.

Falls account for up to 20% of all industrial accidents in the USA. As per the Swedish information system, 17% of occupational accidents per year are related to falls (Razavi, 2016). Recent estimates included in the Global Burden of Diseases (GBD) study showed that neurological disorders such as Alzheimer's and other dementias, epilepsy and headache disorders, multiple sclerosis and Parkinson's disease comprise 3% of worldwide diseases. Migraine and epilepsy represent one-third and one-fourth of the neurological diseases, respectively. Dementia and Parkinson's disease are listed within the top 15 disorders that had the most considerable increase in patients in the last decade (Thakur et al., 2016). Parkinson's disease falls under the category of neurological disorders, which are known to affect the movement and gait patterns due to the degeneration of the motor areas in the brain responsible for generation of smooth, coordinated and rhythmic motor patterns (Miller & Henley, 2017). Parkinson's disease is found to be the fastest growing in disability, deaths and prevalence. Individuals affected from Parkinson's disease in the whole world have increased from 2.5 million in 1990 to 6.1 million in 2016, which is more than a 100% increase. It has caused about 3.2 million disability-adjusted life years (DALY) and about 211,296 deaths in 2016 (Ray Dorsey et al., 2018). In India, it has been reported in some separate cases with prevalence rates of 27, 16.1 and 14.1 out of 100,000 in Bangalore, rural Bengal and rural Kashmir, respectively (Radhakrishnan & Goyal, 2018). The symptoms of Parkinson's disease include poor balance, tremors and stiffness, as well as depression and dementia. It can be grouped under the acronym TRAP: Tremor at rest, Rigidity, Akinesia and Postural Instability (Blochberger & Jones, 2011). The disease progresses slowly, and it might take years for the symptoms to appear and people can have years of independent life after being diagnosed. So, an early diagnosis can further increase the independent life years through proper medication. Thus, the human posture and its stability are required to be studied to understand the effect of the changes of external and internal environments. This would provide insight into the factors leading to balance impairment of both pathological and non-pathological nature. For pathologies such as neurological disorders, human balance can be used as a biomarker and continuous deviation of postural assessment parameters from its normal range can be employed for alerting the subject to seek medical consultation. It can also be employed in tracking treatment protocols and determining the effectiveness of treatment by observing the changes in gait and posture after intervention.

Stability can be assessed in two different directions, namely in the M/L direction in the frontal plane and in the (A/P) direction in the sagittal plane. In the A/P direction, during quiet standing, the COM of the body is stabilized with respect to the BOS by increasing and decreasing ankle planterflexor activations. This is termed as *ankle strategy*. The stability in the M/L direction during quiet standing is, however, maintained through the hip abductors/adductors (Winter, 1995). The clinical gait and posture assessment is generally done through visual observation and is rated on various scales such as the BEST, Falls Efficacy Scale (FES), and Timed Up and Go (TUG) test. However, this approach has two main shortcomings: (i) It's based on visual observation and hence depends on the expertise and the experience of the medical professional performing the gait assessment. It is, thus, qualitative and not quantitative. (ii) The collection of very little information limits the possibility of detecting the onset of gait and posture impairments and also understanding the disorganization of gait and posture control (Beauchet et al., 2017). Thus, a more quantitative approach is of the need for gait assessment, which can enable us to understand various gait disorders and also design and follow different preventive and curative interventions. These measurements can not only help us to identify the effects of gait and posture disorders and the progress of the treatment protocols, but also help us to identify the causes of the walking pattern (Vaughan et al., 1982).

The various gait parameters that can be employed as biomarkers are the spatiotemporal variables such as stance time, stride length, stride duration, step length, step width, step duration, cadence, walking velocity and degree of toe-out. There are also kinetic variables, viz. ground reaction forces (GRF) and COP, which can be used as a biomarker for gait and posture assessment. These parameters can be measured and analyzed through both wearable sensors and sophisticated setups, which have their own advantages and limitations. The wearable sensors provide us the ability to continuously monitor the changes noticed from the biomarkers and hence access the gait and posture continuously. The more sophisticated setup consists of IR cameras, force plates, EMG sensors, etc., which can record all the kinematic and kinetic parameters of human motion with great accuracy. These data can be used for the purpose of medical diagnosis and also the development of healthy and pathological datasets, which can be employed for training AI models. It can be executed using wearable sensors and augment healthcare professionals in their decision making by providing real-time monitoring of gait and posture variables and alerting of any possible deviations from the healthy range.

9.2 CURRENT CLINICAL BALANCE ASSESSMENT TECHNIQUES

Balance assessment was introduced in the 19th century by neurologist Romberg, who related posture control with some neurological dysfunctions. He developed the Romberg test (Romberg, 1840–1846) that can be used to diagnose damage to the spinal cord and ataxia, that deprives the subjects of its vision and he/she relies only on the somatosensory and vestibular information to maintain the balance.

Some of the other tests that followed are sharpened Romberg test, Tinetti test, the clinical test for sensory interaction in balance (CTSIB), balance error scoring system (BESS) and the Mini-Balance Evaluation Systems Test (Mini-BESTest). The sharpened Romberg test (Lee, 1998) is an adaptation of the Romberg test making it more difficult by reducing the BOS. Questionnaire item-based tests such as the Tinetti test (Tinetti et al., 1990), which is also known as performance-oriented mobility assessment (POMA), and Berg test (Berg et al., 1992) are used to assess fall risk in elderly and patients with stroke, brain injury or multiple sclerosis. In some balance tests such as the BESS and CTSIB (Shumway-Cook & Horak, 1986), foam pads are used, where the somatosensory system is manipulated, thus reducing the balance ability of the subject. The dynamic balance of a subject that includes postural responses, anticipatory transitions and sensory orientation while standing on an inclined or compliant BOS can be assessed through the 14-item balance scale Mini-BESTest. It can also be employed to assess the dynamic stability during gait. This test has a greater differentiability than the Berg Balance Scale (BBS) to classify people suffered with stroke into fast and slow walkers (Madhavan & Bishnoi, 2017). In addition to the above tests, there are also questionnaire-based assessments such as FES developed and validated by the Prevention of Falls Network Europe. It is a psychometric approach and is a self-report questionnaire. It gives us a self-assessment of one's concern about falls for a range of activities of daily life on a 4-point scale with 4 being highly concerned and 1 being not concerned. The original questionnaire contains 16 items on which subject assesses oneself, while the shortened questionnaire contains seven items (Delbaere et al., 2010).

The above-reported tests are qualitative in nature and hence make it difficult to follow up patients and to compare conditions. Thus, quantitative tests can be performed through a force platform and measuring the vertical GRF and the moments about all three axes, thus providing the subject's

COP. This kinetic data can quantify the clinical tests and make the process of comparing the condition of multiple subjects easier. These data from a large number of datasets can be employed to train AI models to predict the onset of pathological conditions and augment the clinician's ability to administer treatment protocols and also track their effectiveness.

9.3 POSTURE CONTROL AND ANALYSIS

Posture and stability during upright standing is possible through a combination of mechanical, sensory and motor processing strategies. Postural stability can be defined as the ability to control the velocity and amplitude of the center of gravity's (COG) displacement while quiet standing. Stability is higher when the COG displacement's amplitudes and velocities are smaller (Stodolka et al., 2016). The stability can be categorized into two types: static stability and dynamic stability. Static posture or postural equilibrium implies that the COG of the whole body is maintained over the BOS through the forces and moments acting on the body (Iqbal, 2011).

9.3.1 Postural control

The neurophysiological processes, i.e., musculoskeletal system and the central nervous system (CNS), are involved in the movement regulation and postural control. The musculoskeletal system comprises of the skeleton driven by the musculo-tendon actuators and the sensory system. The CNS comprises of: (i) the peripheral nervous system comprising of the afferent and efferent pathways and (ii) the brain and spinal cord. These processes collectively make up the neuro-musculoskeletal control system (NMSCS) that plans, organizes, executes and regulates the motor modalities in the body (Iqbal, 2011). The body, thus, maintains its position, orientation in space and balance with respect to the external environment through visual, vestibular and somatosensory information. This information is received through the receptor located in muscles, tendon, skin and joints and is processed by the brain (Stodolka et al., 2016). The vision is the system through which we can observe our environment, and it plans our locomotion and assists us to avoid obstacles in our way. The vestibular system recognizes the linear and angular accelerations and acts as our 'gyro'. The somatosensory system is a collection of sensors that recognize the velocity and position of all body segments, their contact with external objects and the orientation of the gravity (Winter, 1995). COM and COP are the important determinants of postural stability, which is affected by several factors such as visibility, terrain, head-arm-and-trunk (HAT) movements, heartbeat, breathing and lateral adjustments. The combined effect of these disturbances results in the displacement of the COM of the body from its intended position within the BOS. These disturbances mostly affect the COM position in A/P direction as most of the DOFs associated with postural adjustments (hip, knee and ankle joints) lie in the sagittal plane. The COM of a body is located about 5 cm anterior to the ankle joint and thus requires support that is provided by the constantly activated tibialis and/or soleus muscles in the lower leg. The muscles generate the necessary planter-flexion torque that counters the gravity and maintains balance (Iqbal, 2011). The COP is the projection of the vertical GRF distribution on the ground plane within the BOS. To maintain postural stability under static conditions, the COM of the body should be restricted within the BOS. The ability of a person to terminate or restore static balance during an impending fall depends on how that person perceives various physical constraints arising from environmental, anatomical and physiological origins (Iqbal, 2011). Postural stabilization is thus achieved through both active and passive mechanisms at the muscular and spinal level and also through visual and vestibular processes. A change in any of the physical constraints will cause one or more of the sensory receptors to respond and generate CNS commands resulting in active torques by muscle contraction. This will result in change of COM position and hence the COP position. In addition to active torques from muscle contractions, the intrinsic stiffness and viscosity of muscle and the surrounding ligaments and tendons also generate a passive torque that contributes to static stabilization. The displacement of the COM leads to the change of COP in the ground. COP position can be evaluated from the forces and moments of those forces obtained from the force plates and thus can be used to assess the quality of quiet standing.

9.3.2 Postural analysis

The static stability of a person can be assessed by comparing the postural sway. For a subject to be in static stability, there is only one major requirement, which is to keep the COG within the BOS (Razavi, 2016). During quiet standing, a person experiences a postural sway. It is because COP is not exactly below the COG. Considering the sagittal plane, as shown in Figure 9.1, in time instant 1, the angular velocity ω is considered to be clockwise and the COG is a little ahead of COP. The vertical reaction force R is equal and opposite to the body weight W, and both remain constant during quiet standing. W and R act at a distance of g and p, respectively, from the ankle joint. Considering the body pivoting about the ankle like an inverted pendulum, a clockwise moment equal to W_g and a counterclockwise moment equal to R_p act on the body such that

$$R_p - W_g = I\alpha$$

where I is the moment of inertia of the total body about the ankle joint and α is the angular acceleration of the body.

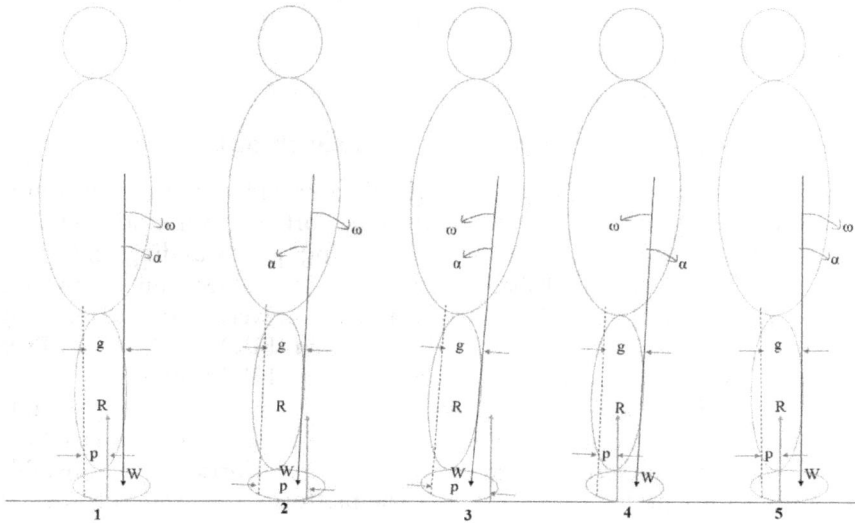

Figure 9.1 Forces and torques acting on a subject during quiet standing.

If $W_g > R_p$, clockwise angular acceleration and hence a forward 'sway' is experienced by the body. This is corrected by increasing one's COP by increasing the ankle planter-flexion activation such that in time instant 2, the COP is anterior, i.e., ahead of the COG. This results in $R_p > W_g$, and, thus, α changes direction and starts decreasing ω until, at time instant 3, α will reverse ω causing both α and ω to be counterclockwise. This causes the body to experience a backward sway. When this posterior shift of the COG is detected by the CNS, it responds by decreasing the planter-flexor activations and hence the COP decreases and it is done until the position of the COG is again anterior to the COP. At time instant 4, α reverses to clockwise direction, and after a certain time period, ω will again decrease and reverse. This will cause the body to again return to its original position as shown in time instant 5. Thus, in the sagittal plane, COP moves in the A/P direction with respect to the COG. The corrective movement of the COP might not be enough to reverse ω if the COG moved within a few millimeters of the toes. This would cause the subject to move a limb forward to break the forward fall (Winter, 1995). Winter (1995) reported COP and COG of a subject with respect to time. The subject was instructed to stand as still as possible on a force plate. It was observed that COG and COP fluctuates in quiet stance and COP excursions oscillate on both sides of the COG and have higher amplitude and frequency. The COP movement can be in two directions, i.e., M/L and A/P, and thus, we can obtain and assess the postural sway in two planes, the sagittal and the frontal plane. Since the static stability or balance is maintained by three sensory inputs, i.e., the visual, vestibular and somatosensory processes, a change in environment causing any of the senses to respond will result in loss of balance and change of postural sway extremes.

9.3.3 Postural analysis of an open-source database

An analysis was performed based on the data provided in an open-source database (Goldberger et al., 2000) by the work of Santos and Duarte (2016), where a reference range for COP during quiet standing under different conditions was established. They studied 163 subjects under multiple conditions, where the standing surface and vision were manipulated. The different conditions are Firm Ground-Eyes Open (FIRM_EO), Foam-Eyes Open (FOAM_EO), Firm Ground-Eyes Closed (FIRM_EC) and Foam-Eyes Closed (FOAM_EC). The subjects stood on a commercially available force platform directly for the rigid surface conditions and over a 6 cm high foam block by Airex AG placed over the force platform for the unstable conditions for a period of 60 seconds. The platform data were recorded at a sampling frequency of 100 Hz, and the system outputs were the forces and moments (F_x, F_y, F_z, M_x, M_y and M_z). The open-source data provided COP in X- and Y-directions, where the X-direction is the A/P direction, with positive X in the anterior direction, and the Y-direction is the M/L direction, with positive Y signifying the right side of the subject. The data were provided as a time series data over a period of 60 seconds with 100 Hz and hence with 6000 entries. Out of the 163 subjects, 116 were females and 47 were males. Their age varied from 18 to 85 years with an average of 48.09 years, body weight was in the range 44–75.9 kg with an average of 62.26 kg, height was in the range 140–189.8 cm with an average of 162.28 cm, and BMI was in the range 17.2–31.9 with an average of 23.75. All the subjects were interviewed to know about their conditions and to evaluate them on clinical balance tests, namely the Mini-BESTest and FES. The 16 of the 163 subjects were assessed to have at least one severe disability or more. It includes one with intellectual disability, one with visual and hearing deficits, one with musculoskeletal and visual deficits, three with only musculoskeletal deficits, two with only visual deficits and eight with hearing and vestibular deficits.

9.3.3.1 COP reference range for all subjects

The reference range was calculated by averaging the time series data of 163 subjects while keeping the time series intact, and then, sample standard deviation is calculated for each point of the time series. Figure 9.2 illustrates the reference range of the COP varying over a period of time in the A/P direction during quiet standing in different conditions. The four conditions considered here give us the contribution of each sensory organ in the

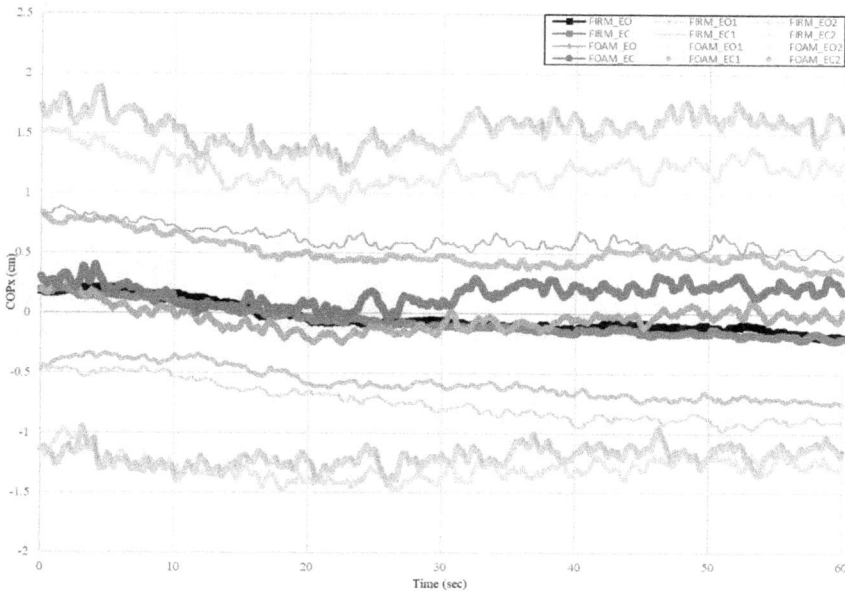

Figure 9.2 Reference range of COP in the X-direction, i.e., A/P direction in different conditions.

postural stability. A subject is most stable in the FIRM_EO condition, and all the three sensory organs work simultaneously to give an upright posture. In the condition of FIRM_EC, where the visual sense is eliminated, the postural stability is achieved only by vestibular and somatosensory perception and hence the effect of visual sense is assessed. In the condition of FOAM_EO, the somatosensory perception is manipulated, and in the condition FOAM_EC, both the vision and somatosensory perception is affected, thus employing mostly the vestibular sense for postural control. Thus, even though the mean COP for all the four conditions is nearer to the origin line, the standard deviation range is the highest for FOAM_EC and follows the decreasing order of FOAM_EO, FIRM_EC and FIRM_EO. The higher range of FOAM_EO than FIRM_EC can lead to infer that the contribution of somatosensory perception is greater than the contribution of vision, while maintaining a quiet standing posture.

Similar observation is also observed from Figure 9.3, which illustrates the reference range in the M/L direction. It can be observed from Figures 9.2 and 9.3 that the reference range in the A/P direction is larger than in the M/L direction, and hence, it is inferred that human quiet standing is more unstable in the A/P direction. This observation also further confirms the fact that most of the DOFs during postural adjustments lie in the sagittal plane in A/P direction (Iqbal, 2011). Higher DOFs cause the body to

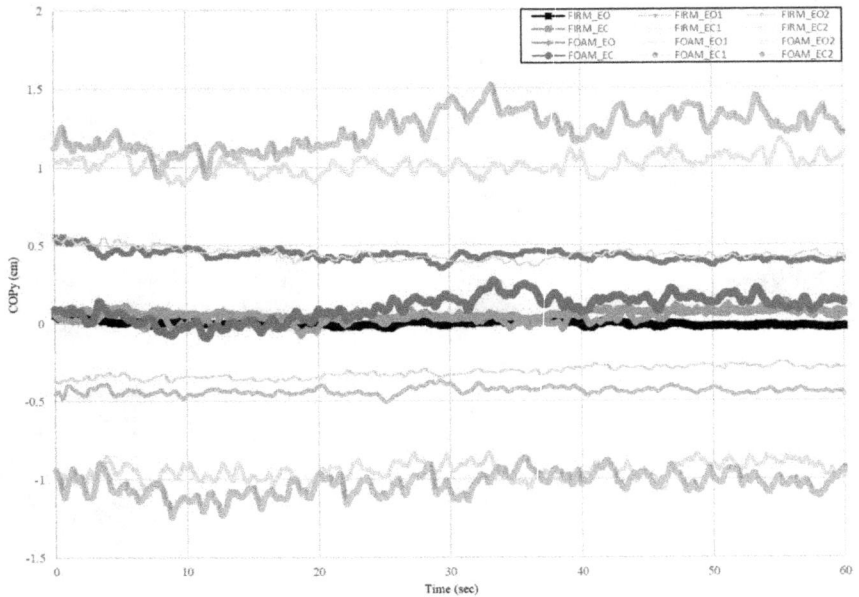

Figure 9.3 Reference range of COP in the Y-direction, i.e., M/L direction in different conditions.

experience more torque and hence a large number of muscles activate continuously to balance them, resulting in the effective sway.

9.3.3.2 Gender-specific COP reference range

Figure 9.4a–d shows the reference range of the COP in the X-direction, i.e., the A/P direction separated for male and female subjects. The reference range is calculated in four different conditions, i.e., FIRM_EO, FIRM_EC, FOAM_EO and FOAM_EC. The male reference range is calculated using 47 subjects, and the female reference range is calculated using 116 subjects. It can be observed that the range is higher for the male than for the female in all the conditions. A similar behavior can be seen when the COP was represented by normalizing with the height of the subjects as shown in Figure 9.5a–d. Thus, we can infer that the static stability of females is better than that of males. Since the behavior is reciprocated when the COP is normalized with height, thus giving the effect of weight, which generates the torque, it may be inferred that this is because of some other factors such as muscle strength that is causing this behavior in the A/P direction. In addition, it can be observed that in case of FOAM_EO condition, the

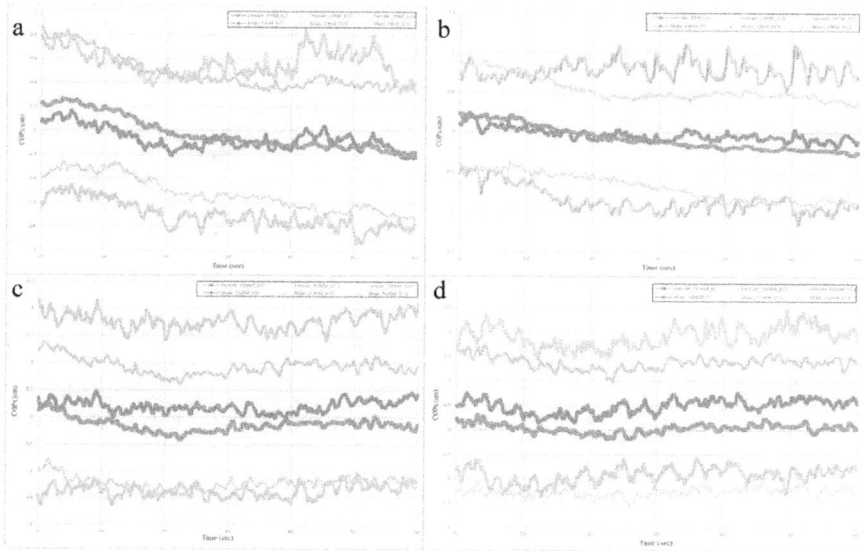

Figure 9.4 (a–d) COP reference range in the X-direction, i.e., A/P direction for male and female in different conditions.

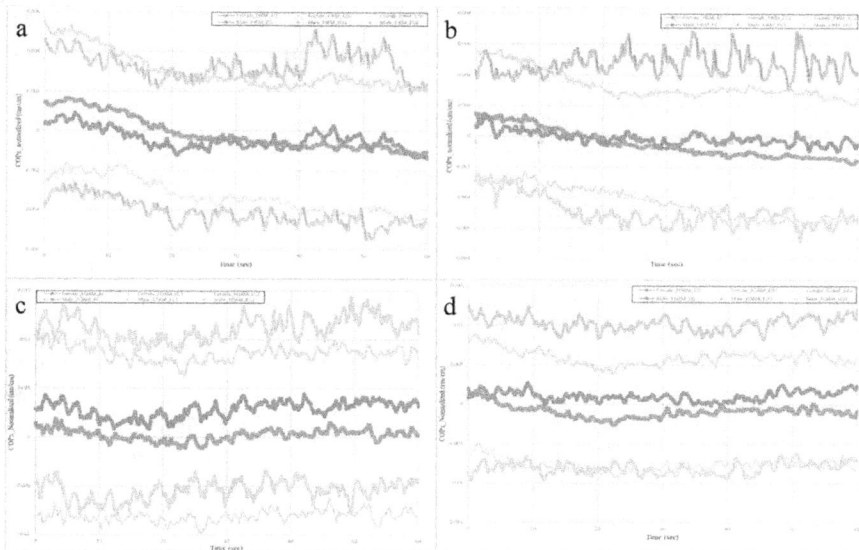

Figure 9.5 (a–d) Height-normalized COP reference range in the X-direction, i.e., A/P direction for male and female in different conditions.

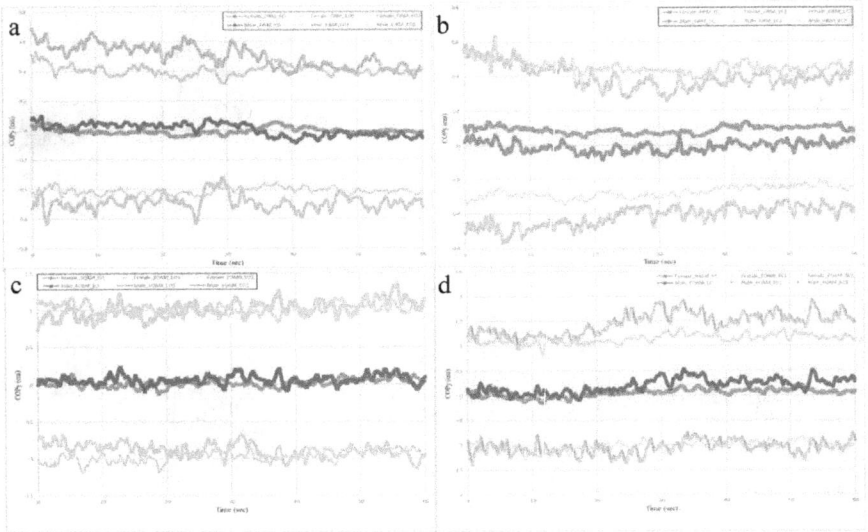

Figure 9.6 (a–d) COP reference range in the Y-direction, i.e., M/L direction for male and female in different conditions.

FOAM_EO1, i.e., the anterior direction limit, is lower for females than for males and the posterior direction limit is similar for both males and females. Similar observation can be seen in FOAM_EC condition, where the anterior limit is lower for females than for males and the posterior limit remains the same. The FOAM condition manipulates the somatosensory system of the subject. This observation, thus, suggests better muscle control for anterior direction movement in females than in males.

Figure 9.6a–d shows the reference range of the COP in the Y-direction, i.e., the M/L direction separated for male and female subjects. The reference range is calculated in four different conditions, i.e., FIRM_EO, FIRM_EC, FOAM_EO and FOAM_EC. The male reference range is calculated using 47 subjects, and the female reference range is calculated using 116 subjects. It can be observed that the range is found to be similar for both males and females in all the conditions. This behavior is also seen when the COP is normalized with the subjects' height as shown in Figure 9.7a–d. This suggests that the static stability in the M/L direction is gender independent.

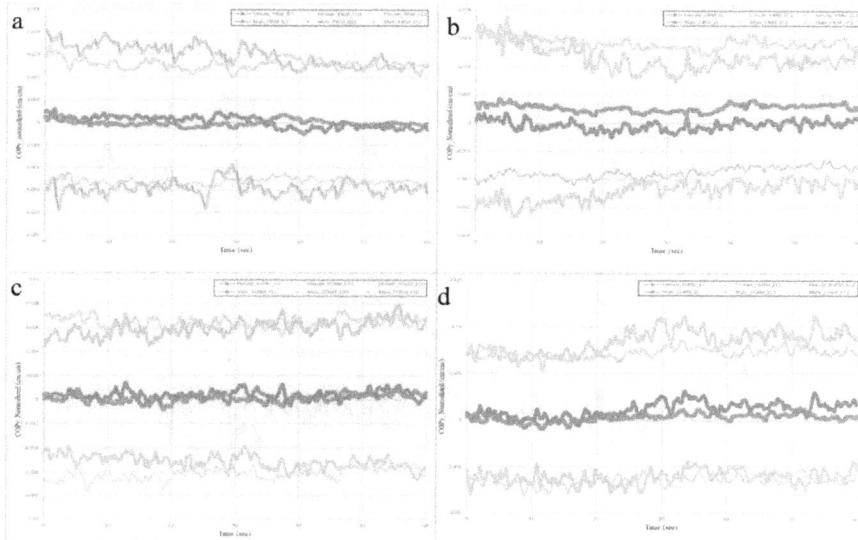

Figure 9.7 (a–d) Height-normalized COP reference range in the Y-direction, i.e., M/L direction for male and female in different conditions.

9.3.3.3 COP of subjects with certain pathology

The establishment of a reference range for COP can be helpful in diagnosing pathological conditions and also tracking the effectiveness of any intensive treatment provided. Thus, COP of a subject with Parkinson's disorder and a subject with hearing disability on the left side was superimposed over the reference ranges calculated in the previous sections in different conditions.

It can be observed from Figure 9.8 that both disorders, which are different in their causes and overall effects, have a significant distinguishable difference than the reference range with its high amplitude, which is a differentiating trait that can be employed for diagnosing the severity of the disorders.

Similarly, Figure 9.9 shows the sway of COP in the Y-direction, i.e., the M/L direction in different conditions. In addition to the higher amplitudes of the signals for both the pathological conditions, it can also be noted that the COP is majorly in the positive side for the hearing (left) impaired subject, which is the right side of the subject. It can thus be inferred that the loss of hearing in the left side has also contributed to loss of perception on that side, and hence to compensate for a fear of falling, the COP is shifting toward the right, i.e., the sound side.

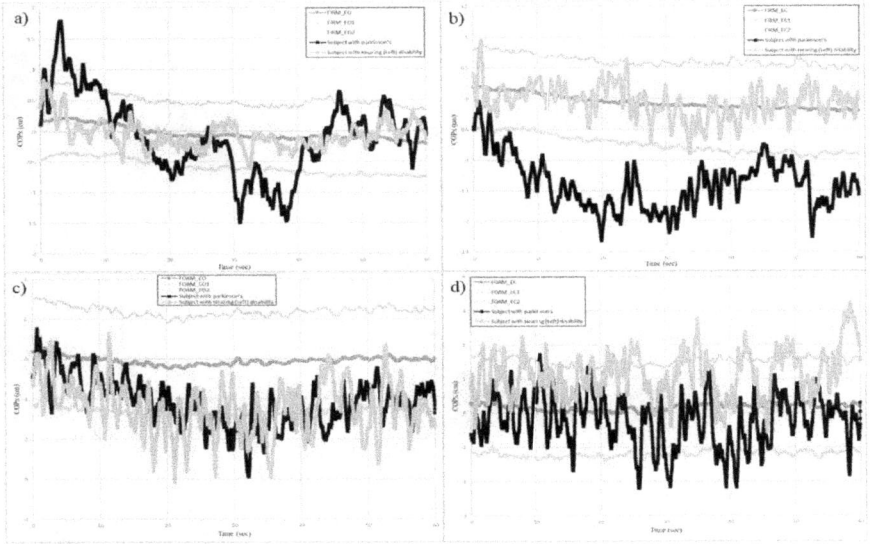

Figure 9.8 (a–d) COP in the X-direction, i.e., A/P direction for pathological subjects.

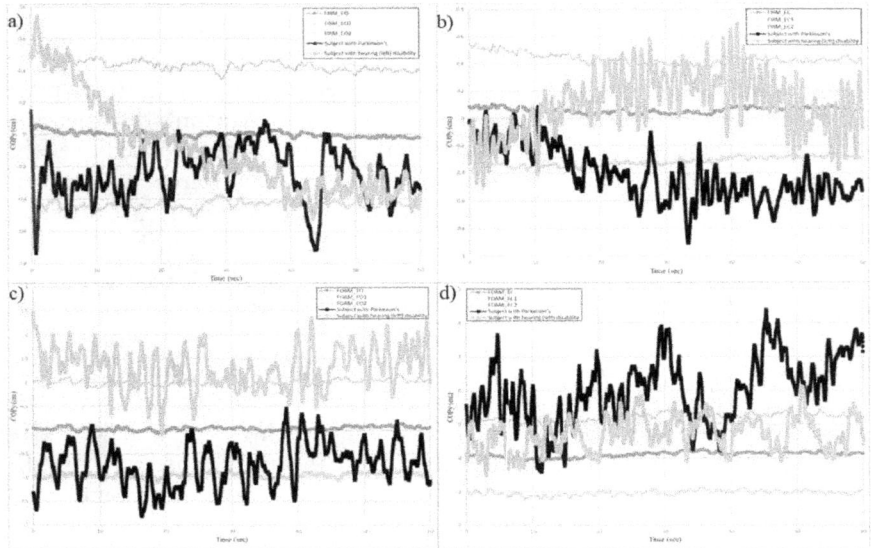

Figure 9.9 (a–d) COP in the Y-direction, i.e., M/L direction for pathological subjects.

9.4 CONCLUSIONS AND FUTURE WORK

This study provides a reference range for COP in two axes, namely in the A/P direction and in the M/L direction. The major conclusions obtained from the study are listed below:

- The contribution of somatosensory perception is greater than the contribution of vision while maintaining a quiet standing.
- Human quiet standing can be concluded to be more unsettle in the A/P direction than in the M/L direction judging from the larger reference range in the A/P direction for COP in all the conditions.
- Female static stability was also found to be better than that in males in the A/P direction. Female subjects in the sample set had lower height and weight.
- In the M/L direction, the static stability reference ranges in all different conditions for both male and female remain the same.
- The static stability is better for females than for males in the A/P direction.
- In the M/L direction, the static stability is found to be gender-neutral.
- The deviation of COP is demonstrated for pathological subjects in both amplitude and absolute value from the sample population. The pathological conditions considered were Parkinson's disease and hearing disability in left side.

However, this study doesn't consider various other factors that may influence the COP position sway such as foot length, footwear, and other illnesses. These features can be used in a classification algorithm, which would be able to incorporate all the features of the subject's condition and give an informed decision if a subject has the possibility of any balance-related disorders. It can also provide better results on which factors have a higher degree of influence on the postural sway. These types of classification algorithms perfected from experimental data can then be executed through wearable sensors to provide real-time monitoring and the onset of several balance-related disorders.

ACKNOWLEDGMENT

The authors acknowledge the support provided by NECBH (BT/COE/34/SP28408/2018), II&SI, IIT Guwahati.

REFERENCES

Beauchet, O., Allali, G., Sekhon, H., Verghese, J., Guilain, S., Steinmetz, J.-P., Kressig, R. W., Barden, J. M., Szturm, T., Launay, C. P., Grenier, S., Bherer, L., Liu-Ambrose, T., Chester, V. L., Callisaya, M. L., Srikanth, V., Léonard, G., De Cock, A.-M., Sawa, R., ... Helbostad, J. L. (2017). Guidelines for assessment of gait and reference values for spatiotemporal gait parameters in older adults: The biomathics and canadian gait consortiums initiative. *Frontiers in Human Neuroscience, 11*, 353. https://doi.org/10.3389/fnhum.2017.00353.

Berg, K. O., Wood-Dauphinee, S. L., Williams, J. I., & Maki, B. (1992). Measuring balance in the elderly: Validation of an instrument. *Canadian Journal of Public Health = Revue Canadienne de Sante Publique, 83*(Suppl 2), S7–S11.

Blochberger, A., & Jones, S. (2011). Parkinson's disease clinical features and diagnosis. *Clinical Pharmacist, 3*(11), 361–366. https://doi.org/10.1136/jnnp.2007.131045.

Delbaere, K., Close, J. C. T., Mikolaizak, A. S., Sachdev, P. S., Brodaty, H., & Lord, S. R. (2010). The falls efficacy scale international (FES-I). A comprehensive longitudinal validation study. *Age and Ageing, 39*(2), 210–216. https://doi.org/10.1093/ageing/afp225.

Egoyan, A., & Moistsrapishvili, K. (2013). Equilibrium and stability of the upright human body. *The General Science Journal*, 2–4.

Goldberger, A., Amaral, L., Glass, L., Hausdorff, J., Ivanov, P. C., Mark, R., ... Stanley, H. E. (2000). PhysioBank, PhysioToolkit, and PhysioNet: Components of a new research resource for complex physiologic signals. *Circulation, 101*(23), e215–e220.

Iqbal, K. (2011). Mechanisms and models of postural stability and control. *Proceedings of the Annual International Conference of the IEEE Engineering in Medicine and Biology Society, EMBS*, August 2011, pp. 7837–7840. https://doi.org/10.1109/IEMBS.2011.6091931.

Lee, C. T. (1998). Sharpening the sharpened romberg. *SPUMS Journal, 28*(3), 125–132.

Madhavan, S., & Bishnoi, A. (2017). Comparison of the mini-balance evaluations systems test with the berg balance scale in relationship to walking speed and motor recovery post stroke. *Topics in Stroke Rehabilitation*. https://doi.org/10.1080/10749357.2017.1366097.

Miller, F., & Henley, J. (2017). Diagnostic gait analysis use in the treatment protocol for cerebral palsy BT. *Handbook of Human Motion* (B. Müller, S. I. Wolf, G.-P. Brueggemann, Z. Deng, A. McIntosh, F. Miller, & W. S. Selbie (eds.); pp. 1–15). Springer International Publishing. https://doi.org/10.1007/978-3-319-30808-1_48-1.

Radhakrishnan, D. M., & Goyal, V. (2018). Parkinson's disease: A review. *Neurology India, 66*(7), S26–S35. https://doi.org/10.4103/0028-3886.226451.

Ray Dorsey, E., Elbaz, A., Nichols, E., Abd-Allah, F., Abdelalim, A., Adsuar, J. C., Ansha, M. G., Brayne, C., Choi, J. Y. J., Collado-Mateo, D., Dahodwala, N., Do, H. P., Edessa, D., Endres, M., Fereshtehnejad, S. M., Foreman, K. J., Gankpe, F. G., Gupta, R., Hankey, G. J., ... Murray, C. J. L. (2018). Global, regional, and national burden of Parkinson's disease, 1990–2016: A systematic analysis for the Global Burden of Disease Study 2016. *The Lancet Neurology*, *17*(11), 939–953. https://doi.org/10.1016/S1474-4422(18)30295-3.

Razavi, H. (2016). A comparison between static and dynamic stability in postural sway and fall risks. *Journal of Ergonomics*, *07*(01), 1–7. https://doi.org/10.4172/2165-7556.1000186.

Romberg, M. H. (1840–1846). Lehrbuch der Nerven-Krankheiten des Menschen. Duncker, Berlin.

Santos, D. A., & Duarte, M. (2016). A public data set of human balance evaluations. *Peer J*. https://doi.org/10.7717/peerj.2648.

Shumway-Cook, A., & Horak, F. B. (1986). Assessing the influence of sensory interaction of balance. Suggestion from the field. *Physical Therapy*, *66*(10), 1548–1550. https://doi.org/10.1093/ptj/66.10.1548.

Stodolka, J., Golema, M., & Migasiewicz, J. (2016). Balance maintenance in the upright body position: Analysis of autocorrelation. *Journal of Human Kinetics*, *50*(1), 45–52. https://doi.org/10.1515/hukin-2015-0140.

Thakur, K., Albanese, E., Giannakopoulos, P., Jette, N., Linde, M., Prince, M., Steiner, T., & Dua, T. (2016). Cost-effectiveness and affordability of interventions, policies, and platforms for the prevention and treatment of mental, neurological, and substance use disorders. *Disease Control Priorities*, Third Edition (Volume 4): Mental, Neurological, and Substance Use Disorders, 87. https://doi.org/10.1596/978-1-4648-0426-7_ch12.

Tinetti, M. E., Richman, D., & Powell, L. (1990). Falls efficacy as a measure of fear of falling. *Journal of Gerontology*, *45*(6), P239–P243. https://doi.org/10.1093/geronj/45.6.p239.

Vaughan, C. L., Hay, J. G., & Andrews, J. G. (1982). Closed loop problems in biomechanics. Part I--a classification system. *Journal of Biomechanics*, *15*(3), 197–200. https://doi.org/10.1016/0021-9290(82)90252-4.

Winter, D. A. (1995). Human balance and posture control during standing and walking. *Gait & Posture*, *3*(4), 193–214. https://doi.org/10.1016/0966-6362(96)82849-9.

Chapter 10

Turing test to validate perceptually reduced model for needle insertion simulation

Ravali Gourishetti and M. Manivannan

Indian Institute of Technology Madras

CONTENTS

10.1 INTRODUCTION

With the advent of surgical robotics, the study of human-robot interaction (HRI) has become prominent. In recent times, one of the significant applications of HRI has been in healthcare, specifically medical simulations and simulators. In modern clinical practices where minimally invasive procedures have become essential medical techniques, the needle insertion procedure is a vital element [1]. In most of the medical residencies, the present training technique for needle insertion procedures by the novice is the apprenticeship method, which can have the patient's safety at risk [2]. A survey [3] shows high failure rates, especially in anesthesia procedures (about 32% of lumbar procedures and 27% of thoracic procedures) even by the traditionally trained doctors. Medical simulators are among the best solutions for the novice to learn and enhance their skills, considering the patient's safety.

DOI: 10.1201/9781003344810-10

Medical simulators, specifically needle simulators, have several benefits over traditional training methods, such as training the physicians to experience both common and rare cases by changing the tissue properties [4]. The research- and prototype-based needle simulators reported in the literature are lumbar epidural puncture [5–7] and regional anesthesia [8,9]. Although these simulations have benefited several healthcare areas, they have never considered human perception in general and sensory thresholds in particular in their models. These existing models focus on the mechanical properties of the tools and tissues for modeling the interactions. In contrast, we developed a novel analytical model of needle insertion that considers human perception thresholds that precisely capture the needle-tissue interaction forces in linear heterogeneous tissues, the perceptually reduced model (PRM).

The current state-of-the-art needle insertion simulations are reviewed in detail [10]. The needle insertion simulation procedures include three major modeling stages: modeling of needle deflection [11–15], modeling of tissue deformation [16–18], and modeling of needle-tissue interaction forces [15,19–21]. The majority of the models mentioned above have been developed using heuristic and phenomenological models, which are not validated and are not generalizable. These literature models have not considered the biomechanical and psychophysical concepts during their development.

10.1.1 Biomechanics of needle insertion

The needle insertion simulation procedures include three major modeling stages as shown in Figure 10.1. Biomechanical concepts play a key role in modeling the three stages of a needle insertion procedure, i.e., needle deflection model, tissue deformation model, and needle-tissue interaction model. In the literature, three techniques used for modeling these three stages are mass-damper models [22–24], beam-based models [14,19,20], and finite element models [25–27].

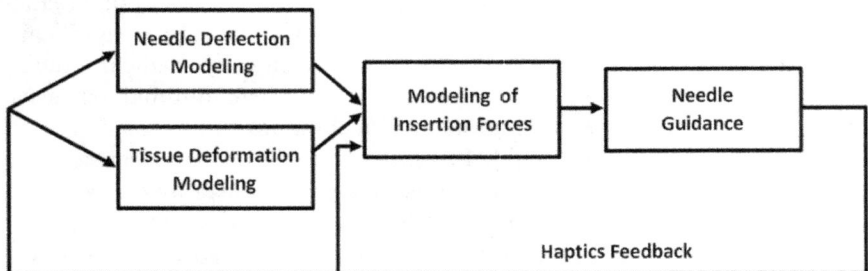

Figure 10.1 Schematic of needle insertion simulation: The needle-tissue interaction is modeled with three stages, namely needle deflection modeling, tissue deformation modeling, and the interaction is modeled as insertion forces. The haptic feedback is provided at each stage of the model [10].

In tissue models, deformations of the tissues for different forces, maximum compression strength, and yield strength are evaluated. In needle-tissue interaction models, the bending and twisting deformations in the needle structure during needle insertion and the relations between the rupture force, compression force, and the puncture force and the deformation of the tissue are evaluated.

10.1.2 Role of psychophysics in needle insertion procedures

The force feedback perceived during needle insertion must be measured and included in the model as the trainee controls these forces. Therefore, including the human perceptual parameters in the models of needle simulators can reduce the models' complexity. The psychophysical parameters such as human force discrimination, force thresholds, tissue stiffness discrimination, force bandwidth, and velocity discrimination can be used in the model design. The parameters such as just noticeable difference (JND) of joint rotations and range of motion can be used to develop the needle simulators [10]. Thus, these psychophysical parameters would help improve the design of simulators and simplify the tissue interaction models [28].

Although the medical community recognizes the importance and effectiveness of needle simulators, the confidence of this training method by the residents, helping them perform the real procedures with minimal errors, is questionable until they are validated. The main objective of this chapter is to develop and validate the PRM to observe the effectiveness of the perceptual filter in two stages of the Turing test experiment. The first stage of the experiment is to verify the effectiveness of the perceptual filter by comparing the PRM and biomechanical model without the perceptual filter. The second stage is to compare the simulated model and physical phantom tissue (PPT).

10.2 METHODOLOGY

10.2.1 Experimental system to measure needle-tissue interaction forces

We developed an acquisition system to measure needle-tissue interaction forces. The constraints required for the interaction force measurements, design of the force acquisition system, and measured force output for each layer are detailed below:

A. Constraints for needle-tissue interaction force measurement
    The basic constraints required for the needle-tissue interaction force measurement are dependent on the influence of three parameters [29]. They are as follows:

Table 10.1 Measured mechanical properties of the eight layers of phantom tissues

Layer No.	Thickness (mm)	Stiffness (N/m²)	Yield strength (MPa)	Young's modulus (MPa)
1	5.6	560	0.89	0.63
2	1.8	143	0.69	0.21
3	1.6	330	0.72	0.45
4	3.6	356	0.54	0.48
5	5.7	400	0.64	0.51
6	8.9	421	1.1	0.52
7	4.5	1146	1.1	1.23
8	3.6	0	0	0

- Method of needle insertion: manual/automated, a variation of insertion velocities.
- Needle characteristics:
  - Shape: bevel, conical, Tuohy, sharp.
  - Diameter: various possible diameters.
- Tissue characteristics: phantom material selection, single- and multi-layered, the thickness of the tissue.

We measured the interaction forces with some of the constraints mentioned above, such as automated needle insertion with different constant velocities (3, 6, 9, 12, and 15 mm/s), with bevel and sharp needles for various diameters (5, 6, and 7 gauge), on individual tissue layers shown in Table 10.1 and multi-layered (eight layers, explicitly considering the epidural anesthesia simulation).

B. **Interaction force acquisition**

Figure 10.2 shows the force acquisition measurement setup. The acquisition system consists of a linear actuator instrumented with force and displacement sensors – the precision light sensor for displacement measurement with a resolution of 0.1 mm and repeatability of 1.8%. An FSR for force measurement with a resolution of 0.05 N and repeatability of 2.4% was mounted on the actuator. The repeatability of the sensors was a measure of the mean of three trials. The force and displacement data were acquired using an Arduino Uno at a rate of 500 samples/s.

C. **Phantom preparation and its characterization**

We prepared PPT with two-component silicone gel and agar materials. We prepared these phantom tissues with various thicknesses to represent each layer of the human tissue and combine different proportions of silicone gel and agar for reproducing the physical properties. The physical properties and their characterization of all the eight layers are as shown in Table 10.1. The biomechanical properties of tissues such as elasticity, yield strength, and Young's modulus are

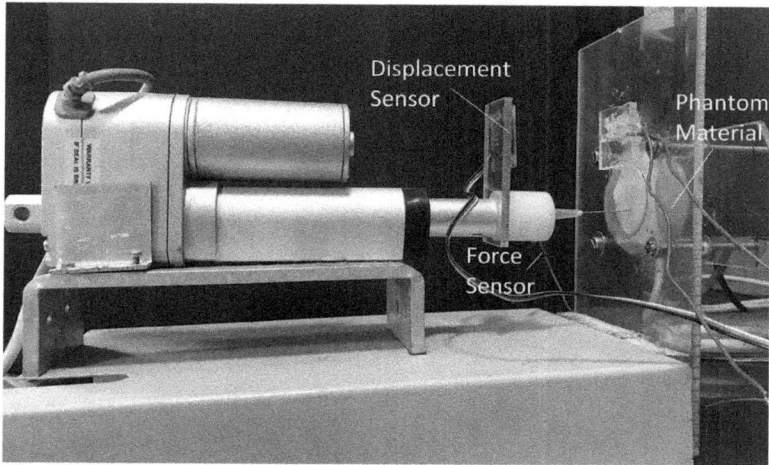

Figure 10.2 Experimental setup: A linear actuator is used for needle insertion force measurements on phantom tissues. The setup measures force only in the translational direction of the needle. Forces at the needle base and the needle displacement are measured using Interlink FSR and precision light sensor, respectively. The linear actuator is controlled using a motor driver board and is programmed to move with different velocities (3–15 mm/s with an interval of 3 mm/s).

measured using IC-5KN UTM. These parameters for all eight layers are individually measured by compression tests.

D. **Needle insertion force measurement**

A set of measurements were acquired with the above-said constraints using the force acquisition system, as shown in Figure 10.2. A sample average plot of experimental data for a needle diameter of 1.83 mm at a velocity of 9 mm/s is as shown in Figure 10.3. A typical force profile has three phases: (i) tissue compression phase, up to 5 mm where there is an increase in the force, (ii) tissue puncture phase, up to 6.4 mm where a small dip in the force occurs as the tissue cracks and the needle penetration begins, and (iii) the frictional phase, up to 33.5 mm where it shows the friction between the outer needle structure and the tissues surrounding it. The measured forces are used for system identification of the biomechanical model of needle-tissue interaction.

10.2.2 Needle-tissue interaction force modeling

Modeling the needle-tissue interaction has been the topic of significant research efforts [30,31]. The needle-tissue interaction forces during needle insertion into soft tissues are classified into three forces corresponding to the three phases mentioned above:

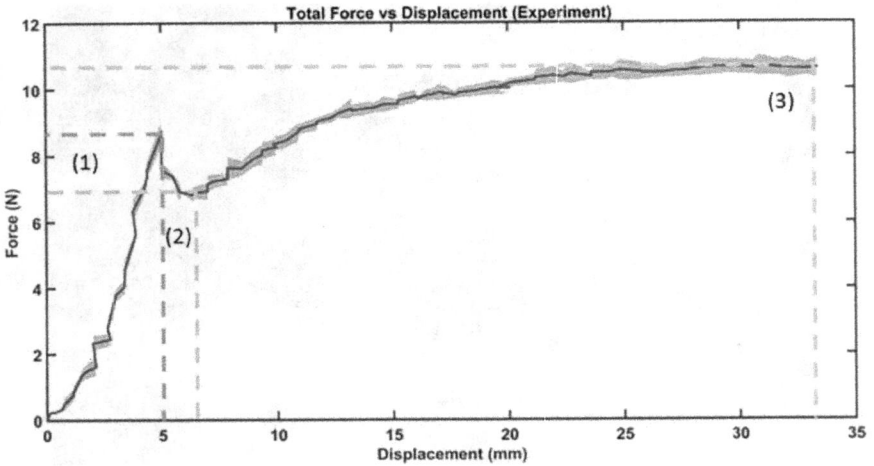

Figure 10.3 A typical average plot of measured data with the eight layers for needle diameter of 1.83 mm at a velocity of 9 mm/s. (1) The compression phase, (2) the puncture phase, and (3) the frictional phase.

1. Tissue compression force, F_c: The tissue compression force refers to the force in the compression phase of the force profile. It is termed as an elastic force, where the tissue regains its shape. It starts when the needle tip and the tissue surface are in contact; the tissue is deformed at the contact surface and continues until the contact force reaches its maximum (force at the yield point), and then the tissue gets punctured $(0 < F_c < F_{c\,max})$.

2. Tissue puncture force, F_p: The puncture force refers to the second phase of the force profile, and it starts at the yield point when the crack is initiated. The puncture force continues until the needle tip completely penetrates the tissue.

3. Frictional force, F_f: The frictional force refers to the force in the third phase of the force profile, and it starts with the penetration of the needle tip and continues until the entire tissue is penetrated. A frictional force acts tangential to the needle shaft and resists the relative motion of the needle into the tissue.

In this section, the dynamics of needle interaction with tissue is studied, and three biomechanical-based models are developed for three phases to estimate needle-tissue interaction forces using the experimental data.

A. **Modeling tissue compression force** (F_c)

To predict the force-deformation response of needle-tissue interaction during the compression phase, a four-parameter Burger's model, which exhibits linear viscoelastic behavior [32], is employed. The model has the following response equation:

$$F + p_1 * \dot{F} + p_2 * \ddot{F} = q_1 * \dot{x} + q_2 * \ddot{x}$$

where

$$p_1 = \lambda_1\left[1 + \frac{E_1}{E_2}\right] + \lambda_2; p_1 = \lambda_1 * \lambda_2$$

$$q_1 = \lambda_1 * E_1; q_2 = \lambda_2 * \eta_1$$

$$\lambda_1 = \frac{\eta_1}{E_1}; \lambda_2 = \frac{\eta_2}{E_2}$$

where F is the contact force, E_1 and E_2 are tissue stiffnesses, η_1 and η_2 are tissue damping coefficients, x is the needle tip displacement, and dot denotes differentiation with respect to time t.

B. Modeling tissue puncture force (F_p)

The tissue puncturing phase is further divided into two events:

- Crack initiation: When the contact force at the needle tip reaches its maximum, the tissue in the proximity of the needle tip (failure zone) is severely damaged. The molecular bonds in the failure zone break, and a crack is formed in the tissue.
- Needle propagation: It starts at the end of the crack initiation phase and continues until the entire needle tip completely penetrates the tissue as shown in Figure 10.4.

Crack initiation:

The axial force applied by the needle tip during the crack initiation (F_{ci}) is estimated by

$$F_{ci} = 2 * \sigma_Y * A_t * \sin\left(\frac{\alpha}{2}\right)$$

where A_t is the contact area between the needle tip and the tissue, α is the angle between edges of the needle tip and the tissue, and σ_Y is the stress in the tissue surface.

Needle propagation:

The dynamic force for needle propagation (F_{np}) is expressed as [30]:

$$F_{np} = \frac{4 * F_c * \tan\left(\frac{\alpha}{2}\right)}{3 * w_c}$$

where w_c is the crack thickness equal to the needle outer diameter.

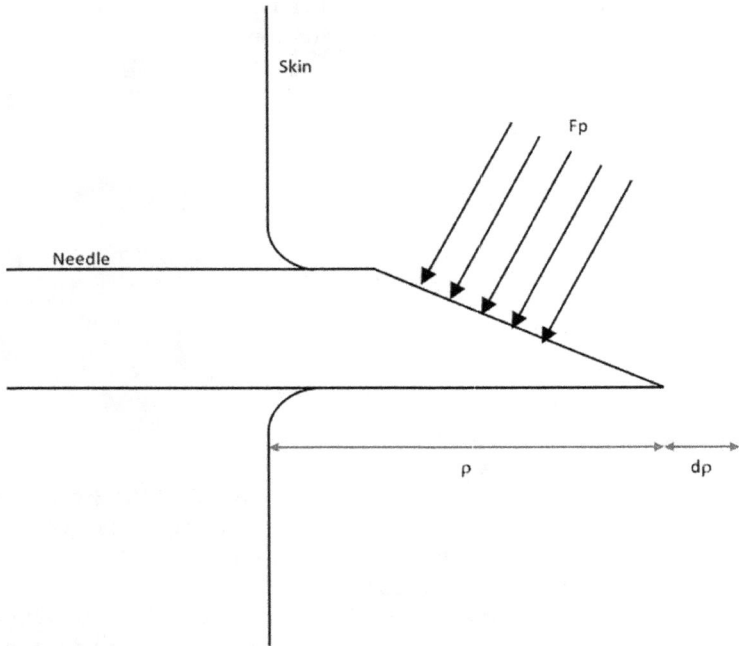

Figure 10.4 Crack propagation in tissue puncture. Needle tip-tissue interface during puncture represented by a force distribution with magnitude of F_p. p is the needle tip length, and d_p is the incremental crack growth.

The total needle puncture force (F_p) is expressed as:

$$F_p = F_{ci} + F_{np}$$

C. Modeling frictional force (F_f)

The frictional force is modeled as an extension of the seven-parameter model [10] that has a dependency on the velocity of needle insertion and the diameter of needle. The frictional force is modeled as follows:

When sticking,

$$F_f(x) = \sigma_0 x$$

When sliding,

$$F_f(v,t) = \left(F_c + F_s(\gamma, t_d) \frac{1}{\left(\dfrac{1+v(t-\tau_e)}{v_s} \right)^2} \right) \mathrm{sgn}(v) + F_v v + \pi * (d_2 - d_1) * x * \sigma$$

where

$$F_s\left(\gamma, t_d\right) = F_{s,a} + \left(F_{s,\infty} - F_{s,a}\frac{t_d}{\left(t_d + \gamma\right)}\right)$$

where σ_0 is the tangential stiffness of the static contact, F_c is the Coulomb friction, F_s is the Stribeck friction, τ_e is the temporal parameter of the rising static friction, v_s is the characteristic velocity of the Stribeck friction, $F_{s,a}$ and $F_{s,\infty}$ are the Stribeck friction at the end of the previous sliding period and after a long time at rest, respectively, t_d is the dwell time, which is the time spent at a certain stage of the process, σ is the empirical constant, and d_2 and d_1 are the outer and inner diameters of the needle, respectively. In this model, the Stribeck friction parameter is considered with velocity v after a certain time γ.

10.2.3 Human perception filtering

As a human is involved in the process of needle insertion, the forces he/she encounters during the needle-tissue interaction are the physical stimulus and the sensation of these forces. The force feedback, which is perceived during the needle insertion, must be measured and included in the model as the trainee controls these forces. A block diagram of the needle-tissue interaction model is shown in Figure 10.5. Incorporating a human perception filter over the biomechanical models for needle-tissue interaction enhances the model by reducing the computational complexity without changing the perception of forces experienced by the trainee. Force and stiffness thresholds are used for perceptual filtering over the biomechanical model.

Since it is uncommon in medical simulators to have sensors connected to the subject to quantitatively measure all the required thresholds and differential thresholds for each parameter, we consider the psychophysical measures from the literature. Psychophysical parameters involved during the needle insertion procedure are stated in Table 10.2. Some of the psychophysical parameters (force and stiffness thresholds) used in the perceptual filter reduce the number of layers (say, from 8 to 5) to be simulated for needle insertion, thereby reducing the computational complexity, and others (orientation and velocity thresholds) help in enhancing the needle simulator. Parameter identification of different layers of the tissues and the psychophysical parameters relevant to the needle insertion procedure [10] help in modifying the needle-tissue interaction force model accordingly.

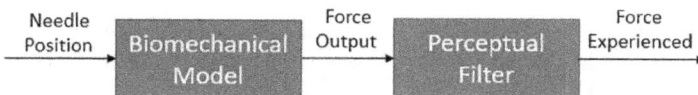

Figure 10.5 Block diagram of needle-tissue interaction model with the perceptual filter.

Table 10.2 Psychophysical parameters related to the needle insertion procedure

Psychophysical parameters	Measure	Value
Threshold forces	Control resolution for single finger	0.05–0.5 N [33]
	Contact force resolution	5%–15% [34]
	Force JND for index finger	10% [34]
	Force detection threshold for multi-finger interaction	28.9 mN [35]
Tissue stiffness	Stiffness JND	8% [36]
Orientation of the needle	JND of rotation for hand [37]	
	Finger joints	2.5°
	Wrist and elbow joints	2°
	Shoulder joint	0.8°
Threshold velocity [37]	Velocity JND at finger tip	0.1 m/s
	Velocity JND at wrist	1 m/s

As stated, the two parameters force and stiffness thresholds are used for the perceptual filtering over the biomechanical model. Considering each parameter individually, as a first note, the different force thresholds from Table 10.2: The threshold force for multi-finger interaction is 28.9 mN and the force control resolution is 0.05–0.5 N. The tissue layers that require the force application/control less than these threshold forces are filtered in the model (8 layers to 5 layers) since they are not perceived by the human as a different tissue layer from the current tissue layer.

It is very similar to the telephonic communication where high-frequency audio signals which are not perceived by the human are filtered, and only the voice band signals (300–3400 Hz) are transmitted [38] without having any loss of perception in the long-distance hearing.

The next parameter considered is stiffness, where the consecutive tissues with stiffness variation less than the stiffness JND of human (8%) can be filtered in the model. The stiffness for each layer is estimated using UTM as stated in Section 10.3. Based on these mechanical properties (stiffness), the consecutive tissues with a lesser difference are filtered.

10.2.4 Experimental validation: Turing test

The PRM is validated using two stages of Turing test experiments. The Turing test is originally a test proposed by Alan Turing [39] to replace the question, "Can machines think?" The test is also known as the imitation game and has various versions due to the ambiguity of the description of the author. The most related version in the context of this research is the version that is played by two people and a machine. There are three roles, namely person A, person B, and interrogator. The gender of the people playing the game is irrelevant. The machine takes the role of either person A or person B. An actual human takes the remaining role of A or B, and the other human will take the role of the investigator (also known as C). The true identity of persons A and B is not known to the investigator. The objective of persons A and B is to converse with the investigator to make them believe that they are human (as an individual is human). The main aim of the interrogator is to determine whether person A or B is human. The notion of imitation is that the machine imitates the human-like behavior such that the investigator gets fooled into believing that it is a human.

A. Modification to the imitation game

Although there exist many debates about the nature of the test and its implementations, the goal was clear that the machine must simulate qualities pertaining to the human. Hence, this concept has been used in other fields such as biotechnology [40] for comparing an artificial entity to a real-life entity. In the first stage of our experiment, the imitation game compares the PPT model to the simulated PRM in the Omni Phantom (a force feedback device). Hence, the PPT and the simulated PRM models assume the roles A and B, respectively, while the subject who is testing the model assumes the role of investigator. The goal of the simulated model is to trick the participant into making them believe that it is a PPT model. In the context of our filtered model, the imitation game is used to compare the PRM to the unfiltered biomechanical model. Hence, the two models assume the roles A and B, while the subject who is testing the model assumes the role of investigator. The goal of the PRM is to trick the participant into making them believe that it is a biomechanical model without the perceptual filter.

B. Participants

Twenty voluntary participants (6 females and 14 males) have performed both stages of the experiments, each on a different day. All the participants were right-handed, and they are naive about these studies.

C. Experiment: Comparison of PPT and PRM models

The first stage of the Turing test aims to observe the perceptual difference between the PRM and PPT by a participant.

Experimental setup:

Two Omni Phantoms are placed on the opposite sides on a rotating board to prevent external biases during the imitation game, as shown in Figures 10.6 and 10.7. The board can rotate such that the models (PRM and PPT) can be switched with minimum effort. One of the Omni Phantoms is programmed with the PRM and acts as a force feedback device, while the other has a PPT placed near the end effector. The force feedback device with the PPT is not programmed and is merely present to create consistency during the experiment. Both the Omni Phantom end effectors are connected with needles. The participant is blindfolded for the test such that they do not see the PPT present in the device.

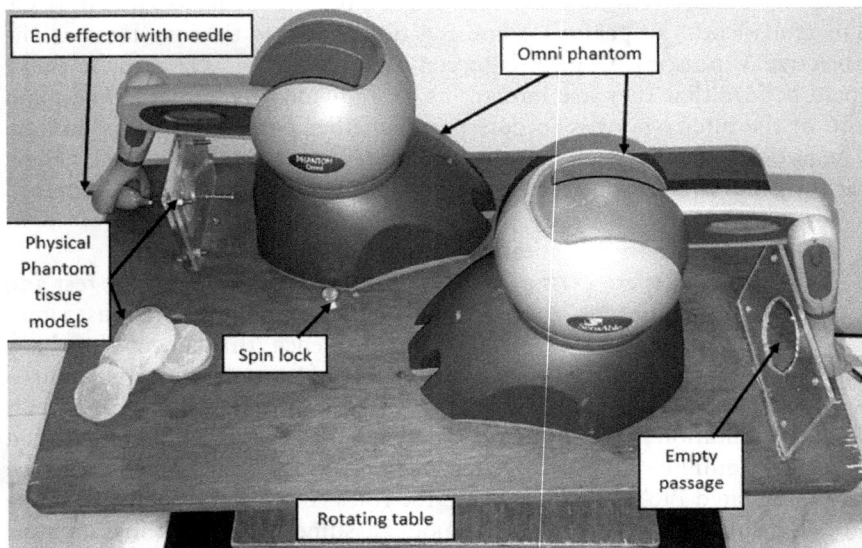

Figure 10.6 The Turing test setup for experiment I includes a rotating table with two Omni Phantom devices placed on it. The device on the left side is programmed with PRM, and the simulated forces have to be experienced, whereas the device on the right side has PPT, and the force is experienced from the PPT.

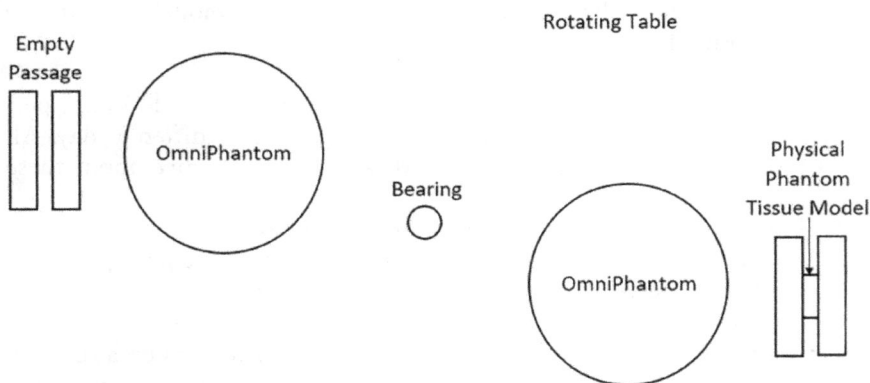

Figure 10.7 Schematic of the top view of the experimental setup.

Experimental protocol:

The participants were blindfolded and seated in a comfortable position in front of the apparatus and wearing earplugs to avoid visual and audio cues. The end effector of the Omni Phantom (either A or B at random) was then given to the participant's hand. The participant then performed the needle insertion procedure on either the PRM or PPT in random order. The haptic feedback was provided to the participant by either PRM or PPT. After the first test, the participant performs the same experiment on the other PPT with different properties. To switch from force feedback device 1 to force feedback device 2 seamlessly, the board was be rotated such that the next phantom then faces the participant. The participant was not changing their position for the interchange of models to prevent external biases on the participant during the interchange of models. After the participant experienced each model, the participant is asked: "Is the model a PPT or a PRM?" The answer of the participant is then noted as "A" or "B". The participants were initially provided with the experience of both the simulated model and the PPT feedback until they were confident in their choice. Each layer was repeated for six trials (PRM and PPT were repeated three times each). There were five sessions of the experiment on all the five different tissue layers. The number of times the participant punctures the tissue is not restricted. At the end of the study, after all the five sessions, participants were asked to fill out a questionnaire regarding their experience and confidence in their responses. Typically, each session takes about a maximum of 5 minutes. The entire experiment lasts for about 40–50 minutes.

D. **Experiment: Comparison of PRM and biomechanical model without perceptual filter**

We modified the imitation game to compare PRM with the biomechanical model without the perceptual filter. The objective of this experiment is to observe the perceptual difference in the participant for the two models.

Experimental setup:

The experiment includes the needle insertion with the simulated model under two criteria: (i) the model with the perceptual filter (PRM) and (ii) the model without the perceptual filter. Both the unfiltered and filtered models are simulated, and the force feedback is provided to the participant using the Omni Phantom. The experimental setup remained the same as the first stage of the experiment except that there is no PPT on the second Omni Phantom, but it is programmed with the biomechanical model without the perceptual filter.

Experimental protocol:

The experimental concept of the Turing test remains the same as in experiment stage 1. After the participant experiences each model, he/she is asked the question: "Is the model a perceptually filtered model or an unfiltered model?" The answer of the participant is then noted as "A" or "B". This experiment is repeated for three trials in each condition.

E. **Data analysis for both the experiments**

The basic statistical measure used for the imitation game is the pass rate, which is a percentage based on the guesses made by the participants. The equation as per Collins et al. [41] is shown below.

$$\text{Pass Rate} = 1 - \left(\frac{\text{Right Guesses} - \text{Wrong Guesses}}{\text{Total Guesses}} \right)$$

The pass rate equals one when the confusion is 100%; i.e., the right guesses are equal to the wrong guesses. As the pass rate approaches one, the simulation approaches closer in confusing the participants.

10.3 RESULTS AND DISCUSSION

10.3.1 Experiment 1: comparison with physical phantom

The average time taken by the participants to experience the perceptually filtered model and the PPT for them to be confident is 4.25 minutes (ranging from 2.5 to 6.25 minutes).

The results analyzed for 20 participants for five layers are shown in Table 10.3. From the table, the average pass rate for five layers of the needle insertion are 1.04, 1.97, 1.12, 1.02, and 1.19, which are close to one. There is no significant

Table 10.3 Pass rate for various layers for 20 participants

Subject #	Layer 1	Layer 2	Layer 3	Layer 4	Layer 5
1	0.67	1	1	1	1.33
2	1	1	1.33	1.33	0.67
3	0.67	0.67	1.33	0.67	1.67
4	1	1.33	1.67	1.33	1
5	1	1	1	0.67	1
6	1.33	0.67	0.67	1.33	1.33
7	0.67	1.67	0.67	1	0.67
8	1.67	1.33	1	1	1.33
9	1	1	1.33	0.67	1.67
10	1	1	0.67	1	0.67
11	1.67	0.67	1.67	1.33	1.33
12	1.33	1.33	1	0.67	1
13	0.67	1	1.33	1	1.33
14	1	1.33	1	1.33	1.67
15	1	1	1.33	0.67	1.671
16	1	1	0.67	1.67	0.67
17	1.67	0.67	1.67	1	1.33
18	1.33	1.33	1.33	1.33	1
19	0.67	1	0.67	0.67	1.33
20	1	1.33	1.67	1.33	1.67
Average	1.04	1.07	1.12	1.02	1.19

difference between the number of participants who attained a pass rate greater than one and the number of participants with a pass rate less than or equal to one. According to the Turing test rules, as explained in Section 10.3, the PRM for each layer successfully fools the participants as perceived PPT.

We analyzed the participants' responses to the questionnaire (provided in the supplementary material) in a Likert scale rating their experience and confidence in differentiating the PRM and PPT. Seventeen of twenty participants either strongly agreed or agreed that they were confident in their responses in differentiating the PRM from the PPT. However, from Table 10.3, it is evident that they could identify the PRM from PPT for only 50% of the trials. Therefore, it can be considered that the participants have been thoroughly confused in differentiating the PRM and PPT, thereby showing the success of the PRM. Three participants had neither agreed nor disagreed that they were confident, as shown in Figure 10.8. This can also imply that the three participants were 50% confident in their response and were not confident in differentiating the PRM from PPT.

Participants were also asked to state if they liked the force feedback experience when they think of it as the PRM and another question on the force feedback experienced when they think of it as the PPT. Eleven participants could not tell if they liked it when they think they had experienced a PPT or the PRM, as shown in Figure 10.8. Nine participants were almost equally distributed on liking the PPT to that of the PRM. The participants' confusion to decide on PPT to the PRM can be the cause for their response to be neutral feedback.

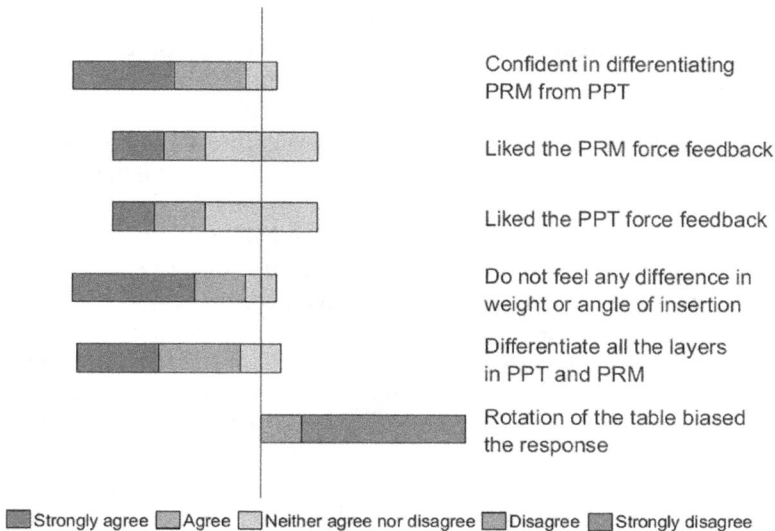

Figure 10.8 Level of agreement with the six questions of the stage 1 questionnaire from twenty participants.

Participants were either strongly agreeing or agreeing on the statement that they do not physically feel any difference in weight or angle of insertion for all the trials, except three participants. The three participants were neither agreeing nor disagreeing, as shown in Figure 10.8. This question is to make sure that the system remained stable and the same for all the trials.

The level of agreement for each layer in the corresponding session for differentiating both PPT and PRM is shown in Figure 10.8. Sixteen participants either strongly agreed or agreed with the above statement. Four participants neither agreed nor disagreed that they could differentiate between layers. The responses of four participants might be neutral as some of the layers have minute differences in the mechanical properties, and we only considered the average human perception thresholds in the perceptual filter parameters for model reduction.

We also confirmed if the participants were comfortable with the system, and they did not feel that knowing the rotation of the table has biased their response. All the participants strongly disagreed or disagreed with this statement that the rotation of the table has a biased response, as shown in Figure 10.8.

10.3.2 Stage 2 experiment

The results from the experiment of stage 2 show that the addition of the perceptual filter over the biomechanical model did not change the experience of the needle insertion procedure on the participant. This filtering could reduce the time complexity of the model and also reduced the computational cost for the simulator. The average pass rate of 20 subjects is 1.04. Therefore, the simulated model with and without the perceptual filter is undifferentiated according to the Turing test rules.

We analyzed the participants' responses to the questionnaire regarding their experience and confidence in differentiating the PRM and the biomechanical model without the perceptual filter. Thirteen participants either strongly agreed or agreed that they were confident in their responses in differentiating the PRM from the biomechanical model without the perceptual filter. Seven participants neither agree nor disagree that they were confident, as shown in Figure 10.9. However, from the average pass rate, 1.04, it is evident that they could identify the PRM from the biomechanical model without the perceptual filter for only 50% of the trials. Therefore, it can be considered the participants have been thoroughly confused in differentiating the two models, thereby showing that the PRM can be used for simulating the needle insertion forces by reducing the computational complexity caused due to the model without the perceptual filter.

Participants were also asked to state if they liked the force feedback experience when they think of it as the PRM and another question on the force feedback experienced when they think of it as the unfiltered biomechanical model. Eight participants neither agreed nor disagreed with the earlier question, and twelve participants had a neutral response to the later question, as shown in Figure 10.9. Twelve participants were almost equally distributed on strongly agreeing and agreeing that they like the force feedback when they think of it as the PRM. Eight participants either strongly agreed or agreed that they like the biomechanical model without the perceptual filter. This shows that a larger group of participants liked the PRM compared to that of the model without the filter.

Sixteen participants were either strongly agreeing or agreeing with the statement that they do not physically feel any difference in weight or angle of insertion for all the trials. Four participants were neither agreeing nor disagreeing, as shown in Figure 10.9. We could observe that the participants' response was not biased because of the weight or the physical feel.

Participants were also asked to state that the force feedback helped them differentiate the five layers when they think of it as PRM. Thirteen participants either strongly agreed or agreed that they could differentiate the five layers, and four participants neither agreed nor disagreed that they could differentiate the five layers. Three participants disagreed that they could differentiate the five layers in PRM, as shown in Figure 10.9. We also questioned the participants if they can differentiate the eight layers in the biomechanical model without the filter. Five participants either strongly agreed or agreed that they could differentiate the eight layers, two participants had a neutral response, and thirteen participants either disagreed or strongly disagreed that they could differentiate the eight layers, as shown in Figure 10.9.

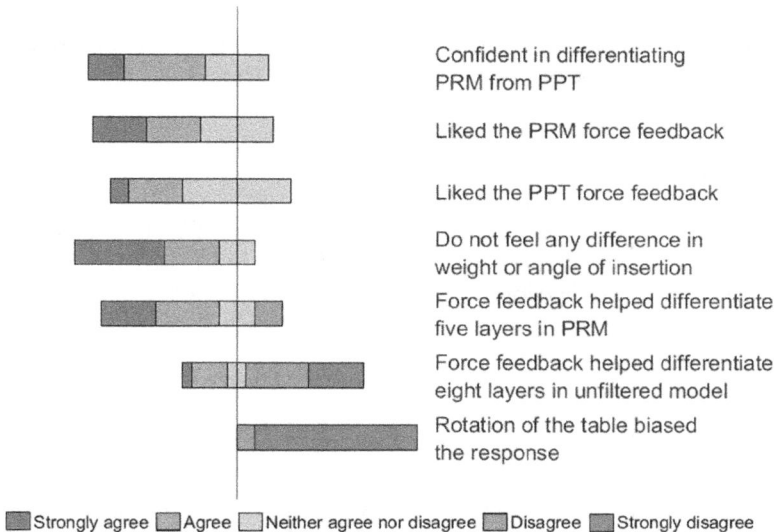

Figure 10.9 Level of agreement with the seven questions of the stage 2 questionnaire from twenty participants.

Similar to stage 1 of the experiment, we also confirmed if the participants were comfortable with the system, and they did not feel that knowing the rotation of the table has biased their response. All the participants strongly disagreed or disagreed with this statement that the rotation of the table has a biased response, as shown in Figure 10.9.

10.4 CONCLUSIONS AND FUTURE SCOPE

The primary objective of this work was to validate the developed analytical models of needle insertion, including the biomechanical and psychophysical concepts that precisely capture the needle-tissue interaction forces. The models were validated in two stages of Turing test experiments with human intervention. Needle insertion into soft tissues was classified into three phases: tissue compression, tissue puncture, and friction. The analytical model for the three phases and the perceptual filter were used to relate the interaction forces to the tissue deformation. The perceptual filter's main advantage is that it reduces computation complexity and can be used in telesurgical applications. The objective of the first experiment was to observe the perceptual difference in the participant for the unfiltered and filtered model response, whereas the second was to observe the perceptual difference between the simulated and the physical phantom models in the participant. The Turing test results showed that the model could replicate the PPTs with reasonable accuracy, and also, the perceptual reduction did not affect the experience of the model. The proposed needle-tissue interaction force models can be used more often in improving realism and performance and enabling future applications in needle simulators in heterogeneous tissue.

ACKNOWLEDGMENTS

The authors thank the mechanical workshop team, IIT Madras, for helping in the development of the rotating table and Joseph H. R. Isaac for helping in the software development and also for making suggestions on this manuscript. Further, we are thankful to the subjects who participated in the experiment.

REFERENCES

1. Alterovitz, R., Lim, A., Goldberg, K., Chirikjian, G. S., and Okamura, A. M., Steering flexible needles under Markov motion uncertainty, In *2005 IEEE/RSJ International Conference on Intelligent Robots and Systems*, Edmonton, AB, Canada, pp. 1570–1575, (2005, 02-06 August).

2. Gorman, P., Krummel, T., Webster, R., Smith, M., and Hutchens, D., A prototype haptic lumbar puncture simulator, *Studies in Health Technology and Informatics*, 70, 106–109, (2000). PMID: 10977521.

3. Ready, L. B., American Society of Regional Anesthesia 1999 Gaston Labat Lecture–Acute pain: Lessons learned from 25,000 patients, *Regional Anesthesia and Pain Medicine*, 24(6), 499, (1999).

4. Taschereau, R., Pouliot, J., Roy, J., and Tremblay, D., Seed misplacement and stabilizing needles in transperineal permanent prostate implants, *Radiotherapy, and Oncology*, 55(1), 59–63, (2000).

5. Shin, S., Park, W., Cho, H., Park, S., and Kim, L., Needle insertion simulator with haptic feedback, In *International Conference on Human-Computer Interaction*, Orlando, Florida, USA pp. 119–124, (2011, 9-14 Jul).

6. Daykin, A. P., and Bacon, R. J., An epidural injection simulator, *Anaesthesia*, 45(3), 235–236, (1990).

7. Dang, T., Annaswamy, T. M., and Srinivasan, M. A., Development and evaluation of an epidural injection simulator with force feedback for medical training, *Studies in Health Technology and Informatics*, 81, 97–102, (2001). PMID: 11317827

8. Bibin, L., Lécuyer, A., Burkhardt, J. M., Delbos, A., and Bonnet, M., SAILOR: a 3-D medical simulator of loco-regional anesthesia based on desktop virtual reality and pseudo-haptic feedback, In *Proceedings of the 2008 ACM Symposium on Virtual Reality Software and Technology*, Bordeaux France, pp. 97–100, (2008, 27-29 October).

9. Grottke, O., Ntouba, A., Ullrich, S., Liao, W., Fried, E., Prescher, A., Deserno, T.M., Kuhlen, T., and Rossaint, R., Virtual reality-based simulator for training in regional anesthesia, *British Journal of Anesthesia*, 103(4), 594–600, (2009).

10. Ravali, G., and Manivannan, M., Haptic feedback in needle insertion modeling and simulation, *IEEE Reviews in Biomedical Engineering*, 10, 63–77, (2017).

11. Goksel, O., Dehghan, E., and Salcudean, S. E., Modeling and simulation of flexible needles, *Medical Engineering and Physics*, 31(9), 1069–1078, (2009).

12. Kataoka, H., Washio, T., Audette, M., and Mizuhara, K., A model for relations between needle deflection, force, and thickness on needle penetration, In *International Conference on Medical Image Computing and Computer-Assisted Intervention*, Netherlands, pp. 966–974, (2001, 14–17 October).

13. Abolhassani, N., Patel, R., and Moallem, M., Needle insertion into soft tissue: A survey, *Medical Engineering, and Physics*, 29(4), 413–431, (2007).

14. Lehmann, T., Tavakoli, M., Usmani, N., and Sloboda, R., Force-sensor-based estimation of needle tip deflection in brachytherapy, *Journal of Sensors*, (2013). Volume 2013, Article ID 263153, pages 1–10. http://dx.doi.org/10.1155/2013/263153

15. Asadian, A., Kermani, M. R., and Patel, R. V., A compact dynamic force model for needle-tissue interaction, In *2010 Annual International Conference of the IEEE Engineering in Medicine and Biology*, Argentina, pp. 2292–2295, (2010).

16. Querleux, B., *Computational Biophysics of the Skin*, Jenny Stanford Publishing, Singapore, (2016).

17. DiMaio, S. P., and Salcudean, S. E., Needle insertion modeling and simulation, *IEEE Transactions on Robotics and Automation*, 19(5), 864–875, (2003).
18. Goksel, O., Salcudean, S. E., and DiMaio, S. P., 3D simulation of needle-tissue interaction with application to prostate brachytherapy, *Computer-Aided Surgery*, 11(6), 279–288, (2006).
19. Glozman, D., and Shoham, M., Flexible needle steering for percutaneous therapies, *Computer-Aided Surgery*, 11(4), 194–201, (2006).
20. Yan, K., Ng, W. S., Ling, K. V., Yu, Y., Podder, T., Liu, T. I., and Cheng, C. W. S., Needle steering modeling and analysis using unconstrained modal analysis, In *The First IEEE/RAS-EMBS International Conference on Biomedical Robotics and Biomechatronics*, Pisa, Italy, 87–92, (2006).
21. Barbé, L., Bayle, B., de Mathelin, M., and Gangi, A., Needle insertions modeling: Identifiability and limitations, *Biomedical Signal Processing and Control*, 2(3), 191–198, (2007).
22. Padthe, A. K., Oh, J., and Bernstein, D. S., On the LuGre model and friction-induced hysteresis, In *2006 American Control Conference*, Minneapolis, MN, USA, 6 pp, (2006).
23. Torabi, M., Hauser, K., Alterovitz, R., Duindam, V., and Goldberg, K., Guiding medical needles using single-point tissue manipulation, In *2009 IEEE International Conference on Robotics and Automation*, Kobe, Japan, pp. 2705–2710, (2009).
24. Simone, C., and Okamura, A. M., Modeling of needle insertion forces for robot-assisted percutaneous therapy, In *Proceedings 2002 IEEE International Conference on Robotics and Automation (Cat. No. 02CH37292)*, Washington, DC, USA, Vol. 2, pp. 2085–2091, (2002).
25. Chentanez, N., Alterovitz, R., Ritchie, D., Cho, L., Hauser, K. K., Goldberg, K., Shewchuk, J. R., and O'Brien, J. F., Interactive simulation of surgical needle insertion and steering, *ACM*, Cambridge, USA, 28(3), 1–10, (2009).
26. Goksel, O., Sapchuk, K., and Salcudean, S. E., Haptic simulator for prostate brachytherapy with simulated needle and probe interaction, *IEEE Transactions on Haptics*, 4(3), 188–198, (2011).
27. DiMaio, S. P., and Salcudean, S. E., Interactive simulation of needle insertion models, *IEEE Transactions on Biomedical Engineering*, 52(7), 1167–1179, (2005).
28. Batteau, L. M., Liu, A., Maintz, J. A., Bhasin, Y., and Bowyer, M. W., A study on the perception of haptics in surgical simulation, In *International Symposium on Medical Simulation*, Cambridge, USA, pp. 185–192, (2004).
29. van Gerwen, D. J., Dankelman, J., and van den Dobbelsteen, J. J., Needle–tissue interaction forces–A survey of experimental data, *Medical Engineering and Physics*, 34(6), 665–680, (2012).
30. Khadem, M., Rossa, C., Sloboda, R. S., Usmani, N., and Tavakoli, M., Mechanics of tissue cutting during needle insertion in biological tissue, *IEEE Robotics and Automation Letters*, 1(2), 800–807, (2016).
31. Mahvash, M., and Dupont, P. E., Mechanics of dynamic needle insertion into a biological material, *IEEE Transactions on Biomedical Engineering*, 57(4), 934–943, (2009).

32. Pyatigorets, A. V., and Mogilevskaya, S. G., Evaluation of effective transverse mechanical properties of transversely isotropic viscoelastic composite materials, *Journal of Composite Materials*, 45(25), 2641–2658, (2011).
33. Tan, H. Z., Srinivasan, M. A., Eberman, B., and Cheng, B., Human factors for the design of force-reflecting haptic interfaces, *Dynamic Systems and Control*, 55(1), 353–359, (1994).
34. Jones, L. A., Matching forces: constant errors and differential thresholds, *Perception*, 18(5), 681–687, (1989).
35. King, H. H., Donlin, R., and Hannaford, B., Perceptual thresholds for single vs. multi-finger haptic interaction, In *2010 IEEE Haptics Symposium*, Waltham, MA, pp. 95–99, (2010).
36. Pang, X. D., Tan, H. Z., and Durlach, N. I., Manual discrimination of force using active finger motion, *Perception and psychophysics*, 49(6), 531–540, (1991).
37. Brooks, T. L., Telerobotic response requirements, *In 1990 IEEE International Conference on Systems, Man, and Cybernetics Conference Proceedings*, Los Angeles, CA, USA, pp. 113–120, (1990).
38. Jayant, N., Johnston, J., and Safranek, R., Signal compression based on models of human perception, *Proceedings of the IEEE*, 81(10), 1385–1422, (1993).
39. Turing, A. M., Computing machinery and intelligence, *Mind*, LIX(236), 433–460, (1950).
40. Cronin, L., Krasnogor, N., Davis, B. G., Alexander, C., Robertson, N., Steinke, J. H., Schroeder, S. L., et al., The imitation game—a computational chemical approach to recognizing life, *Nature Biotechnology*, 24(10), 1203, (2006).
41. Collins, H., Evans, R., Weinel, M., Lyttleton-Smith, J., Bartlett, A., and Hall, M., The Imitation Game and the nature of mixed methods, *Journal of Mixed Methods Research*, 11(4), 510–527, (2017).

Chapter 11

Microfluidics-based isolation of circulating tumor cells

Anju R. Babu, Adharsh Raj M. K.,
and Bansod Sneha Bharat

National Institute of Technology Rourkela

CONTENTS

11.1 INTRODUCTION

Circulating tumor cells (CTCs) are floating tumor cells distinguished as epithelial cancer cells that traverse through the blood and lead to the formation of secondary tumor (Krebs et al., 2010). The analysis of CTCs provides an easily repeated procedure to isolate and analyze the tumor cells having potential for metastasis. Conventional imaging techniques are not much sensitive to identifying the tumors during the early stage of development (Hüsemann et al., 2008). However, some studies show that CTCs can be detected from blood samples in the early stages of cancer development (Lloyd et al., 2006). CTC count in the blood usually increases with cancer progression; however, its concentration is deficient as compared to other blood components (Mohan et al., 2017). Depending on the malignant potential of cancer, CTC count varies as follows: low CTC count for mild malignancy (<3 CTCs/mL), moderate CTC count for intermediate malignancy (3–20 CTCs/mL), and higher count for high-risk cancers (>20 CTCs/mL) (Ried et al., 2017). The lower concentration of CTCs is the major limitation during the isolation

DOI: 10.1201/9781003344810-11

procedure (Ranuncolo, 2017). Various methods such as immunobead assay, functional assay, microdevices, and microfluidic platform-based separation have been developed to overcome these limitations (Rushton et al., 2021).

Microfluidic devices are miniaturized devices containing chambers and channels that can manipulate and control fluid samples (Tiwari et al., 2020). Compared to the other biomarker detection processes, microfluidic approaches have advantages such as the requirement of less volume of samples and reagents, less completion time, and high portability (Streets & Huang, 2013). In the isolation of CTCs, microfluidic technologies are mainly based on affinity-based and label-free separations (Lei, 2020). Antibody-coated microfluidic channels are designed for affinity-based methods to bind the specific antigens that are present on the surface of CTCs or blood cells, and label-free methods use the physical and electrical properties of the CTCs (Dong et al., 2013). The microfluidic platforms should essentially have properties such as resistance to the chemical reagents used for separation, required physical and electrical properties, dielectric strength, and adhesive properties for integrating electrodes (Mark et al., 2010). Polymer-based microfluidics platforms are commonly used because their optical properties are similar to glass microfluidic devices, and their fabrication process is not complicated (Scott & Ali, 2021).

In Section 11.2, we review the metastasis process and the secondary tumor site formation, followed by an overview of CTCs. These cancer cells flow through the blood or lymph and reach different body sites and trigger the formation of secondary tumors. Isolation and analysis of CTCs give the progress of metastasis, and results are used to monitor the prognosis of cancer patients. In Section 11.3, we discuss affinity-based microfluidic technologies for the isolation of CTCs. Positive and negative selection processes are briefly introduced under affinity-based separation. Next, we discuss the label-free microfluidic strategies to isolate CTCs. Isolation based on the physical and electrical characteristics of CTCs is introduced in this section.

11.2 METASTASIS

The process by which cancers spread from the primary formed regions to the secondary sites in the body is termed metastasis (Coleman & Eccles, 2006). The spreading of tumor cells mainly occurs through the bloodstream in a series of steps, and Figure 11.1 shows an overview of the metastatic process. First, tumor cells shed from the primary site and dissolve the basement membrane, and the detached cells intravasate into lymph or blood vessels (Van Zijl et al., 2011). Platelets in the blood protect CTCs from the immune system, and these cells reach different body regions by invading the blood vessel walls (Harouaka et al., 2013). Cancer cells grew in the secondary site initially as a tiny tumor, followed by new blood vessel formation and complete secondary tumor growth.

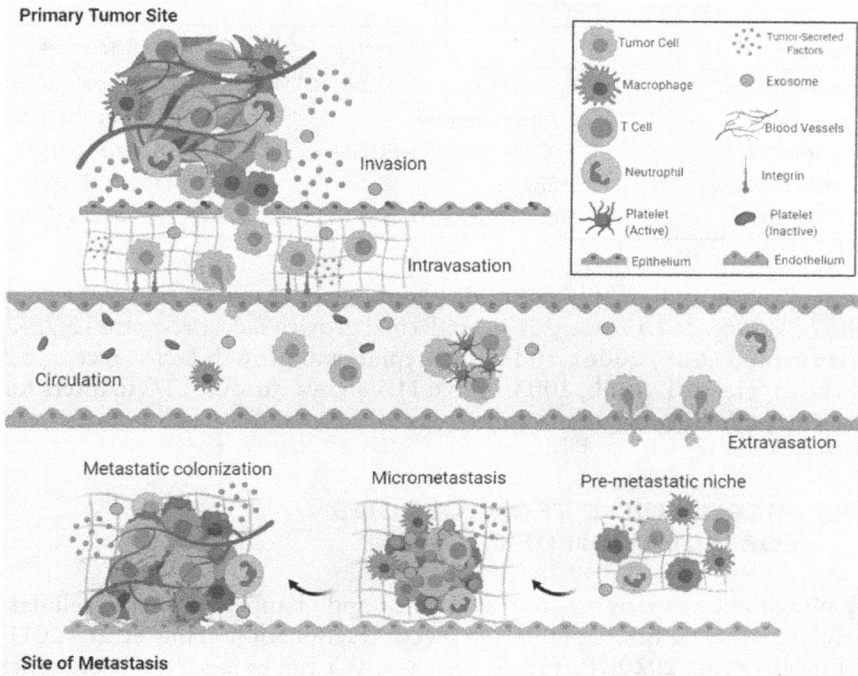

Figure 11.1 Metastatic process of cancer cells (Fares et al., 2020).

11.2.1 Circulating tumor cells

CTCs are the cells detached from primary tumor sites into lymph or blood vessels (Yap et al., 2014). Enumeration and analysis of molecular characteristics of CTCs give rise to potential applications such as prediction of accurate prognosis, measuring the response of particular drugs on tumor growth, assessing genotypic and phenotypic features, and assessing treatment resistance mechanisms (Krebs et al., 2010). If the concentration of CTCs in the blood is high, there is an increased risk of metastasis and reduced patient prognosis. In the study of Cristofanilli et al., it is discovered that patients with less concentration of CTCs in blood lived longer than patients with higher CTCs (Cristofanilli, 2006). The main disadvantage of the analysis of CTCs is the lower concentration of cells as compared to other blood cells. However, the isolation is possible based on the chemical, physical, and electrical characteristics of the CTCs (Sharma et al., 2018). Epithelial cell adhesion molecule (EpCAM) and cytokeratin (CK) are the common tumor-specific surface proteins present on the CTCs, and the antibodies corresponding to these proteins are used for the isolation of CTCs from the sample (Habli et al., 2020). Along with EpCAM and CK,

Table 11.1 CTC markers for different cancers

Origin of cancer	CTC marker	References
General cancer	EpCAM+ or cytokeratin+, CD45−	Deng et al. (2008)
Lung cancer	Folate receptor+	Gallo et al. (2017)
Breast cancer	EpCAM+, HER2+, EGFR+	Lee et al. (2013)
Gastric cancer	HER2+	Yang et al. (2019)
Brain cancer	Ki67+, EGFR+ or EBI+	Krol et al. (2018)

there are other commonly used CTC markers for different cancers such as Ki67 (Klöppel & La Rosa, 2018), epidermal growth factor receptor (EGFR) (Normanno et al., 2006), and human epidermal growth factor receptor 2 (HER2) (Hendriks et al., 2003). Table 11.1 shows various CTC markers for the corresponding origin of cancer.

11.3 MICROFLUIDIC TECHNOLOGIES FOR ISOLATION OF CTCs

A microfluidic device contains structures and channels of below-cellular-level size and is best suitable for blood fractionation (Hou et al., 2011; Clinically et al., 2020). Rare cells such as CTCs can be separated from other hematologic components by manipulating small quantities of blood samples in the microchannels. CTCs are captured on microfluidic channels based on two technologies: affinity-based and label-free strategies (Lin et al., 2020).

11.3.1 Affinity-based strategies

The main principle of isolating particular cells from the sample in this technique is by the affinity of antigen present on the cell surface to the antibodies coated on the microfluidic channels (Murlidhar et al., 2016). There are two selection processes: positive selection and negative selection processes. The interaction between the antigen present on the surface of CTCs and the corresponding antibody coated on the microchannels is the principle of separation in the positive selection process (Witek et al., 2017). In the negative selection process, the interaction mainly occurs between white blood cells (WBCs) or other blood cells to the antibodies coated on the microchannels (Casavant et al., 2013).

11.3.1.1 Positive selection process

In the positive selection process, the affinity of antigens present on the CTCs toward the coated antibodies on the surface of microfluidic channels is used to isolate the cells. In the positive selection process, the two commonly used markers are EpCAM and CK (Barriere et al., 2014). These biomarkers are used to differentiate hematopoietic and epithelial origin cells (van der Toom et al., 2016). Epithelial tumors are commonly found in prostate cancer (Frank & Miranti, 2013), breast cancer (Wu et al., 2016), and lung cancer patients (Bhora et al., 2014). CTCs detached from these tumors have the expression of EpCAM antigen on the surface and are attracted by the anti-EpCAM antibodies coated on the microfluidic channels. Epithelial-to-mesenchymal transition of CTCs causes the cells to be undiscoverable by the anti-EpCAM antibodies. Many CTCs lose their epithelial markers during this transition (Li et al., 2020). This mesenchymal marker can be detected using microfluidic channels coated with N-cadherin and vimentin antibodies (Liu, 2013).

11.3.1.2 Negative selection process

During the dissemination of tumor cells, CTCs often undergo some phenotypic changes such as epithelial-to-mesenchymal transition (Jie et al., 2017). Then the use of antibodies for the epithelial cell markers is not suitable for the separation of CTCs. The surface protein expression changes during this transition, and the positive selection-based isolation using anti-EpCAM antibodies becomes meaningless (Hyun et al., 2016). This limitation can be resolved using a negative selection process of CTCs. In the negative selection process, the affinity of the surface markers of WBCs and other blood cells to the corresponding antibodies is used to reject these cells and isolate CTCs. Microfluidic devices are functionalized with anti-CD45-like antibodies, and CTCs are separated by the depletion of other blood cells from the sample (Casavant et al., 2013). Leukocytes are effectively eliminated using a dual-patterned immunofiltration (DIF) device developed by Bu et al. (2016). The anti-CD45 antibody is patterned on dual layers in a DIF device to enhance the binding chance of leukocytes.

Masking of CTCs by the platelets is a major limitation of affinity-based separation, and cell survival in the bloodstream is enhanced by this interaction. Jiang et al. (2017) introduced a two-stage microfluidic device to isolate the platelet-covered CTCs. Initially, size-based separation of platelets are done, and the platelet-covered CTCs are isolated from the remaining sample using a herringbone chip (HB-chip) (Stott et al., 2010).

11.3.2 Label-free strategies

As mentioned in Section 11.3.1, affinity-based methods are based on the affinity of the antigen expressions on the surface of CTCs or hematopoietic cells toward the corresponding chemical substances coated on the surface of the microfluidic device. The antibodies used for the isolation process are very expensive, and these specific antibodies should be known in advance for detecting the particular tumor cells (Habli et al., 2020). Since these methods use chemicals, they may interfere with the further downstream assay. Another disadvantage of the affinity-based method is the heterogenicity of CTCs. Biomarker expression changes when EMT transmission occurs (Bulfoni et al., 2016). Negative enrichment using antibodies such as anti-CD45 or label-free technique can be used to overcome this limitation.

Label-free technologies avoid the use of expensive antibodies, and the removal of chemical substances ensures further downstream assay (Yousuff et al., 2017). Prior knowledge of antigen-antibody interaction of specific tumor cells is not required for this method. Physical properties such as size, deformability, density, and surface charge of CTCs and other blood cells are used in isolation (Sajeesh & Sen, 2014). CTCs show different physical characteristics from other blood cell types, and this is manipulated to get proper separation from the bloodstream (Cima et al., 2013). Passive filtration is done using weir, pillar, cross-flow, and membrane-type filters, and deformability-based isolation methods are based on the stiffness property of CTCs. Deterministic lateral displacement techniques are based on the size and deformability of CTCs, and the electrical property of CTC is used in dielectrophoresis techniques. This section deals with size-based passive filtration, deformability-based sorting, deterministic lateral displacement, and dielectrophoresis.

11.3.2.1 Size-based passive filtration

Size-based passive filtration is a more straightforward method for the separation of CTCs. While considering the diameter of CTCs (13–15 μm), other blood cells such as RBCs (7–9 μm) and WBCs (8–15 μm) are having lesser diameters. This difference in size is used as the principle of microfilter fabrications to capture CTCs from blood and easy passage of other blood cells. Clogging is a challenge for these size-based passive filtration methods, and it leads to irregular flow of samples. Another drawback of size-based separation is the similarity in the diameter of leukocytes and CTCs, and this overlapping of size reduces the separation efficiency. Commonly used microfilters in microfluidic devices are weir, pillar, cross-flow, and membrane-type filters (Gossett et al., 2010).

Weir-type microfilters shown in Figure 11.2a contain a small planar slit for capturing large CTCs. Since the channel is in the micro-size range, the main driving force for the fluid flow is capillary force. The sample flows through the slits, the CTCs get captured, and other blood cells leave the slits. In pillar-type filters (Figure 11.2b), a microfilter pattern of micro-posts is created in the fluid flow channels. The design and placement of micro-posts depend on the size of the CTCs. Particles with a diameter higher than the gap between micro-posts captured and other cells easily flow to the other end. The main disadvantages of weir- and pillar-type

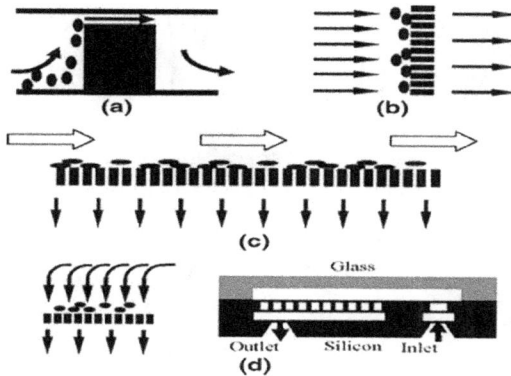

Figure 11.2 (a) Weir-type microfilter. (b) Pillar-type microfilter. (c) Cross-flow-type microfilter. (d) Membrane-type microfilter (Gossett et al., 2010).

filters are the higher rate of clogging (Sano & Davalos, 2012). Cross-flow filters (Figure 11.2c) are similar to the weir and pillar types; however, the flow direction is perpendicular to the pillars or slits. Cross-flow filters reduce clogging as compared to previous models. Small-sized blood cells pass through the gaps, and large CTCs filter out. The filtered CTCs flow along with the primary flow, and small cells are collected in separate outlets. Membrane-type filters (Figure 11.2d) consist of a filtering membrane with well-sized pores designed to separate the cells with a larger size than the critical pore size.

11.3.2.2 Deformability (stiffness)-based sorting

Another strategy to separate the overlapped leukocytes and CTCs is based on the difference in deformability or stiffness of cells (Kim et al., 2015). The nuclear-cytoplasmic ratio (N/C) of a cell is defined as the ratio of nuclear area to cytoplasmic area (Zhou et al., 2020). The higher the ratio is, the lower the deformability of the cell. The N/C proportion of CTCs and leukocytes is around 0.8 and 0.55, respectively, thus indicating that the leukocytes are more deformable than CTCs (Ferreira et al., 2016). Preira et al. (2013) designed a gradual microfluidic filter where circulating cells pass through a series of narrow comb-like constrictions. Single constriction is sensitive to clogging and blocking of cells and is not adopted to analyze numerous cells. To avoid this, a microfilter is designed as a parallel arranged set of constrictions of similar size. The cross section of the constriction or the cut-off dimension of constrictions is unique. A wide range of cell deformability-based separations cannot be achieved through a single layer of the comb-like microfluidic filter. To amplify the separation process, a series of filters are used.

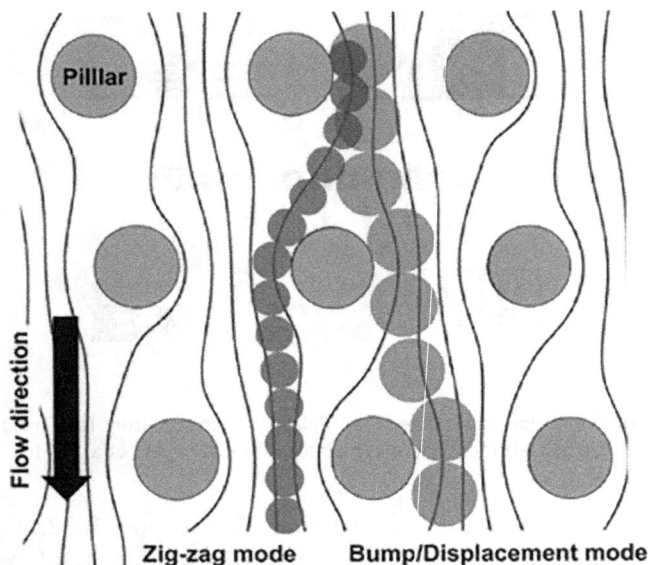

Figure 11.3 Displacement mode and zigzag mode separation in DLD (Salafi et al., 2019).

11.3.2.3 Deterministic lateral displacement

Using deterministic lateral displacement (DLD), high-resolution cell separation based on size, deformability, shape, and electrical properties can be implemented. This passive filtration device contains micropillars with different conditions such as circular, triangular, or other forms (McGrath et al., 2014). When the sample is given to the pillar gaps, the cells less than the critical size of the given DLD channel travel in zigzag mode and the cells that are more prominent than the necessary size are laterally displaced to the following streamline (Salafi et al., 2019).

Figure 11.3 shows the flow of cells through the DLD channel. The critical size between lateral displacement and zigzag mode is called DLD-required diameter. The micropillar shapes also influence the critical diameter parameter.

11.3.2.4 Dielectrophoresis

In a non-uniform electric field, a neutral particle experiences a dielectrophoresis force (DEP force) due to polarization (Zhang et al., 2019). When a blood sample flows across a non-uniform electric field, cells with different dielectric properties experience this translational force. Polarized cells in the blood sample move either toward or away from the maximum field strength depending on the degree of polarization acquired in the applied

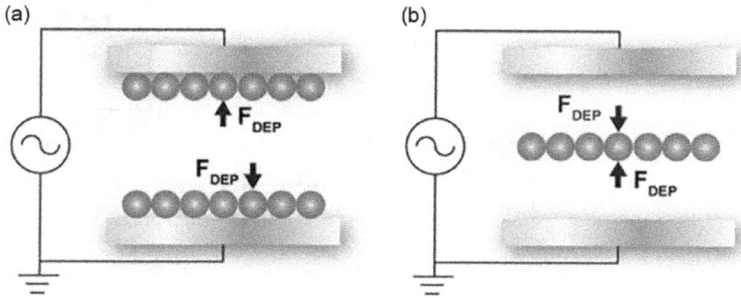

Figure 11.4 (a) Positive DEP-based separation of cells in which the more polarized cells move toward the wall region where the field strength is high. (b) Negative DEP-based separation of cells in which the less polarized cells flow in the central region where the field strength is lesser than the wall region (Gossett et al., 2010).

electric field (Yousuff et al., 2017). CTCs have distinct dielectric properties from the normal cells of blood samples (Gascoyne & Shim, 2014). DEP-based separation utilizes differences in these properties to isolate CTCs from other blood cells (Gossett et al., 2010). There are two types of DEPs for the separation of CTCs by deflecting or attracting the cells toward the higher field that is applied across the microfluidic channels: positive dielectrophoresis (p-DEP) and negative dielectrophoresis (n-DEP), as shown in Figure 11.4 (Chen et al., 2020). In the presence of a non-uniform electric field, both cells and the medium can be polarized. In p-DEP, the cells are more polarizable as compared to the medium and the net force drives the cells toward the high electric field area (Lee et al., 2016). In n-DEP, the medium is more polarizable than cells and the net force drives the medium toward the high electric field area (Yang et al., 2013).

This composite electrode can be easily integrated into the PDMS microchannel as the cohesive force of attraction between the conducting PDMS electrode and the PDMS microchannels strengthens the bond. Based on the dielectric characteristics of CTCs, various dielectrophoretic models have been developed for the separation CTCs. Figure 11.5 shows the ApoStream device based on DEP developed by Gupta et al. (2012). In this device, the CTCs are attracted by positive DEP, and negative DEP removes the remaining medium. The sample is injected at a low flow rate to ensure the cell stay within the effective DEP field. The CTCs are pulled by the DEP force toward the chamber floor (Gupta et al., 2012). Cancer cells flowing closer to the chamber are collected through one outlet valve, and the remaining samples flowing in height are collected out through the second outlet valve.

The non-small cell lung cancer (NSCLC) cells are isolated using a Y-Y-shaped dielectrophoretic-based microfluidic channel designed by Zhang et al. (2021). The device consists of successive triangle structures connected

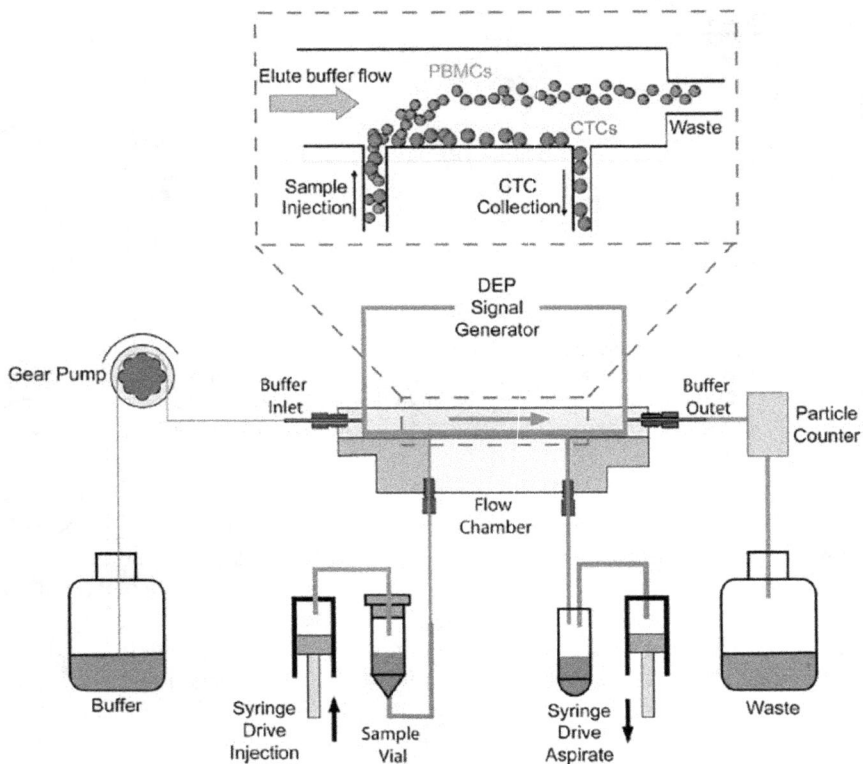

Figure 11.5 ApoStream device based on DEP (Gupta et al., 2012).

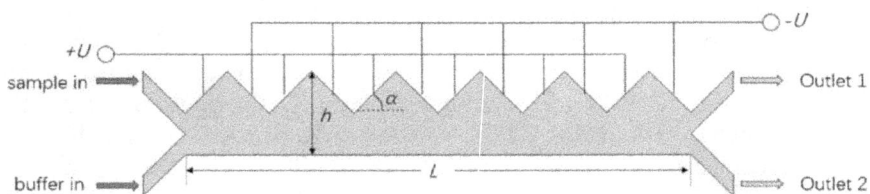

Figure 11.6 Y-Y-shaped microfluidic device with successive triangular microstructures (Zhang et al., 2021).

with electrodes for generating an alternating electric field. This arrangement provides an opposite charge on the alternate sides of the triangular structures. Figure 11.6 shows the designed microfluidic device with two inlet and outlet channels. Sample and buffer were introduced through the inlet valves and mixed up inside the microchannels. When the cells are passing through the channels, DEP forces translate the cells from their initial path. CTCs will be repelled due to large size and separated through the second outlet, and other cells will escape through the first outlet.

11.4 CONCLUSIONS

In this chapter, we discussed various microfluidic technologies for the isolation of CTCs. Monitoring of potential metastasis during the cancer development and prognosis of the patients is done by analyzing the CTCs. Miniaturized microfluidic devices have advantages over other isolation technologies such as the requirement of less volume of liquid samples and reagents, low-cost fabrication, less completion time, and high portability. Different affinity-based and label-free isolation technologies are developed for the efficient separation of CTCs from the blood sample. Antibody-coated microfluidic channels give highly specific isolation of CTCs. Positive selection processes and negative selection processes work on the principle of this antigen-antibody interaction. Label-free microfluidic channels are another separation technique. The basic principle of such separation is based on the physical and electrical characteristics of CTCs. This chapter also discusses different microfluidic devices based on these affinity-based and label-free isolation technologies.

REFERENCES

Barriere, G., Fici, P., Gallerani, G., Fabbri, F., Zoli, W., & Rigaud, M. (2014). Circulating tumor cells and epithelial, mesenchymal and stemness markers: Characterization of cell subpopulations. *Annals of Translational Medicine*, 2(11), 1–8. https://doi.org/10.3978/j.issn.2305–5839.2014.10.04.

Bhora, F. Y., Chen, D. J., Detterbeck, F. C., Asamura, H., Falkson, C., Filosso, P. L., Giaccone, G., Huang, J., Kim, J., Kondo, K., Lucchi, M., Marino, M., Marom, E. M., Nicholson, A. G., Okumura, M., Ruffini, E., Van Schil, P., Goldstraw, P., Rami-Porta, R., ... Blackstone, E. (2014). The ITMIG/IASLC thymic epithelial tumors staging project: A proposed lymph node map for thymic epithelial tumors in the forthcoming 8th edition of the TNM classification of malignant tumors. *Journal of Thoracic Oncology*, 9(9), S88–S96. https://doi.org/10.1097/JTO.0000000000000293.

Bu, J., Kang, Y. T., Kim, Y. J., Cho, Y. H., Chang, H. J., Kim, H., Moon, B. I., & Kim, H. G. (2016). Dual-patterned immunofiltration (DIF) device for the rapid efficient negative selection of heterogeneous circulating tumor cells. *Lab on a Chip*, 16(24), 4759–4769. https://doi.org/10.1039/c6lc01179a.

Bulfoni, M., Turetta, M., Del Ben, F., Di Loreto, C., Beltrami, A. P., & Cesselli, D. (2016). Dissecting the heterogeneity of circulating tumor cells in metastatic breast cancer: Going far beyond the needle in the Haystack. *International Journal of Molecular Sciences*, 17(10), 1–25. https://doi.org/10.3390/ijms17101775.

Casavant, B. P., Mosher, R., Warrick, J. W., Maccoux, L. J., Berry, S. M. F., Becker, J. T., Chen, V., Lang, J. M., McNeel, D. G., & Beebe, D. J. (2013). A negative selection methodology using a microfluidic platform for the isolation and enumeration of circulating tumor cells. *Methods*, 64(2), 137–143. https://doi.org/10.1016/j.ymeth.2013.05.027.

Chen, L., Liu, X., Zheng, X., Zhang, X., Yang, J., Tian, T., & Liao, Y. (2020). Dielectrophoretic separation of particles using microfluidic chip with composite three-dimensional electrode. *Micromachines*, 11(7). https://doi.org/10.3390/mi11070700.

Cima, I., Wen Yee, C., Iliescu, F. S., Min Phyo, W., Hon Lim, K., Iliescu, C., & Han Tan, M. (2013). Label-free isolation of circulating tumor cells in microfluidic devices: Current research and perspectives. *Biomicrofluidics*, 7(1). https://doi.org/10.1063/1.4780062.

Clinically, I., Circulating, R., & Cells, T. (2020). Epithelial cell adhesion molecule : An anchor to to isolate clinically relevant circulating tumor cells. *Cells*, 9, 1836.

Coleman, R. E., & Eccles, S. A. (2006). General mechanisms of metastasis. *Textbook of Bone Metastases*, 1–25. https://doi.org/10.1002/0470011610.ch1.

Cristofanilli, M. (2006). Circulating tumor cells, disease progression, and survival in metastatic breast cancer. *Seminars in Oncology*, 33(Suppl. 9), 9–14. https://doi.org/10.1053/j.seminoncol.2006.03.016.

Deng, G., Herrler, M., Burgess, D., Manna, E., Krag, D., & Burke, J. F. (2008). Research article Enrichment with anti-cytokeratin alone or combined with anti-EpCAM antibodies significantly increases the sensitivity for circulating tumor cell detection in metastatic breast cancer patients. *10*(4), 1–11. https://doi.org/10.1186/bcr2131.

Dong, Y., Skelley, A. M., Merdek, K. D., Sprott, K. M., Jiang, C., Pierceall, W. E., Lin, J., Stocum, M., Carney, W. P., & Smirnov, D. A. (2013). Microfluidics and circulating tumor cells. *Journal of Molecular Diagnostics*, 15(2), 149–157. https://doi.org/10.1016/j.jmoldx.2012.09.004.

Fares, J., Fares, M. Y., Khachfe, H. H., Salhab, H. A., & Fares, Y. (2020). Molecular principles of metastasis: a hallmark of cancer revisited. *Signal Transduction and Targeted Therapy*, 5(1), 1–17. https://doi.org/10.1038/s41392-020-0134-x.

Ferreira, M. M., Ramani, V. C., & Jeffrey, S. S. (2016). Circulating tumor cell technologies. *Molecular Oncology*, 10(3), 374–394.

Frank, S. B., & Miranti, C. K. (2013). Disruption of prostate epithelial differentiation pathways and prostate cancer development. *Frontiers in Oncology*, 3(October), 1–23. https://doi.org/10.3389/fonc.2013.00273.

Gallo, M., De Luca, A., Maiello, M. R., Alessio, A. D., Esposito, C., Chicchinelli, N., Forgione, L., Piccirillo, M. C., Rocco, G., Botti, G., & Normanno, N. (2017). Clinical utility of circulating tumor cells in patients with non-small-cell lung cancer. *6*(2), 486–498. https://doi.org/10.21037/tlcr.2017.05.07.

Gascoyne, P. R. C., & Shim, S. (2014). Isolation of circulating tumor cells by dielectrophoresis. *Cancers*, 6(1), 545–579. https://doi.org/10.3390/cancers6010545.

Gossett, D. R., Weaver, W. M., MacH, A. J., Hur, S. C., Tse, H. T. K., Lee, W., Amini, H., & Di Carlo, D. (2010). Label-free cell separation and sorting in microfluidic systems. *Analytical and Bioanalytical Chemistry*, 397(8), 3249–3267. https://doi.org/10.1007/s00216-010-3721-9.

Gupta, V., Jafferji, I., Garza, M., Melnikova, V. O., Hasegawa, D. K., Pethig, R., & Davis, D. W. (2012). ApoStream, a new dielectrophoretic device for anti-body independent isolation and recovery of viable cancer cells from blood. *Biomicrofluidics, 024133*, 1–14.

Habli, Z., Alchamaa, W., Saab, R., Kadara, H., & Khraiche, M. L. (2020). Circulating tumor cell detection technologies and clinical utility: Challenges and opportunities. *Cancers, 12*(7), 1–30. https://doi.org/10.3390/cancers12071930.

Harouaka, R. A., Nisic, M., & Zheng, S. Y. (2013). Circulating tumor cell enrichment based on physical properties. *Journal of Laboratory Automation, 18*(6), 455–468. https://doi.org/10.1177/2211068213494391.

Hendriks, B. S., Opresko, L. K., Wiley, H. S., & Lauffenburger, D. (2003). Coregulation of epidermal growth factor receptor/human epidermal growth factor receptor 2 (HER2) levels and locations: Quantitative analysis of HER2 overexpression effects. *Cancer Research, 63*(5), 1130–1137.

Hou, H. W., Bhagat, A. A. S., Lee, W. C., Huang, S., Han, J., & Lim, C. T. (2011). Microfluidic devices for blood fractionation. *Micromachines, 2*(3), 319–343. https://doi.org/10.3390/mi2030319.

Hüsemann, Y., Geigl, J. B., Schubert, F., Musiani, P., Meyer, M., Burghart, E., Forni, G., Eils, R., Fehm, T., Riethmüller, G., & Klein, C. A. (2008). Systemic spread is an early step in breast cancer. *Cancer Cell, 13*(1), 58–68. https://doi.org/10.1016/j.ccr.2007.12.003.

Hyun, K. A., Goo, K. B., Han, H., Sohn, J., Choi, W., Kim, S. I., Jung, H. I., & Kim, Y. S. (2016). Epithelial-to-mesenchymal transition leads to loss of EpCAM and different physical properties in circulating tumor cells from metastatic breast cancer. *Oncotarget, 7*(17), 24677–24687. https://doi.org/10.18632/oncotarget.8250.

Jiang, X., Wong, K. H. K., Khankhel, A. H., Zeinali, M., Reategui, E., Phillips, M. J., Luo, X., Aceto, N., Fachin, F., Hoang, A. N., Kim, W., Jensen, A. E., Sequist, L. V., Maheswaran, S., Haber, D. A., Stott, S. L., & Toner, M. (2017). Microfluidic isolation of platelet-covered circulating tumor cells. *Lab on a Chip, 17*(20), 3498–3503. https://doi.org/10.1039/c7lc00654c.

Jie, X. X., Zhang, X. Y., & Xu, C. J. (2017). Epithelial-to-mesenchymal transition, circulating tumor cells and cancer metastasis: Mechanisms and clinical applications. *Oncotarget, 8*(46), 81558–81571. https://doi.org/10.18632/oncotarget.18277.

Kim, J., Lee, H., & Shin, S. (2015). Advances in the measurement of red blood cell deformability: A brief review. *Journal of Cellular Biotechnology, 1*(1), 63–79. https://doi.org/10.3233/jcb-15007.

Klöppel, G., & La Rosa, S. (2018). Ki67 labeling index: Assessment and prognostic role in gastroenteropancreatic neuroendocrine neoplasms. *Virchows Archiv, 472*(3), 341–349. https://doi.org/10.1007/s00428-017-2258-0.

Krebs, M. G., Hou, J. M., Ward, T. H., Blackhall, F. H., & Dive, C. (2010). Circulating tumour cells: Their utility in cancer management and predicting outcomes. *Therapeutic Advances in Medical Oncology, 2*(6), 351–365. https://doi.org/10.1177/1758834010378414.

Krol, I., Castro-giner, F., Maurer, M., Szczerba, B. M., Scherrer, R., Coleman, N., Carreira, S., Bachmann, F., Anderson, S., Engelhardt, M., Lane, H., Ronald, T., Evans, J., Plummer, R., Kristeleit, R., Lopez, J., & Aceto, N. (2018). Detection of circulating tumour cell clusters in human glioblastoma. *British Journal of Cancer, 119*(4), 487–491.

Lee, D., Hwang, B., & Kim, B. (2016). The potential of a dielectrophoresis activated cell sorter (DACS) as a next generation cell sorter. *Micro and Nano Systems Letters*, 4(1). https://doi.org/10.1186/s40486-016-0028-4.

Lee, H. J., Cho, H. Y., Oh, J. H., Namkoong, K., Lee, J. G., Park, J. M., Lee, S. S., Huh, N., & Choi, J. W. (2013). Simultaneous capture and in situ analysis of circulating tumor cells using multiple hybrid nanoparticles. *Biosensors and Bioelectronics*, 47, 508–514. https://doi.org/10.1016/j.bios.2013.03.040.

Lei, K. F. (2020). A review on microdevices for isolating circulating tumor cells. *Micromachines*, 11(5), 1–19. https://doi.org/10.3390/mi11050531.

Li, X., Li, Y., Shao, W., Li, Z., Zhao, R., & Ye, Z. (2020). Strategies for enrichment of circulating tumor cells. *Translational Cancer Research*, 9(3), 2012–2025. https://doi.org/10.21037/tcr.2020.01.17.

Lin, Z., Luo, G., Du, W., Kong, T., Liu, C., & Liu, Z. (2020). Recent advances in microfluidic platforms applied in cancer metastasis: Circulating Tumor Cells' (CTCs) isolation and tumor-on-a-chip. *Small*, 16(9), 1–21. https://doi.org/10.1002/smll.201903899.

Liu, H. (2013). Dysfunction of large-conductance Ca^{2+}-activated K^+ channels in vascular: Risks developed in fetal origins. *Hypertension Research*, 36(2), 115–116. https://doi.org/10.1038/hr.2012.179.

Lloyd, J. M., McIver, C. M., Stephenson, S. A., Hewett, P. J., Rieger, N., & Hardingham, J. E. (2006). Identification of early-stage colorectal cancer patients at risk of relapse post-resection by immunobead reverse transcription-PCR analysis of peritoneal lavage fluid for malignant cells. *Clinical Cancer Research*, 12(2), 417–423. https://doi.org/10.1158/1078-0432.CCR-05-1473.

Mark, D., Haeberle, S., Roth, G., Stetten, F. V., & Zengerle, R. (2010). Microfluidic lab-on-a-chip platforms: Requirements, characteristics and applications. *Chemical Society Reviews*, 39(3), 1153–1182. https://doi.org/10.1039/b820557b.

McGrath, J., Jimenez, M., & Bridle, H. (2014). Deterministic lateral displacement for particle separation: A review. *Lab on a Chip*, 14(21), 4139–4158. https://doi.org/10.1039/c4lc00939h.

Mohan, S., Chemi, F., & Brady, G. (2017). Challenges and unanswered questions for the next decade of circulating tumour cell research in lung cancer. *Translational Lung Cancer Research*, 6(4), 454–472. https://doi.org/10.21037/tlcr.2017.06.04.

Murlidhar, V., Rivera-Báez, L., & Nagrath, S. (2016). Affinity versus label-free isolation of circulating tumor cells: Who wins? *Small (Weinheim an Der Bergstrasse, Germany)*, 12(33), 4450–4463. https://doi.org/10.1002/smll.201601394.

Normanno, N., De Luca, A., Bianco, C., Strizzi, L., Mancino, M., Maiello, M. R., Carotenuto, A., De Feo, G., Caponigro, F., & Salomon, D. S. (2006). Epidermal growth factor receptor (EGFR) signaling in cancer. *Gene*, 366(1), 2–16. https://doi.org/10.1016/j.gene.2005.10.018.

Preira, P., Grandne, V., Forel, J. M., Gabriele, S., Camara, M., & Theodoly, O. (2013). Passive circulating cell sorting by deformability using a microfluidic gradual filter. *Lab on a Chip*, 13(1), 161–170. https://doi.org/10.1039/c2lc40847c.

Ranuncolo, S. M. (2017). Liquid biopsy in liquid tumors. *Journal of Cancer Therapy*, 08(03), 302–320. https://doi.org/10.4236/jct.2017.83026.

Ried, K., Eng, P., & Sali, A. (2017). Screening for circulating tumour cells allows early detection of cancer and monitoring of treatment effectiveness: An observational study. *Asian Pacific Journal of Cancer Prevention, 18*(8), 2275–2285. https://doi.org/10.22034/APJCP.2017.18.8.2275.

Rushton, A. J., Nteliopoulos, G., Shaw, J. A., & Coombes, R. C. (2021). A review of circulating tumour cell enrichment technologies. *Cancers, 13*(5), 1–33. https://doi.org/10.3390/cancers13050970

Sajeesh, P., & Sen, A. K. (2014). Particle separation and sorting in microfluidic devices: A review. *Microfluidics and Nanofluidics, 17*(1), 1–52. https://doi.org/10.1007/s10404-013-1291-9.

Salafi, T., Zhang, Y., & Zhang, Y. (2019). A review on deterministic lateral displacement for particle separation and detection. In *Nano-Micro Letters* (Vol. 11, Issue 1). Springer, Singapore. https://doi.org/10.1007/s40820-019-0308-7.

Sano, M. B., & Davalos, R. V. (2012). Microfluidic techniques for the detection, manipulation and isolation of rare cells. In *MEMS for Biomedical Applications*. Woodhead Publishing Limited. https://doi.org/10.1533/97808 57096272.3.337.

Scott, S. M., & Ali, Z. (2021). Fabrication methods for microfluidic devices: An overview. *Micromachines, 12*(3). https://doi.org/10.3390/mi12030319.

Sharma, S., Zhuang, R., Long, M., Pavlovic, M., Kang, Y., Ilyas, A., & Asghar, W. (2018). Circulating tumor cell isolation, culture, and downstream molecular analysis. *Biotechnology Advances, 36*(4), 1063–1078. https://doi.org/10.1016/j.biotechadv.2018.03.007.

Stott, S. L., Hsu, C. H., Tsukrov, D. I., Yu, M., Miyamoto, D. T., Waltman, B. A., Michael Rothenberg, S., Shah, A. M., Smas, M. E., Korir, G. K., Floyd, F. P., Gilman, A. J., Lord, J. B., Winokur, D., Springer, S., Irimia, D., Nagrath, S., Sequist, L. V., Lee, R. J., … Toner, M. (2010). Isolation of circulating tumor cells using a microvortex-generating herringbone-chip. *Proceedings of the National Academy of Sciences of the United States of America, 107*(43), 18392–18397. https://doi.org/10.1073/pnas.1012539107.

Streets, A. M., & Huang, Y. (2013). Chip in a lab: Microfluidics for next generation life science research. *Biomicrofluidics, 7*(1), 1–23. https://doi.org/10.1063/1.4789751.

Tiwari, S. K., Bhat, S., & Mahato, K. K. (2020). Design and fabrication of low-cost microfluidic channel for biomedical application. *Scientific Reports, 10*(1), 1–14. https://doi.org/10.1038/s41598-020-65995-x.

van der Toom, E. E., Verdone, J. E., Gorin, M. A., & Pienta, K. J. (2016). Technical challenges in the isolation and analysis of circulating tumor cells. *Oncotarget, 7*(38), 62754–62766. https://doi.org/10.18632/oncotarget.11191.

Van Zijl, F., Krupitza, G., & Mikulits, W. (2011). Initial steps of metastasis: Cell invasion and endothelial transmigration. *Mutation Research - Reviews in Mutation Research, 728*(1–2), 23–34. https://doi.org/10.1016/j.mrrev.2011.05.002.

Witek, M. A., Aufforth, R. D., Wang, H., Kamande, J. W., Jackson, J. M., Pullagurla, S. R., Hupert, M. L., Usary, J., Wysham, W. Z., Hilliard, D., Montgomery, S., Bae-Jump, V., Carey, L. A., Gehrig, P. A., Milowsky, M. I., Perou, C. M., Soper, J. T., Whang, Y. E., Yeh, J. J., … Soper, S. A. (2017). Discrete microfluidics for the isolation of circulating tumor cell subpopulations targeting fibroblast activation protein alpha and epithelial cell adhesion molecule. *NPJ Precision Oncology, 1*(1). https://doi.org/10.1038/s41698-017-0028-8.

Wu, Y., Sarkissyan, M., & Vadgama, J. (2016). Epithelial-mesenchymal transition and breast cancer. *Journal of Clinical Medicine, 5*(2), 13. https://doi.org/10.3390/jcm5020013.

Yang, C., Chen, F., Wang, S., Xiong, B., & Xiong, B. (2019). Circulating tumor cells in gastrointestinal cancers: Current status and future perspectives. *9*(December). https://doi.org/10.3389/fonc.2019.01427.

Yang, F., Yang, X., Jiang, H., Butler, W. M., & Wang, G. (2013). Dielectrophoretic separation of prostate cancer cells. *Technology in Cancer Research and Treatment, 12*(1), 61–70. https://doi.org/10.7785/tcrt.2012.500275.

Yap, T. A., Lorente, D., Omlin, A., Olmos, D., & De Bono, J. S. (2014). Circulating tumor cells: A multifunctional biomarker. *Clinical Cancer Research, 20*(10), 2553–2558. https://doi.org/10.1158/1078-0432.CCR-13-2664.

Yousuff, C. M., Ho, E. T. W., Ismail Hussain, K., & Hamid, N. H. B. (2017). Microfluidic platform for cell isolation and manipulation based on cell properties. *Micromachines, 8*(1). https://doi.org/10.3390/mi8010015.

Zhang, H., Chang, H., & Neuzil, P. (2019). DEP-on-a-chip: Dielectrophoresis applied to microfluidic platforms. *Micromachines, 10*(6), 1–22. https://doi.org/10.3390/mi10060423.

Zhang, X., Xu, X., Ren, Y., Yan, Y., & Wu, A. (2021). Numerical simulation of circulating tumor cell separation in a dielectrophoresis based Y-Y shaped microfluidic device. *Separation and Purification Technology, 255*, 117343. https://doi.org/10.1016/j.seppur.2020.117343.

Zhou, J., Tu, C., Liang, Y., Huang, B., Fang, Y., Liang, X., & Ye, X. (2020). The label-free separation and culture of tumor cells in a microfluidic biochip. 1706–1715. https://doi.org/10.1039/c9an02092f.

Chapter 12

Advanced abrasive-based nano-finishing process parameter study for biomedical implants

Chinu Kumari and Sanjay Kumar Chak

Netaji Subhas Institute of Technology (NSIT) New Delhi

CONTENTS

12.1 INTRODUCTION

Freeform and highly finished surfaces are most widely used in aerospace, defense industries, medical implants, imaging, illumination optics, and die and turbine manufacturing industries. The conventional nano-finishing methods are generally 3- or 5-axis CNC milling machining, grinding, lapping, ion beam machining, honing, etc. [1–5]. There are some crucial issues associated with these conventional finishing methods. Under certain circumstances, these methods can be used, but lead to subsurface damage, and workpieces other than cylindrical and plane shapes cannot be finished [6–10]. Furthermore, the above-discussed methods cannot control cutting forces. The complicacies related to these techniques can successfully be overcome by abrasive-based nano-finishing processes (ABNPs). In these advanced ABNPs, the material is finished under gentle circumstances by applying very low forces and here microchips are removed from the material surface. The ABNPs have their applications in almost every field where the surface finish up to the nano-metric level is required.

Abrasive flow machining (AFM) is one of the oldest non-traditional finishing techniques used commonly to finish freeform surfaces [11,12]. Slowness in addition to the unavailability of control over the cutting forces is the major limitation of the primary AFM process. To defeat these troubles, various new inventions were recorded in this field of AFM [13,14]. For more precise finishing, MRF and MRAFF are the other two advanced

DOI: 10.1201/9781003344810-12

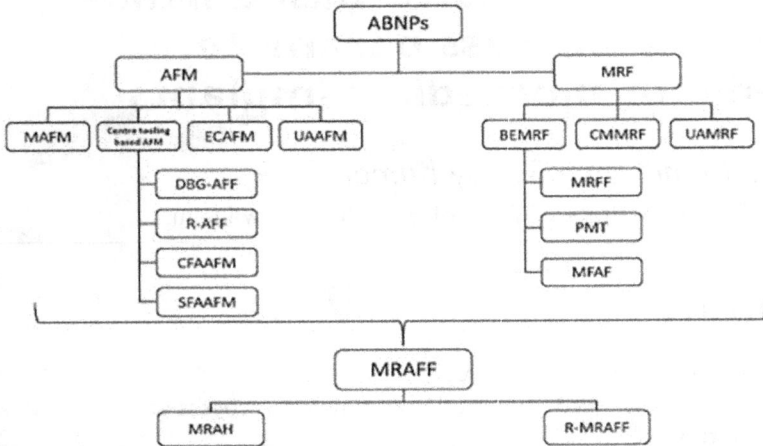

ABNP-Abrasive based finishing process, AFM-Abrasive flow finishing, BEMRF-Ball end magnetorheological finishing, CFAAFM-Centrifugal force assisted abrasive flow machining, DBG-AFF-Drill bit guided abrasive flow finishing, ECAFM-Electrochemical abrasive flow machining, MRF-Magnetorheological finishing, MAFM-Magnetic assisted abrasive flow finishing, MRFF-Magnetorheological fluid based finishing, MFAF-Magnetic field assisted finishing, MRAFF-Magnetorheological abrasive flow finishing, MRAH-Magnetorheological abrasive honing, PMT-Permanent magnet tool, R-AFF-Rotational abrasive flow finishing, R-MRAFF-Rotational magnetorheological finishing, SFAAFM-Spiral flow assisted abrasive flow machining, UAAFM-Ultrasonic assisted abrasive flow machining, UAMRF-Ultrasonic assisted magnetorheological finishing

Figure 12.1 Classification of ABNPs.

magnetically assisted abrasive-based finishing processes that were developed by the researchers [15,16]. The MRF process is very successful in finishing highly precise lenses, ceramics, and semiconductor wafers as compared to other finishing processes. Nano-level surface finish improves the aesthetic appearance and optical properties. The surface finish of order 10–100 nm can be achieved using the MRF processes [17,18]. The MRF processes have many advantages over conventional processes; for example, it has a flexible tool that can change its shape according to the workpiece. To keep the resourcefulness of the AFM process and additional features for controlling the finishing forces, AFM was combined with the MRF process for getting improvement in finishing rate with nano-level finishing [19,20]. These combined processes are called MRAFF processes or hybrid processes, as shown in Figure 12.1. Some new developments of MRAFF are magnetorheological honing (MRAH) process and rotational MRAFF or R-MRAFF process [13]. This chapter discusses the current status and important process parameters of ABNPs, i.e., AFM, MRF, and MRAFF processes.

12.1.1 Advanced abrasive-based finishing processes

Components with surfaces having complex features are broadly used in the optical, turbine blade manufacturing, biomedical, aerospace, and automobile industries. Components used in these fields demand surface finish up to nanometer level for meaningful utilization of the functionality of components. To obtain such high level of surface finish, advanced finishing processes are required. The most commonly used advanced processes are AFM, MRF, and MRAFF processes. These processes are explained below along with their development history and vital process factors/parameters that extensively influence the surface finishing. A comparison of various ABNPs is also provided in Table 12.1.

Abrasive Flow Machining (AFM): Abrasive flow machining (AFM) is one of the micro-finishing processes. In AFM, the material removal takes place due to the impingement of abrasive particles without the control of external force. AFM is one of the best processes for micro-finishing of complex contours on a wide range of materials. The basic principle behind the AFM process is that a semi-solid medium of a polymer-based carrier and abrasives in a specific proportion is extruded under pressure through or across the surface to be machined. The medium acts as a flexible tool (special deformable ability) whenever it is subjected to any restriction. Figure 12.2 shows the experimental setup and the mechanism of material used during the AFM process. This special deformability of the medium is responsible for its movement through any shape of the passage and is classified according to the way of travel of the medium throughout the process. AFM machines are classified according to three different ways: one-way AFM, two-way AFM, and orbital AFM [27,28]. The AFM process provides a superior quality exterior finish for machined surfaces [29–32]. Their three basic elements of AFM processes are the medium, the machine, and the workpiece. The medium determines the kind of abrasion, the machine finds out the amount of abrasion, and the tooling determines the type of experimental setup used. The AFM machines are positive displacement machines in which abrasive-laden media are forced across the workpiece at a predetermined pressure and volume flow rate. The pressure range for these AFM machines is 10–200 bar, and the volume flow rate is up to 225 L/min. Developments in the primary AFM process are continued with time. Due to the lack of control over finishing forces, researchers combined AFM with other finishing process, which increases the flexibility of finishing any irregular shape with improved surface topography. Various researchers have used AFM techniques for finishing different components such as MEMS, industrial components, and biomedical components. But the main drawback of this AFM process is that there is no control over the finishing force. To overcome these problems, magnetorheological processes were developed.

Table 12.1 Comparison among various ABNPs

Characteristics	AFM [21]	MRF [22]	BEMRF [23]	MRFF [24]	MRAFF [25]	R-MRAFF [26]
Principle	Abrasive-laden medium flows over the workpiece	Magnetorheological effect is induced	Ball-end flexible tool is generated at the tool tip	Three kinds of finishing fluids were used for finishing	Reciprocating motion is given to MR fluid	Combined rotational and reciprocating motion is used
Workpiece	Stainless steel	Optical glasses	Silicon chip	Titanium	Stainless steel	Brass
Process parameters	Extrusion pressure, distance from wall	Constituents of MR fluid, material of the workpiece	Working gap, core rotational speed, and magnetizing current	Different types of MR fluid, working gap	No. of finishing cycles, extrusion pressure	Extrusion pressure, abrasive mesh size, finishing time
Finishing achieved	42.9 nm	Up to 10–100 nm	89.9 nm	28 nm	30 nm	26 nm
Application	Micro-range small holes can be finished	Optical lenses of concave and convex curvature	Finishing of any complex 3D surface	Medical implant	Any complex geometry irrespective of its hardness can be finished	Finishing of any complex geometry, especially non-magnetic
Limitations	No control over finishing forces	Can finish only flat and cylindrical surfaces	Very slow process	Non-uniform finishing of all faces	Finishing of soft material is difficult	The change in roughness is not appreciable for non-magnetic workpiece
Future challenges	To control finishing forces during finishing	Finishing of 3D surfaces in least possible time	Reduction in finishing time	Reduction in finishing time and uniformity in surface finish	Simulation of MR polishing fluid and finishing forces	To fabricate the fixture for freeform surfaces to obtain uniform finishing

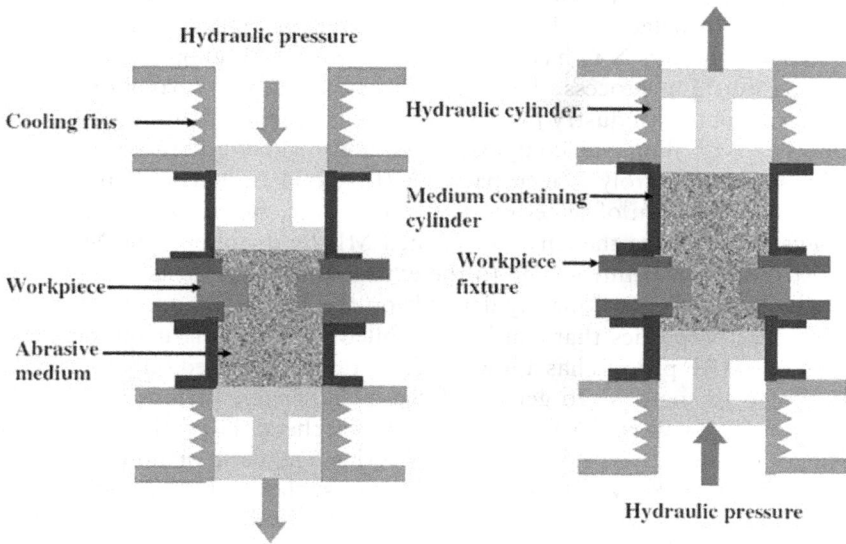

Figure 12.2 AFM's finishing principle and mechanism.

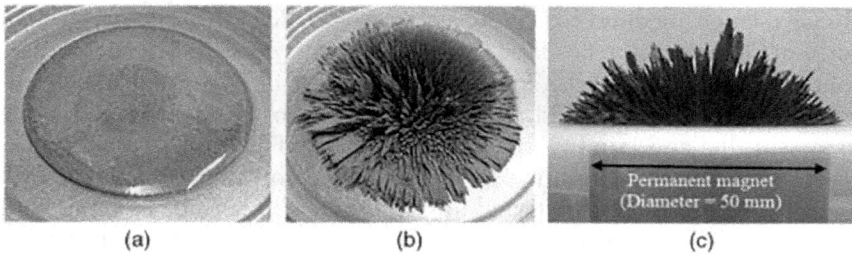

Figure 12.3 Condition of MR fluid (a) without magnetic field and (b) with magnetic field; (c) side view.

Magnetorheological Fluid (MR Fluid): MR fluids are magnetic field-controllable fluids whose rheological behavior depends on the strength of the magnetic field. The rheological properties (viscosity and shear stress) change along with other physical properties. In the "off" state of the magnetic field, MR fluids appear similar to liquid paints as shown in Figure 12.3a and exhibit comparable levels of apparent viscosity (0.1–1 Pa-s at low shear rates) [33,34]. Their apparent viscosity changes significantly (105–106 times) within a few milliseconds when the magnetic field is applied (refer to Figure 12.3b and c).

Magnetorheological Finishing (MRF): The MRF is a deterministic finishing technique used to finish brittle materials such as glass, which tends to fracture while finishing with traditional methods such as grinding. For the brittle optical surfaces such as lens, the Center for Optics Manufacturing (COM), Rochester, NY, has developed an MRF technology to automate the lens finishing process. This process has brought a revolution in the field of the optical industry [35,36]. The basic experimental setup of MRF comprises MR fluid – a composition of non-magnetic abrasive particles and magnetic electrolytic iron particles (EIPs). These particles are mixed in a carrier medium of water or oil [37,38]. Here, surface smoothing was achieved by rotating the lens on stiffened MR fluid ribbon. The MR fluid gets stiff when it is introduced to the external magnetic field. The performance of MRF process mainly depends on the MR fluid and its magneto-rheological properties that can be controlled by a varying magnetic field. The basic MRF process has a low finishing rate and is used only for finishing simple geometries. To get rid of these challenges, various variants of MRF processes were developed by the researchers. The MRF process is used for almost all types of material whether magnetic or non-magnetic. This process is mainly used for optical surfaces, glass, and electronics components [39,40]. This finishing process is able to produce a surface finish of the order of 10–100 nm peak to valley.

Magnetorheological Abrasive Flow Finishing (MRAFF): The AFM processes have the capability to finish any complicated shape that can be difficult to finish by any other conventional machining process. The abrasive-laden medium's rheological properties for controlling the final cutting forces cannot be directed in the AFM process. MRF processes controlled the magnetorheological properties of fluid through the application of the magnetic field. To take advantage of both AFM and MRF processes, Jha and Jain [25] developed an MRAFF process in which backward and forward motion is provided to self-deforming viscoplastic MR fluid. Nano-finishing of external and internal surfaces can be done with precise control over the finishing forces. The results of MRF processes were not found per expectation for non-magnetic materials, and they have a low material removal rate (MRR). To eradicate these difficulties, Khatri et al. [41] invented an innovative process named MRAH for finishing the diamagnetic materials with improved MRR. In this process, in addition to the rotational motion to the specimen, a reciprocating motion was also employed for MR fluid [42]. This process shows ~18% superior outcome in terms of surface finishing in the case of SS relative to other finishing processes. During the experiments, it was also noticed that as the density of magnetic flux was increased, there was a reduction in surface roughness value, but beyond a value of 0.6 T, all CIPs were attracted toward the magnet and there was insufficient bonding with abrasives that leads to meager enhancement in surface topography.

Kumari et al. [43,44] also developed an experimental setup of the MRAH process (Figure 12.4) for finishing the brass workpiece. Owing to combined rotational and reciprocating motion, the helical path was followed by the

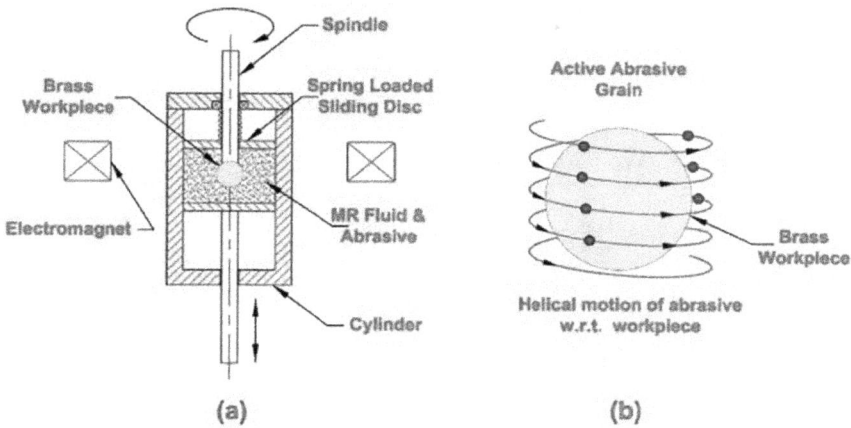

Figure 12.4 (a) Schematic of the MRAH process; (b) movement of the abrasives w.r.t. workpiece.

abrasive grains over the workpiece and, as a result, the path of contact of the abrasive grains with the surface of the workpiece was increased. About 55% improvement in surface roughness was observed during experiments.

12.2 METHODOLOGY

This section describes the important process parameters associated with the ABNPs along with their effects on surface finishing.

12.2.1 Development and process parameters of AFM

AFM is one of the oldest abrasive-based nano-finishing processes, and the main components of AFM are the machine, the tooling, types of abrasives, medium composition, and process settings. Various investigations have been carried out to investigate the effects of process parameters such as extrusion pressure, the number of cycles, viscosity, abrasive concentration, and grain size on the output responses, namely surface finish and material removal during machining [14,45]. All the involved process parameters of AFM are shown in Figure 12.5. Developments in the primary AFM process are continued with time. Due to the lack of control over finishing forces, researchers combined AFM with other finishing processes, which results in an increase in the flexibility of finishing any irregular shape with improved surface topography.

Walia et al. [46] developed a process abbreviated as CFAAFM (centrifugal force-assisted AFM), for escalating the extrusion pressure in addition

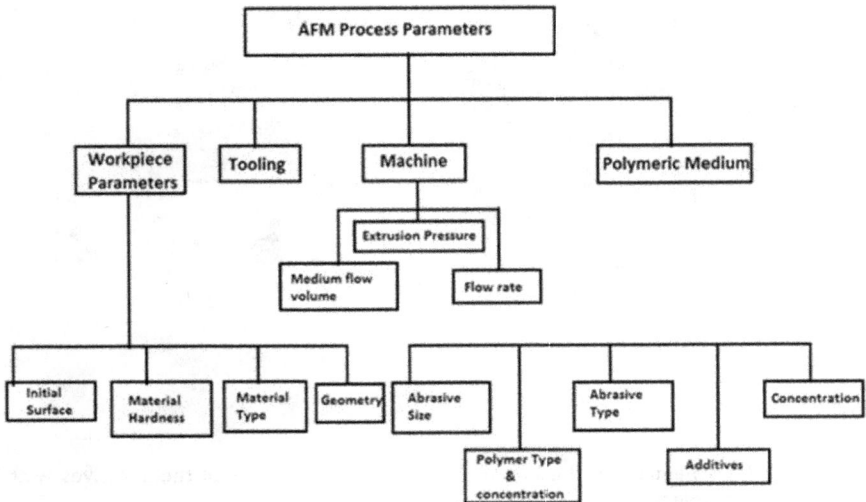

Figure 12.5 Process parameters of AFM.

to centrifugal pressure on abrasive particles during finishing. Extrusion pressure, generating rod's rotational speed, and size of abrasives were the main parameters studied by the researchers. The material removal and % improvement in the finishing value were greater than before with an increase in extrusion pressure and rotational speed of the generating rod. In CFAAFM, the time required to complete the finishing process was also lessened by 70%–80% and the enhancement in surface roughness was around 40% with respect to primary AFM. Sidpara et al. [30] developed another center tooling-based AFM process known as DBG-AFF (drill bit-guided AFM) in which rotary drill bit provides random motion to abrasive particles, resulting in the frequent reshuffling of the medium. Material removal and surface finishing were improved by a factor of 2.35 and 1.6, respectively, as compared to AFF. In DBG-AFF, SFAAFM (spiral flow-assisted AFM), and CFAAFM, the abrasive-laden medium rotates at the center causing considerable flow loss. To overcome this problem, Sankar et al. [29] developed the R-AFF (rotational abrasive flow finishing) process in which abrasive particles follow a helical path as compared to the straight path in AFM. Figure 12.6 depicts the motion of abrasives in addition to cutting forces acting on the workpiece. Owing to this helical motion, abrasives' contact lengths were increased on the workpiece. The authors also studied the effect of SiC particles distribution during the finishing of three MMCs (Al alloy, Al alloy/SiC (15%), and Al alloy/SiC

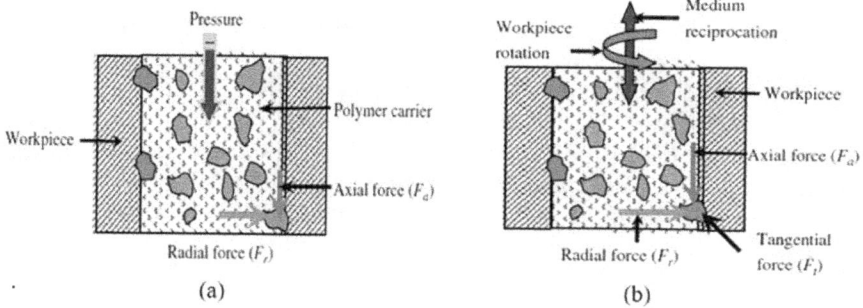

Figure 12.6 Motion of the abrasive particles with forces: (a) AFF and (b) R-AFF.

(10%)) by the R-AFF process. These processes were not found suitable for freeform geometries. To overcome this challenge and to improve the finishing rate of AFM, the ultrasonic-assisted AFM (UAAFM) was invented by Jones et al. [47]. Sharma et al. [32] finished the bevel gears by the UAAFM process. The vibrations were imparted to the specimen, due to which the relative velocity of abrasive particles was increased and the indentation of abrasives on workpiece was at an angle. When the applied frequency was increased, the depth of penetration also increased; consequently, all asperities were machined [48]. In the UAAFM process, 82.01% enhancement in the finishing value of the workpiece surface was observed as compared to the primary AFM process.

Dabrowski et al. [49] developed another hybrid process known as ECAFM (electrochemical-assisted AFM) for increasing the machining efficiency of AFM. Anodic dissolution of the workpiece was associated with micro-cutting abrasion by abrasive particles. One main advantage of this process is that the extrusion pressure required here is low as compared to other processes, so there is no need for cooling arrangements. An improvement of 46.83% in finishing value was achieved in lesser time. In another modification, ultra-fine finishing of the brass workpiece has been achieved by introducing the magnetic field around the tooling. This process is known as MAFM [31,50]. A significant improvement in surface topography value, as well as material removal, was observed under the effect of a 0.2 T magnetic field. The number of cycles required for material removal in the form of microchips from the workpiece surface was less compared to AFM. The finishing achieved from these AFM processes is in the micrometer range, which is not suitable for more precise optical and medical applications in addition to difficulty in finishing three-dimensional and intricate surfaces. These shortcomings motivated the researchers to develop more advanced finishing processes, which are discussed in subsequent sections.

12.2.2 Development and process parameters of MRF

The process parameters associated with this process are depicted in Figure 12.7. Since the basic MRF process had a low finishing rate and its use was limited for the finishing of simple geometries, various variants of MRF processes were developed by the researchers [51].

Singh et al. [52] proposed the BEMRF process to finish the three-dimensional intricate-shaped components. In the BEMRF process, a flexible ball (semi-sphere) of MR fluid was created at the end of the cutting tool, which changes its contour as per the complications of workpieces. Continuous working with an electromagnet is not possible because heating is associated with it. On heating, the viscosity of MR fluid decreases, which causes a reduction in the effectiveness of the MR fluid. Kansal et al. [53] fabricated one PMT (permanent magnet tool) for finishing diamagnetic copper workpieces that were difficult by other advanced finishing processes due to their softness. Here, the surface finish of 28.9 nm was achieved in 7.5 minutes of finishing time. With the enhancement in the working gap, the density of magnetic flux reduces. Barman and Das [54] designed a mu-metal fixture of magnet to concentrate the magnetic lines on the workpieces in the MFAF (magnetic field-assisted finishing) process. The optimum height and diameter of the magnet were 70 and 10 mm, respectively.

Bio-implants used in the medical industry require a roughness value less than 100 nm for more improved performance and longer service life. Using the BEMRF process, it was possible to achieve nano-level finishing, but it has a low finishing rate. Sidpara and Jain [24] achieved the nano-finishing of the biomedical implant (titanium material) using the MRFF

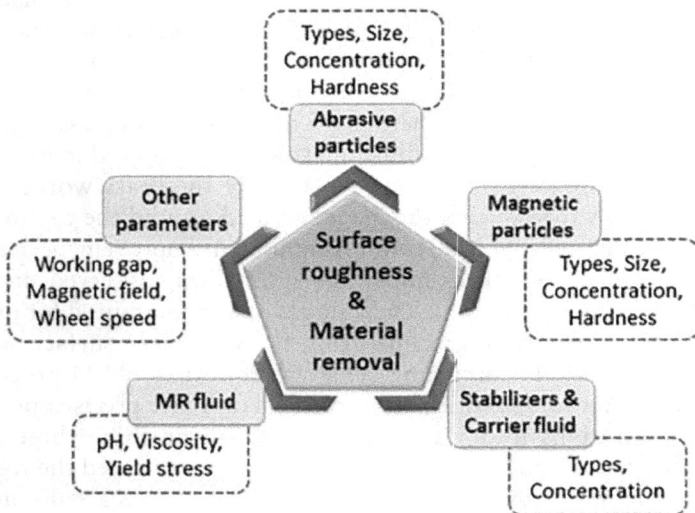

Figure 12.7 Process parameters of MRF.

process. Similar to BEMRF, a flexible ball of finishing fluid was formed in the MRFF process. The knee joint was finished using oil-, chemical-, and water-based finishing. The MRF processes were also hybridized with a combination of conventional electrochemical and ultrasonic vibration processes for finishing the freeform soft material. These processes are known as CMMRF (chemo-mechanical magnetorheological finishing) and UAMRF (ultrasonic-assisted magnetorheological finishing), respectively [55,56].

12.2.3 Development and process parameters of MRAFF

The main components of the MRAFF process are the MR fluid, machine, and magnetic field. Process parameters such as magnetic flux intensity, concentration of CIP, concentration of abrasive and its shape, and the magnetic property of workpiece, and their effect on the surface roughness and MRR have been studied. Figure 12.8 shows the important process parameters associated with the MRAFF process.

The magnetic property of the workpiece was an important parameter studied during the MRAFF process. Ferromagnetic and non-ferromagnetic workpieces were finished by specially prepared magnetorheological polishing (MRP) fluid [57]. Because of the difference in the magnetic property, the magnetic field generated at the tip of the MR finishing tool varied. The magnetic lines of forces were attracted toward the ferromagnetic material, so a very good shape of ball at the tool tip was formed; hence, a good finishing rate was achieved. But in the case of non-magnetic material, almost all magnetic lines of forces were diverted from inner core to outer core; hence,

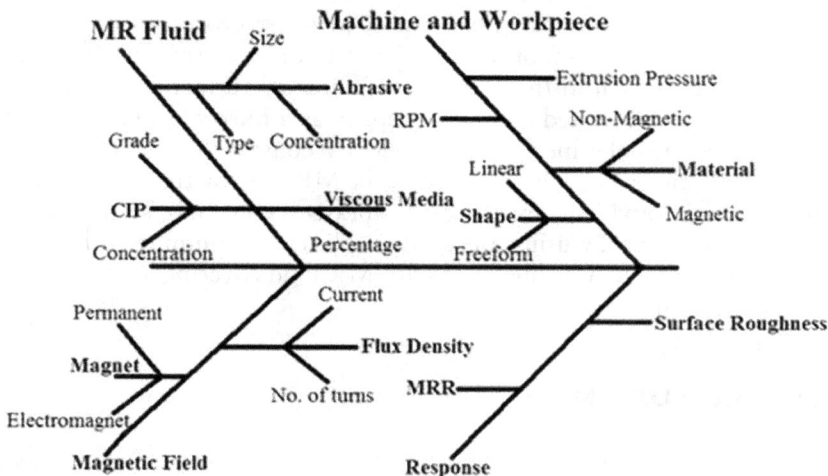

Figure 12.8 Process parameters of MRAFF.

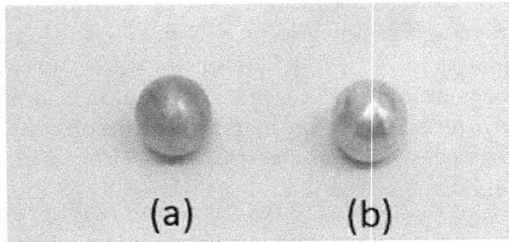

Figure 12.9 Images of (a) unfinished brass ball and (b) finished ball.

the finishing performance decreased. To overcome this problem, MRAH was developed, in which freeform diamagnetic copper alloy was finished. Around 55% improvement in roughness value was obtained with the spherical-shaped brass workpiece, as shown in Figure 12.9. A few more cycles are required to finish non-magnetic materials as compared to magnetic materials. The flexible brush in MRF processes had less contact area to the curved profile as compared to a flat surface. Due to this, there was a large deviation in the roughness value of the knee joint implant during finishing. The investigators invented the setup of the process known as R-MRAFF (rotational magnetorheological abrasive flow finishing), in which the communication time of abrasive particles with the workpiece was increased through the employment of rotation of MR fluid by the use of a rotating magnet [39]. The rotational speed of the magnet was noticed as the most significant parameter during the experiments. A finishing value of 16 nm was achieved with a stainless steel tube. The average finishing rate of R-MRAFF was found to be two times higher than that of the MRFF process. However, one common limitation of both MRFF and R-MRAFF processes was that the medium flow velocity cannot remain constant for freeform surfaces; due to this, a large variation in the surface roughness of all faces was observed. The researchers fabricated a negative replica as a fixture of the knee joint, which maintained the medium flow velocity constant during the process [58,59]. Vibrations were also induced in the MR fluid by the pulsative magnetic field, due to which new and more abrasives come in contact with the freeform knee joint. By using a negative replica, the minimum variation in final roughness value was observed with MR fluid covering a large area on the workpiece that reduces the finishing time.

12.3 CONCLUSIONS

The ABNPs are nano-finishing techniques, in which multiple abrasive grains are implemented as a cutting tool. In this chapter, various published technological papers on MRAFF, MRF, and AFM are reviewed with their particle mechanism during the process. AFM processes are frequently used for finishing complex or intricate 3D geometries for a high level of surface finishing values with tighter tolerances over dimensions. However, the major disadvantage of AFM is its low finishing rate. To get rid of these difficulties, many modifications have been tried. In MAAF processes, the magnetic field governs as well as controls the forces that are involved during the finishing action. The MAAF is a magnetorheological fluid-centered process; thus, most of its parameters are related to MR fluid. The processes BEMRF, MRFF, MFAF, and MRAFF are discussed under magnetorheological finishing processes. In BEMRF processes, the flexible brush at the tool tip adjusts its shape according to the curvature of the workpiece. The MRAFF is the combination of both MRF and AFM processes. R-MRAFF and MRAH are the new developments in the MRAFF process. These ABNPs have revolutionized the field of industrial components, electronics, medical, and optics. Based on the literature review, some research gaps are recognized and discussed:

- In the ABNPs, the material is removed at the atomic level, so it is hard to know the mechanism by FEM or any investigative tool. To understand the cutting mechanism in ABNPs, the MDS likely to be a future research trend [13].
- To reduce the cost and increase mass production, it is required to develop a tool and fixture for numerous components and complex shapes. In magnetic-assisted processes, a magnet fixture needs to be designed for providing uniform magnetic field and concentrating the magnetic lines on freeform surfaces [60].
- The AFM processes rely on the viscoelastic abrasive fluid. Temperature rise and sedimentation are the inconveniences linked with the abrasive-laden medium. The shear viscosity of the medium decreases when the process progresses, due to which the finishing capability of the medium decreases [61]. There is a need to model the temperature change during the process, and their relation with viscosity is important for providing more insight into medium characteristics. To increase the finishing rate, it is also necessary to use a variety of carriers in MR fluid along with some chemical reactions to soften the hard topography with the support of abrasive particles.

REFERENCES

1. Zhong, Z. W. (2008). Recent advances in polishing of advanced materials. *Materials and Manufacturing Processes*, 23, 449–456.
2. Han, R., Sampurno, Y., & Philipossian, A. (2017). Fractional in situ pad conditioning in chemical mechanical planarization. *Tribology Letters*, 65(21), 1–6.

3. Kumari, C., & Chak, S. K. (2018). A review on magnetically assisted abrasive finishing and their critical process parameters. *Manufacturing Review*, 5(13), 1–16.

4. Petare, A. C., & Jain, N. K. (2018). A critical review of past research and advances in abrasive flow finishing process. *The International Journal of Advanced Manufacturing Technology*, 97, 741–782.

5. Hayashi Hayashi, K., & Suzuki, H. (2004). CMP cross-correlation analysis of multi-channel surface-wave. *Exploation Geophysics*, 35, 7–13.

6. Mahajan, K., Pawade, R., & Balasubramaniam, R. (2021). Experimental study of effect of machining parameters on PMMA in diamond turning. In H. K. Dave & D. Nedelcu (Eds.), *Advances in Manufacturing Processes*. Lecture Notes in Mechanical Engineering. Springer, Singapore.

7. Shiou, F. J., Chen, C. C. A., & Li, W. T. (2006). Automated surface finishing of plastic injection mold steel with spherical grinding and ball burnishing processes. *International Journal of Advanced Manufacturing Technology*, 28(1–2), 61–66.

8. Ein-Eli, Y., & Starosvetsky, D. (2007). Review on copper chemical-mechanical polishing (CMP) and post-CMP cleaning in ultra large system integrated (ULSI)-An electrochemical perspective. *Electrochimica Acta*, 52(5), 1825–1838.

9. Pereira, L. C., Arencibia, R. V., Schramm, C. R., & Arantes, L. J. (2018). Assessment of the effect of cutting parameters on roughness in flexible honed cylinders. *International Journal of Advanced Manufacturing Technology*, 95(1–4), 181–196.

10. Bedi, T. C., & Singh, A. K. (2015). Magnetorheological methods for nano finishing-A review. *Particulate Science and Technology: An International Journal*, 34, 412–422.

11. Kozak, J., & Oczos, K. E. (2001). Selected problems of abrasive hybrid machining, *Journal of Materials Processing Technology*, 109(3), 360–366.

12. McCarty, R. W. (1970). Method of honing by extruding (No. 3521412). United States.

13. Jain, V., Sidpara, A., Sankar, M., & Das, M. (2012). Nano-finishing techniques: A review. *Proceedings of the Institution of Mechanical Engineers, Part C*, 226, 327–346.

14. Varghese, V., Ramesh, M. R., & Chakradhar, D. (2018). Experimental investigation and optimization of machining parameters for sustainable machining. *Materials and Manufacturing Processes*, 33(16), 1782–1792.

15. Feng, G., Liu, Q., Guo, W., Xin, Y., & Liang, Q. (2018). Experimental investigations on nanogrinding of RB-SiC wafers. *Materials and Manufacturing Processes*, 33(9), 1030–1035.

16. Sedighi, M., Nasrollahi, M., & Joudaki, J. (2019). Surface integrity in broaching of AA 7075-T651 aluminum alloys. *Machining Science and Technology*, 23(1), 79–94.

17. Fang, L., Zhao, J., Sun, K., Zheng, D., & Ma, D. (2009). Temperature as sensitive monitor for efficiency of work in abrasive flow machining. *Wear*, 266, 678–687.

18. Liu, G., Zhang, X., Zang, X., Li, J., & Su, N. (2018). Study on whole factorial experiment of polishing the micro-hole in non-linear tubes by abrasive flow. *Advances in Mechanical Engineering*, 10(8), 1–15.

19. Kavithaa, T. S., Balashanmugam, N., & Kumar, P. V. S. (2014). Abrasive flow finishing process - a case study. *5th International & 26th All India Manufacturing Technology, Design and Research Conference (AIMTDR 2014)*, pp. 1–5. IIT Guwahati, Assam, India.

20. Jain, R. K., & Jain, V. K. (1999). Simulation of surface generated in abrasive flow machining process. *Robotics and Computer-Integrated Manufacturing, 15*, 403–412.

21. Sarkar, M., & Jain, V. K. (2017). Nanofinishing of freeform surfaces using abrasive flow finishing process. *Proceedings of the Institution of Mechanical Engineers, Part B: Journal of Engineering Manufacture, 231*(9), 1501–1515.

22. Kordonski, W. I., & Jacobs, S. D. (1996). Magnetorheological finishing. *International Journal of Modern Physics B, 10*(23–24), 2837–2848.

23. Saraswathamma, K., Jha, S., & Rao, P. V. (2015). Experimental investigation into Ball end Magnetorheological Finishing of silicon. *Precision Engineering, 42*, 218–223.

24. Sidpara, A. M., & Jain, V. K. (2012). Nanofinishing of freeform surfaces of prosthetic knee joint implant. *Proceedings of the Institution of Mechanical Engineers, Part B: Journal of Engineering Manufacture, 226*(11), 1833–1846.

25. Jha, S., & Jain, V. K. (2004). Design and development of the magnetorheological abrasive flow finishing (MRAFF) process. *International Journal of Machine Tools & Manufacture, 44*, 1019–1029.

26. Kumar, S., Jain, V. K., & Sidpara, A. (2015). Nanofinishing of freeform surfaces (knee joint implant) by rotational-magnetorheological abrasive flow finishing (R-MRAFF) process. *Precision Engineering, 42*, 165–178.

27. Rhoades, L., & Kohut, T. (1991). Reversible unidirectional AFM (No. 5070652). USA.

28. Rhoades, L., Kohut, T., Nokovich, N., & Yanda, D. (1994). Unidirectional abrasive flow machining (No. 5367833). United States.

29. Sankar, M. R., Ramkumar, J., & Jain, V. K. (2009). Experimental investigation and mechanism of material removal in nano finishing of MMCs using abrasive flow finishing (AFF) process. *Wear, 266*, 688–698.

30. Sidpara, A., & Jain, V. K. (2012). Nano-level finishing of single crystal silicon blank using magnetorheological finishing process. *Tribology International, 47*, 159–166.

31. Singh, S., Shan, H. S., & Kumar, P. (2002). Wear behavior of materials in magnetically assisted abrasive flow machining. *Journal of Materials Processing Technology, 128*, 155–161.

32. Sharma, A. K., Venkatesh, G., Rajesha, S., & Kumar, P. (2015). Experimental investigations into ultrasonic-assisted abrasive flow machining (UAAFM) process. *International Journal of Advanced Manufacturing Technology, 80*(1–4), 477–493.

33. Singh, A. K., Jha, S., & Pandey, P. M. P. (2013). Mechanism of material removal in ball end magnetorheological finishing process. *Wear, 302*, 1180–1191.

34. Singh, A. K., Jha, S., & Pandey, P. M. (2012). Nanofinishing of a typical 3D ferromagnetic workpiece using ball end magnetorheological finishing process. *International Journal of Machine Tools and Manufacture, 63*, 21–31.

35. Golini, D., Kordonski, W. I., Dumas, P., & Hogan, S. (1999). Magnetorheological finishing (MRF) in commercial precision optics manufacturing. *Part of the SPIE Conference on Optical Manufacturing and Testing III*, 3782, 80–91.

36. Kordonski, W. I., & Golini, D. (1999). Fundamentals of magnetorheological fluid utilization in high precision finishing. *Electro-Rheological Fluids and Magneto-Rheological Suspensions*, 10(9), 682–692.

37. Paul, P. S., Varadarajan, A. S., & Mohanasundaram, S. (2014). Effect of magnetorheological fluid on tool wear during hard turning with minimal fluid application. *Archives of Civil and Mechanical Engineering*, 15, 124–132.

38. Saraswathamma, K. (2014). Magnetorheological finishing: A review. *International Journal of Current Engineering and Technology*, 30(2), 168–173.

39. Das, M., Jain, V., & Ghoshdastidar, P. S. (2010). Nano-finishing of stainless-steel tubes using rotational magnetorheological abrasive flow finishing process. *Machining Science and Technology: An International Journal*, 14(3), 365–389.

40. Sadiq, A., & Shunmugam, M. S. (2009). Investigation into magnetorheological abrasive honing (MRAH). *International Journal of Machine Tools and Manufacture*, 49(7–8), 554–560.

41. Khatri, N., Manoj, J. X., Mishra, V., Garg, H., & Karar, V. (2018). Experimental and simulation study of nanometric surface roughness generated during Magnetorheological finishing of Silicon. *Materials Today: Proceedings*, 5(2), 6391–6400.

42. Jha, S., Jain, V. K., & Komanduri, R., (2006). Effect of extrusion pressure and number of finishing cycles on surface roughness in magnetorheological abrasive flow finishing (MRAFF) process. *International Journal of Advanced Manufacturing Technology*, 33, 725–729.

43. Kumari, C., Chak, S. K., & Vani, V. V. (2020). Experimental investigations and optimization of machining parameters for Magneto-rheological Abrasive Honing process. *Materials and Manufacturing Processes*, 35(14), 1622–1630.

44. Kumari, C., & Chak, S. K. (2021). Experimental studies on material removal behavior in MRAH based finishing technique. *Materials and Manufacturing Processes*, 36(8), 916–925.

45. Uhlmann, E., Schmiedel, C., & Wendler, J. (2015). CFD simulation of the abrasive flow machining process. *Procedia CIRP*, 31, 209–214.

46. Walia, R. S., Shan, H. S., & Kumar, P. (2006). Abrasive flow machining with additional centrifugal force applied to the media. *Machining Science and Technology*, 10(3), 341–354.

47. Jones, A. R., & Hull, J. B. (1998). Ultrasonic flow polishing. *Ultrasonics*, 36, 97–101.

48. Sankar, M.R., Jain, V. K., Ramkumar, J., Sareen, S. K., & Singh, S. (2019). Medium rheological characterization and performance study during rotational abrasive flow finishing (R-AFF) of Al alloy and Al alloy/SiC MMCs. *The International Journal of Advanced Manufacturing Technology*, 100, 1149–1163.

49. Dabrowski, L., Marciniak, M., & Szewczyk, T. (2006). Analysis of abrasive flow machining with an electrochemical process aid. *Proceedings of the Institution of Mechanical Engineers, Part B: Journal of Engineering Manufacture*, 220, 397–403.

50. Singh, S., & Shan, H. S. (2002). Development of magneto abrasive flow machining process. *International Journal of Machine Tools and Manufacture*, 42, 953–959.

51. Sidpara, A. (2014). Magnetorheological finishing: A perfect solution to nano-finishing requirements. *Optical Engineering*, 53(9), 092002.

52. Singh, A., Jha, J., & Pandey, P. (2011). Design and development of nanofinishing process for 3D surfaces using ball end MR finishing tool. *International Journal of Machine Tools and Manufacture*, 51, 142–151.

53. Kansal, H., Singh, A. K., & Grover, V. (2018). Magnetorheological nano-finishing of diamagnetic material using permanent magnets tool. *Precision Engineering*, 51, 30–39.

54. Barman, A., & Das, M. (2017). Design and fabrication of a novel polishing tool for finishing freeform surfaces in magnetic field assisted finishing (MFAF) process. *Precision Engineering*, 49, 61–68.

55. Ranjan, P., Balasubramaniam, R., & Jain, V. K. (2017). Analysis of magneto-rheological fluid behavior in chemo-mechanical magnetorheological finishing (CMMRF) process. *Precision Engineering*, 49, 122–135.

56. Sihag, N., Kala, P., & Pandey, P. M. (2017). Analysis of surface finish improvement during ultrasonic assisted magnetic abrasive finishing on chemically treated tungsten substrate. *Procedia Manufacturing*, 10, 136–146.

57. Alam, Z., Khan, D. A., & Jha, S. (2019). MR fluid-based novel finishing process for nonplanar copper mirrors. *The International Journal of Advanced Manufacturing Technology*, 101, 995–1006.

58. Nagdeve, L., Jain, V. K., & Ramkumar, J. (2016). Experimental investigations into nano-finishing of freeform surfaces using negative replica of the knee joint. *Procedia CIRP*, 42, 793–798.

59. Nagdeve, L., Sidpara, A., Jain, V. K., & Ramkumar, J. (2018). On the effect of relative size of magnetic particles and abrasive particles in MR fluid-based finishing process. Machining Science and Technology, 22(3), 493–506.

60. Nagdeve, L., Jain, V. K., & Ramkumar, J. (2018). Differential finishing of freeform surfaces (knee joint) using R-MRAFF process and negative replica of workpiece as a fixture. *Machining Science and Technology*, 22(4), 671–695.

61. Cheema, M. S., Venkatesh, G., Dvivedi, A., & Sharma, A. K. (2012). Developments in abrasive flow machining: A review on experimental investigations using abrasive flow machining variants and media. *Proceedings of the Institution of Mechanical Engineers, Part B: Journal of Engineering Manufacture*, 226(12), 1951–1962.

Chapter 13

Thermal and dynamic mechanical analysis of oil palm mesocarp fiber/Kondagogu gum biocomposites

V. Srikanth and K. Raja Narender Reddy
Kakatiya Institute of Technology and Science Warangal

CONTENTS

13.1 INTRODUCTION

Modern technology has brought many benefits for mankind. However, it is evident that the environment is considerably affected and damaged by non-degradable disposable products. Thus, renewable sources of sustainable materials, which are new and very important for the materials industry in the 21st century, are needed not only to address the growing environmental threat, but also to address the uncertainty of oil supply [1,2]. In this scenario, research is in progress for alternate materials with high degree of basic strength and rigidity, and natural and ecological consistency. To make the revolution of biofuels a reality, scientists and engineers must create the necessary technologies [3,4]. A significant number of new biological products have been researched since 1990, such as plant-based biologic resins [5,6]; plant oil bio-resins [7]; maize polylactic acid (PLA); soy protein adhesives; soy polyurethane products; soy and maize oil solvents; vegetable oil lubricants; soy and maize thermal polymers; organic acids; polymers based on oils, such as polyethylene (PE) and polypropylene (PP); or biopolymers such as PLA, polyhydroxyalkanoates, and cellulose esters, mixed with lignocellulosic fiber and biocomposites [8–10]. Nonetheless, because petroleum is a non-renewable resource, greater emphasis is placed on renewable, totally sustainable plant polymers and fibers.

The principal trees of exudate gum include gum arabic, gum karaya, gum tragacanth, Kondagogu gum (KGG), and ghatti. Indian forests constitute a significant source of non-wood forest products harvested by tribals in Telangana and Andhra Pradesh [11]. KGG biopolymers, in particular, are non-toxic. Polysaccharides are derived from the bark of the Indian-native Cochlospermum gossypium tree (family Bixaceae). KGG is extracted from the tree barks. The entire amount of gum is created with in the first 24 hours and it continues for several days [12]. The gum is reinforced in tears. Exudate gums offer a unique set of functions and features that no other synthetic polymer will ever be able to match. The morphological, physicochemical, rheological, compositional, solution, reactive, emulsifying, and metal biomass properties have been described to maximize potential commercial applications [13–15]. KGG is a highly contented gum with major functional groups such as acetyl, hydroxyl, carboxylic, and carbonyl groups [16]. In particular, the synthetic, glass and carbon fiber-enhanced composites, because of their lightweight and excellent performance, are used wildly in the vehicles and aircraft industries. Many researchers tried to replace synthetic and glass fibers with natural fibers in order to solve these problems. Oil palm mesocarp fiber (OPMF) is considered to be one of the highest potential candidates compared to other natural fibers because of its high modulus and strength [17]. Because of its superior properties, OPMF-strengthened composites have attracted many researchers' attention. Currently, there are numerous reports of different preparation conditions such as matrix type and water absorption effects of OPM composites. In particular, OPMF length with surface treatment and OPM material affected the mechanical features of OPM composites [18]. Despite their many benefits, OPM composites' mechanical qualities are underappreciated due to poor interfacial adhesion between the fiber and the matrix [19,20]. Several works on chemical modification has been performed to improve OPMF adhesion to the polymeric matrix [21]. The chemical treatment procedure is one of the most effective methods focused on improving the mechanical properties of composites. The analysis of thermal properties is a critical instrument in the analysis of the relation between the structure and property and the thermal stability of natural fiber composites. Differential scanning calorimetry (DSC) can detect temperature and heat flow connected to material changes depending on time and temperature. The volatile component and moisture content in the composite can also be determined with thermogravimetric analysis (TGA) [22,23]. Tan delta (Tan) analyzes the material's damping capabilities in the glass transition area, offering insight into the interplay between natural fiber reinforcing and polymer patterns in the glass-transition area, whereas this DMA monitors the energy wasted as heat, representing the viscous pattern [24–26].

Research on natural fiber resources must be continued and encouraged. A simple extractive process that does not affect the characteristics of a fiber must be developed. During the current study, the fiber is extracted from oil palm tree and KGG is the newly identified matrix. Alkali treatment process is used to remove the lignin, wax and oil contents in the fiber then hand layup technique process is used to prepare the composites. Subsequently, this research investigated treated and untreated fabricated OPMF/KGG composites and evaluated their viscoelastic properties using DMA and thermal properties using thermogravimetric analysis (TGA). In addition, DSC was also used.

13.2 MATERIALS AND METHODS

13.2.1 Materials

The material was purchased from the Nutriroma Pvt. Ltd., Hyderabad, Telangana State, India, as the matrix KGG grade 1 (Cochlospermum gossypium) powder. Glutaraldehyde (25% purified), glycerol (98% purified), ammonia (25% purified), distilled water, pH paper, HCl, and NaOH were purchased from Rekha chemicals, Hanamkonda, Warangal, Telangana State, India.

13.2.1.1 Alkali treatment

Oil palm mesocarp fiber (OPMF) was collected from 3F Oil Palm Industry in Yernagudem, Devarapalle, West Godavari, Andhra Pradesh, India. Figure 13.1 depicts the extraction of fibers. Initially, a portion of OPMF with an average length of 20–30 mm was treated with 2% aqueous solution of sodium hydroxide (NaOH) at room temperature. To eliminate hemicellulose and other oily impurities, the fibers were soaked in an alkali solution for 24 hours. The fibers were then rinsed many times with water and neutralized with weak acetic acid. Finally, the fibers were rinsed in distilled water and dried for 24–48 hours at room temperature. Dried OPMF was kept at room temperature in a sealed plastic bag until use.

13.2.1.2 Preparation of resin

By using the throwing technique, we show below the development of KGG resin. Figure 13.2 shows the necessary amounts of KGG powder with the weighing balance system are correctly measured and subsequently delivered

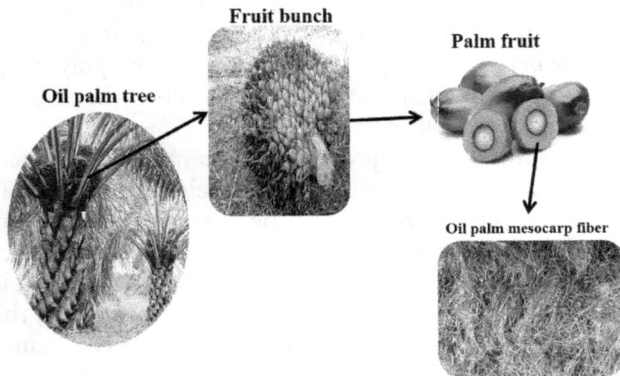

Figure 13.1 Fiber extraction process.

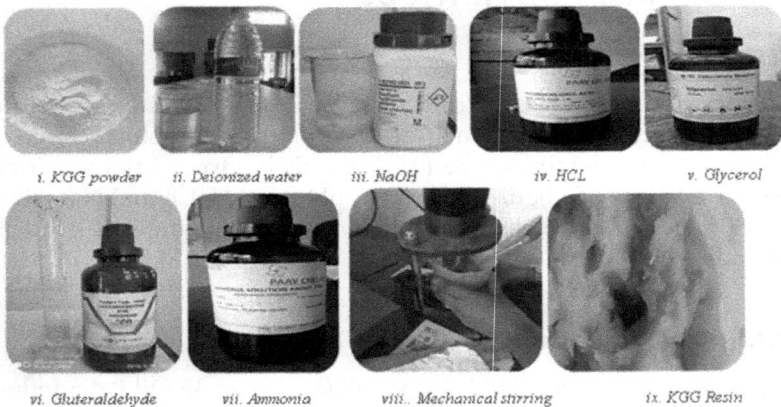

Figure 13.2 Preparation of KGG resin.

in a clean glass beaker and applied to the deionized water (2.5 times KGG). The mixture of material (KGG powder+distilled water) is stirred at room temperature for 20–30 minutes with a mechanical stirrer; afterward, to neutralize the solution of gum, add 1M NaOH and 1M HCl. Then after continuous incubation for 20 minutes, glycerol, glutaraldehyde, and ammonia each 25%–30% by wt. of KGG powder are weighed separately and mixed with the earlier gum solution to obtain a pH of 7–8.

13.2.1.3 Fabrication of biocomposites

A glass mold with dimensions of 150×150×3 mm was utilized to make the composites. The laminates were created with KGG resin; the mold was then filled with a random orientation of mixture of resin and OPMF (4 mm length) with fiber content (5% wt.) and kept at room temperature for 48 hours. The specimens were removed from the mold once the laminates were hardened; samples of suitable dimensions were cut for determining the mechanical and thermal properties, as per ASTM specifications.

13.2.2 Methods

13.2.2.1 Dynamic mechanical analysis (DMA)

DMA was performed using SEIKO SII EXSTAR 6100 DMS (Figure 13.3), Germany make. At a frequency of 1 Hz, the experiment was carried out in three-point bending mode. Under a controlled sinusoidal strain, the temperature was escalated from 25°C to 300°C at a rate of 5°C/min. As per the standard of ASTM D5023, DMA specimens of dimensions 50 mm×10 mm×3 mm are obtained.

13.2.2.2 Differential scanning calorimetry (DSC)

The DSC test was performed on PerkinElmer's TA DSC800 (Figure 13.4) equipment in a nitrogen environment (50 mL/min) at a heating rate of 5°C/min in the temperature range of 25°C–250°C. Samples of approximately 8–20 mg were placed in Al (aluminum) pan for testing using DSC. This study was conducted to determine the glass transition temperature (T_g).

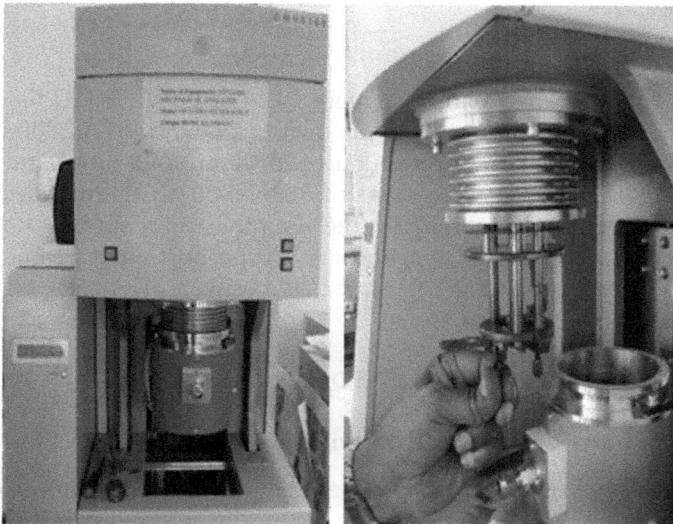

Figure 13.3 Dynamic mechanical analysis test setup.

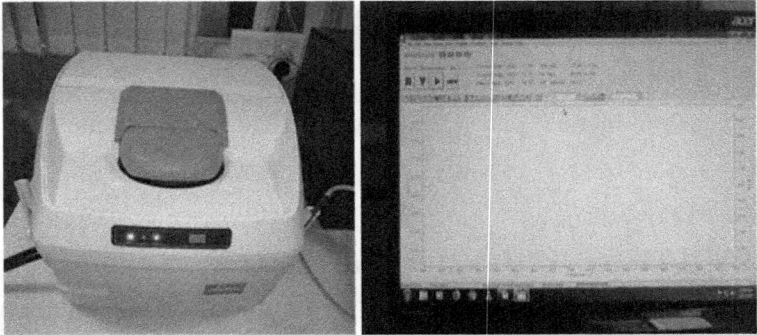

Figure 13.4 Differential scanning calorimetry testing setup.

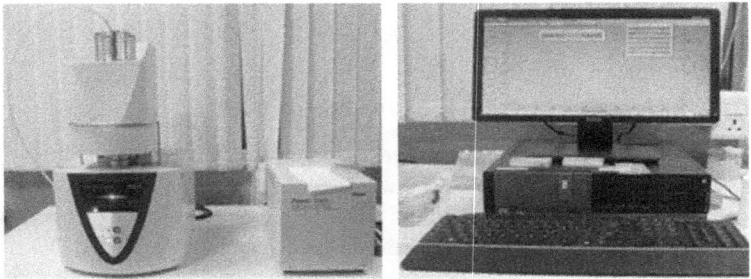

Figure 13.5 Equipment of thermogravimetric analysis.

13.2.2.3 Thermogravimetric analysis (TGA)

The thermogravimetric analysis (Figure 13.5) of OPMF/KGG biocomposites was performed using a thermogravimetric analyzer (STA 2500 Regulus, NETZCH, Germany) at a heating rate of 5°C/min in a nitric atmosphere. At the scheduled temperature range of 30°C–800°C, thermal decomposition of all specimens occurred. In the sample bath, a sample of 5–15 mg was heated. It increased the temperature. The proportion of weight loss as a function of temperature has been calculated using a TGA curve.

13.3 RESULTS AND DISCUSSION

13.3.1 Dynamic mechanical analysis properties

The storage capacity is the cumulative energy that is stored in the material in one operating cycle. It indicates the composite material's rigidity and the load-bearing power. Figure 13.6 shows that the dynamic storage modulus

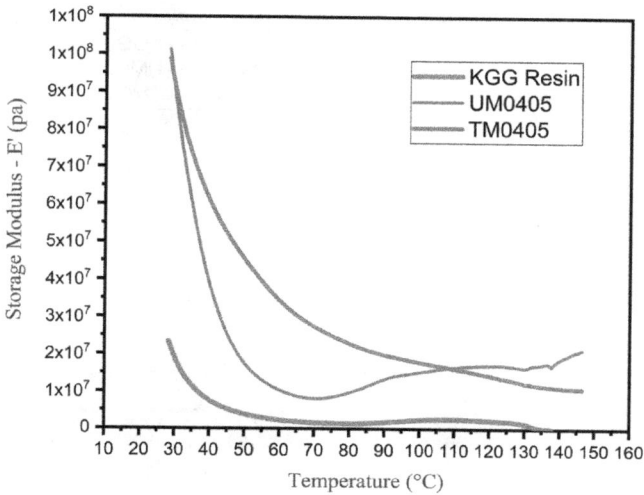

Figure 13.6 Effect of storage modulus on pure KGG resin and surface treatment on OPMF/KGG composites. Note: UM0405; TM0405: UM – untreated meso-carp; TM – treated mesocarp; 04 – length of fiber; 05 – fiber's weight %.

of untreated and alkalized OPMF with KGG resin depends on temperature. Reinforced fiber composites have a higher storage modulus than KGG resin that is not reinforced.

This is because the clean KGG resin, which only contains the matrix, gives the material greater durability, resulting in lower rigidity and therefore a low storage frame. The rigidity of composites increases when OPMF is incorporated into the KGG matrix and results in an improved storage module. In addition, fibers may be inserted into the matrix, which improves the storage modulus at the interface. The optimized OPMF/KGG biocomposites has been found to be lower to 4 mm in length, a 05% wt. biocomposite, in storage modulus for KGG resin (UM0405). In general, however, at a temperature of 69°C (TM0405), the storage cycle is greater than that of pure KGG composites. The treated mesocarp fiber (TM0405) composite's storage modulus is 2.74×10^7 Pa.

Among the OPMF-reinforced composites, when compared to the untreated composites and resin, the treated composites have a better storage modulus. Higher hydrophilicity of the lignocellulosic royal palm fibers induces poor weathering in untreated fiber composites, and an increased moisture level of a fiber-matrix interface helps to create a vacuum, which results in less stiffness and power. When alkaline treatment is applied to the fiber, lignin and hemicellulose are removed from the fiber, providing a rough surface that improves the interaction between the fiber and matrix. Interlocking often induces fibrillation, i.e., the splitting into smaller fibers of the fibers, which will increase the usable surface area of the matrix material

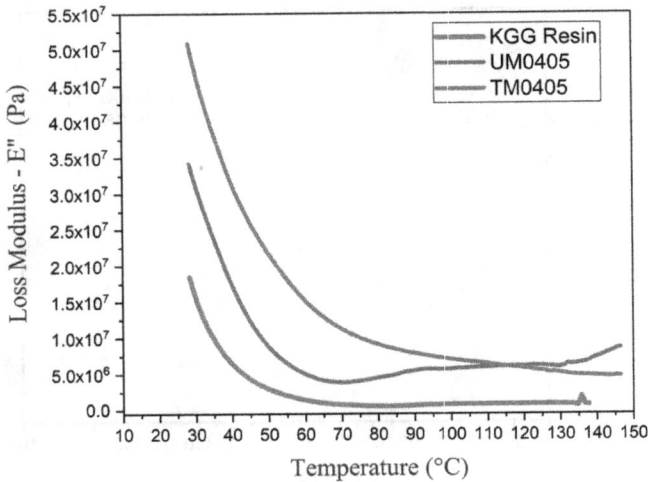

Figure 13.7 **Effect of loss modulus on KGG resin and surface treatment on OPMF/KGG composites.**

available for wetting. The fibers' aspect ratio increases and causes rough topography of the area following fibrillation due to reduced fibers, which provides a stronger interface of the fiber matrix. As a result, improved rigidity and increased storage modulus are achieved.

Loss Modulus

The loss modulus (E') is a dissipated or loss energy metric for heat when diverse systems are evaluated at the same strain deformation, per period of sinusoidal deformation. The material's viscous reaction is more sensitive to the composites' molecular motions. The loss modulus in Figure 13.7 is higher in TM0405 composites compared to UM0405 and KGG alone. The highest value is seen at 76°C, and in all the composites, a large drop in the loss modulus is seen as the interface between fibers and matrices is reduced or the frictional stability between them at higher temperatures decreases. In the transition region, the composite's loss modulus for low fiber material must be low as the internal friction it induces must be increased.

Tan δ

The ratio of the loss modulus to the storage modulus is known as mechanical damping (tan δ), and it is linked to biopolymeric mobility. Tan δ refers to a material's resistance to impact and movement inside a matrix structure made up of tiny groups and chains of molecules. Therefore, molecular mobility will be greater than the peak value of tan δ. Figure 13.8 and Table 13.1 show the variability of the tan δ of pure KGG and the composites depending on the temperature.

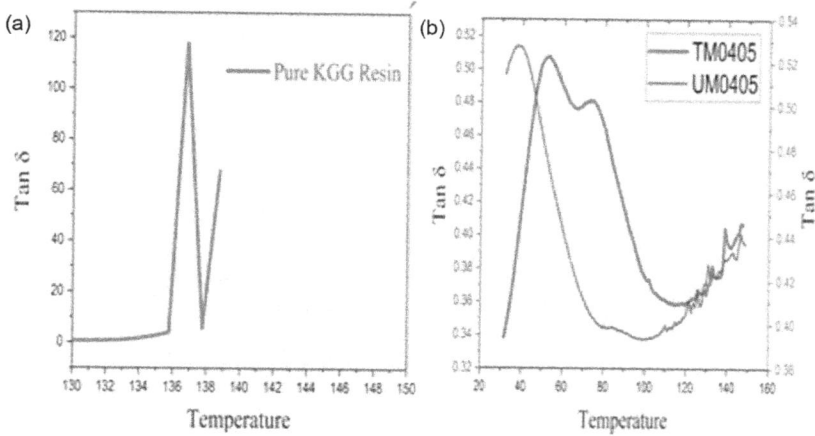

Figure 13.8 Tan δ effect at different temperatures: (a) pure KGG resin; (b) treated and untreated laminates.

Table 13.1 Composites of loss modulus and damping factor

Sample	T_g (°C) obtained from loss modulus curve	Loss modulus (Pa)	Damping factor (tan δ_{max})	Temperature (°C) at tan δ_{max}
KGG resin	50.18	29.39×10^3	117.92	135.5
TM0405	76.03	98.01×10^3	0.50	52.02
UM0405	63.70	43.22×10^3	0.53	333.04

The damping values have been discovered to be lower in the reinforced fibers than in the pure KGG due to the combination of the fibers acting as barriers and stability tests on the matrix chains. The lower damping values in fiber-reinforced composites are also due to the reduction in matrix weight required for vibration energy dissipation. The results show that treated 4 mm length 5% wt. fiber reinforced composite has a lower tan δ value than untreated composites because alkaline treatments create a strong and stiff interface between the fiber and the matrix. The interface field's molecular mobility will be diminished. Surface treatments also enhance the degree of interface connectivity, which prevents molecular mobility leading to low damping values. The treated fibers, relative to the alkaline-treated fiber composites, had greater damping values than unrefined fiber composites, which suggests a lower fiber-matrix interface.

13.3.2 Differential scanning calorimetry (DSC)

Figure 13.9 demonstrates the melting and crystallization behavior, using DSC, of pure KGG resin and optimized OPMF/KGG biocomposites with and without surface treatment. Table 13.2 shows different temperatures

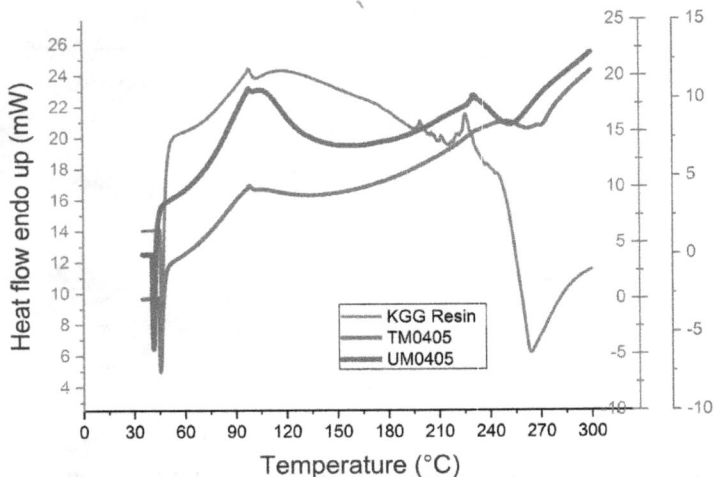

Figure 13.9 DSC curves of resin and OPMF/KGG biocomposites.

Table 13.2 DSC data for pure resin and OPMF/KGG biocomposites

Sample	T_g (°C)	$T_{s,c}$ (°C)	$T_{e,c}$ (°C)	T_c (°C)	$T_{s,m}$ (°C)	$T_{e,m}$ (°C)	T_m (°C)	ΔH_{fusion} (J/g)	ΔH_{Cryst} (J/g)	C_p (J/gc)
KGG resin	46	65	103	99	248	288	263	3162	3377	128
TM0405	46	60	114	99	254	279	262	2167	3975	21.49
UM0405	42	60	108	99	232	284	252	2689	5740	34.45

were observed between 0°C–100°C, 100°C–200°C, and 200°C–300°C in the melting temperature (T_m), crystallization temperature (T_c) and fusion heat (ΔH_m) and thermal degradation of biocomposites at treated, untreated and neat KGG resin compounds. The thermal characteristics vary due to differences in the segments of the fiber cell structure, indicating deterioration over a wide range of temperature. The first step relates to the low-temperature deterioration that turns humidity into vapor. The lowest value for this point suggests that the glass transfer temperature was measured at 46°C, 46°C, and 42°C for pure resin and bio-based composites. Temperature of crystallization of the bio-based composites (T_c) was known to be the temperature at the highest point of the dip. The latent energy of crystallization was also determined from the region of the dip of bio-based composites. Yet most importantly, the dip also suggests that the biocomposites are crystallized. It is because the bio-based composites absorb heat as crystallization happens, which makes crystallization an endothermic process. The crystallization temperature (T_c) of KGG and KGG bio-based composites was at 99°C. The degradation of hemicellulose and a portion of the lignin is reflected in the second stage. Hemicellulose is a polysaccharide similar to cellulose, except that it is made of multiple single sugars that form short chains of monomers. In the field, it also functions as a diverse support for the cell wall. The sharp peaks at 263°C, 262°C, and 252°C show the melting point, respectively, of pure resin, treated, and untreated biocomposites. The final stage refers to a high-temperature zone when cellulose is completely degraded, and most of the lignin in bio-based composites is removed.

13.3.3 Thermogravimetric analysis (TGA)

The TGA can explain how loss of weight changes the physical and chemical characteristics of composites with rising temperature. In thermally sensitive applications, the findings of these tests may be valuable. As shown in Figure 13.10 (a) weight loss with respect to the temperature and Figure 13.10 (b) displays DTG curves (derivative thermogravimetric) are representing the analysis of neat KGG resin and treated, untreated fiber loading conditions of 04/05 (L/W) by length and weight fraction. TGA has evaluated the thermal stability of biocomposites at a temperature of 10°C/min and 25°C~250°C. The following TGA indices were evaluated using continuous temperature and weight loss records: thermal degradation rate (percent weight loss/min), beginning temperature degradation, and residual weight. The temperature weight loss data shown in Figure 13.10a were analyzed to determine the thermal stability of the samples, and the thermal stability of KGG resin is much higher than that of the treated and untreated biocomposites. The thermal stability did not differ significantly between treated and untreated biocomposites. The samples were all thermally stable between 50°C and 62°C. The sample has a much higher thermal stability than other OPMF/KGG biocomposites. Through the TGA curve, a weight loss in three stages was observed. Below 70°C, the degradation happens as a result of the absorbed

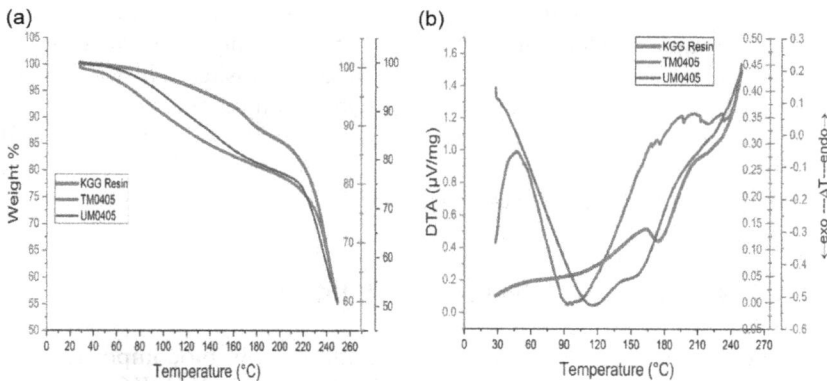

Figure 13.10 Thermogravimetric curves of pure resin and OPMF/KGG biocomposites: (a) weight loss; (b) derivative weight loss.

Table 13.3 TGA of OPMF/KGG biocomposites

Designation	T_{on} (°C)	T_{max} (°C)	Weight loss at min (wt. %)	Weight loss at max (wt. %)
KGG resin	200	250	14.64	55.13
TM0405	206	250	19.27	59.34
UM0405	205	250	23.26	39.70

moisture evaporating. The first state occurs around 70°C–195°C due to lignin degradation; the second state occurs around 200°C–250°C due to cellulose degradation, hemicellulose, and biopolymers; and the third state occurs around 200°C–250°C. Both samples were reported to have a modest weight loss at 140°C. Due to the initial decomposition of cellulose and hemicellulose and the temperature of the sample, the next weight loss of all the samples began at around 205°C. However, for OPMF-treated and untreated with KGG, only one peak for the degradation of cellulose was seen, which is probably because the gums from the fibers were removed. At a temperature of 250°C, samples were found to completely disintegrate into char and all combustible components. It is also clear that the gross weight losses from decompositions in pure KGG resin, treated, and untreated OPMF/KGG biocomposites were 55.5%, 59.68%, and 39.8%, respectively.

A substantial peak can be seen in this region on DTA curve in Figure 13.10b, which could be attributed to hemicellulose thermal depolymerization and cleavage of cellulose's glucosidic linkages. The method is an endothermic one. For all cases, the DTA curve indicates an exothermic slope at the first point of degradation. This rise may be attributed to the effect of volatilization. The development of charred residue is aided by the breakdown of second-stage (second peak) decomposition products. The third endothermal peak on the oxidation and burning of high molecular weight residues is represented by the DTA curve. Most of the composites are decomposed completely at around 250°C. Table 13.3 shows the weight loss with respect to different temperatures in untreated and treated composites. The thermal stability of KGG resin, and treated and untreated composites is demonstrated in the table. KGG resin thermal stability is greater than that of OPMF/KGG biocomposites. KGG resin is stable up to 175°C, while alkali-treated and untreated biocomposites are stable up to 118°C and 94°C, respectively.

13.4 CONCLUSIONS AND FUTURE SCOPE

This study focuses on the successful creation of new biocomposites from sustainable materials based on chemically modified OPMF/KGG biocomposites. The following conclusions are drawn. DMA, DSC, and TGA methods were used to characterize the thermal properties:

- The surface modification impact on the dynamic mechanical analysis of OPMF/KGG biocomposites was discussed. Because of the reinforcement effect of the fibers, the storage and loss moduli of reinforced composites were found to be higher when compared to neat KGG resin, resulting in a strong and stiff interface. However, the tan δ of neat KGG resin is better than that of reinforced composites, and its reveals that pure resin has a high degree of mobility. After surface modification treatments, the storage and loss modulus values increased, while the tan δ values dropped. Alkali treatment was found to be more effective in enhancing the dynamic mechanical properties compared to raw and plain resin.
- The treatment and the addition of OPMF to biocomposites resulted in an increase in the glass transition temperature. It's possible to use DSC to figure out what you're looking for: (i) temperature of glass transition, (ii) glass transition heat jump, (iii) temperature of melting and crystallization, (iv) heat fusion, (v) reaction heat, (vi) purity of sample, (vii) heat capacity measurement, and (viii) characterization of thermoset.
- When compared to neat resin and untreated composites, the addition of a coupling agent (NaOH) improved the thermal properties of treated fiber composites and resulted in lower weight losses in TGA.

REFERENCES

1. S. A. Miller. (2018), Natural fiber textile reinforced bio-based composites: mechanical properties, creep, and environmental impacts, *Journal of Cleaner Production*, 198, 612–623.
2. A. Moudood, A. Rahman, H. M. Khanlou, W. Hall, A. Ochsner, G. Francucci. (2019), Environmental effects on the durability and the mechanical performance of flax fiber/bio-epoxy composites, *Composites Part B*, 171, 284–293.
3. A. K. Mohanty, M. Misra, L. T. Drzal. (2005), *Natural Fibers, Biopolymers, and Biocomposites*, CRC Press is an imprint of Taylor & Francis Group, USA.
4. Mohanty. A.K., Misra, M., Hinrichsen, G. (2000), Biofibers, biodegradable polymers and biocomposites: An overview. *Macromolecular Materials and Engineering*, 276, 1–24.
5. R. R. Koshy, S. K. Mary, S. Thomas, L. A. Pothan. (2015), Environment friendly green composites based on soy protein isolate - A review, *Food Hydrocolloids*, 50, 174–192.
6. X. Huang, A. Netravali. (2009), Biodegradable green composites made using bamboo micro/nano-fibrils and chemically modified soy protein resin, *Composites Science and Technology*, 69, 1009–1015.
7. D. Jagadeesh, D. Jeevan Prasad Reddy, A. Varada Rajulu. (2011), Preparation and properties of biodegradable films from wheat protein isolate, *Journal of Polymers and Environment*, 19, 248–253.
8. D. Jagadeesh, D. Jeevan Prasad Reddy, A. Varada Rajulu, R. Li (2011), Green composites from wheat protein isolate and hildegardia populifolia natural fabric, *Polymer Composites*, 32, 398–406.

9. S. Avancha, A. K. Behera, R. Sen, B. Adhikari. (2013), Physical and mechanical characterization of jute reinforced soy composites, *Journal of Reinforced Plastics and Composites*, 32, 1380–1390.

10. R. B. Sashidhar, D. Raju, R. Karuna. (2015), Tree Gum: Gum Kondagogu. In: Ramawat K., Mérillon JM. (eds) *Polysaccharides*. Springer, Cham, 185–217.

11. V. T. P. Vinod, R. B. Sashidhar, K. I. Suresh, B. Rama Rao, U. V. R. Vijaya Saradhi, T. Prabhakar Rao. (2008), Morphological, physico-chemical and structural characterization of gum Kondagogu (Cochlospermum gossypium): A tree gum from India, *Food Hydrocolloids*, 22, 899–915.

12. V. T. P. Vinod, R. B. Sashidhar, V. U. M. Sarma, U. V. R. Vijaya Saradhi. (2008), Compositional analysis and rheological properties of gum kondagogu (Cochlospermum gossypium): A tree gum from India, *Journal of Agricultural and Food Chemistry*, 56, 2199–2207.

13. V. T. P. Vinod, R. B. Sashidhar. (2009), Solution and conformational properties of gum kondagogu (Cochlospermum gossypium) – A natural product with immense potential as a food additive, *Food Chemistry*, 116, 686–692.

14. V. T. P. Vinod, R. B. Sashidhar, B. Sreedhar, B. Rama Rao, T. Nageswara Rao, J. T. Abraham. (2009), Interaction of Pb^{2+} and Cd^{2+} with gum kondagogu (Cochlospermum gossypium): A natural carbohydrate polymer with biosorbent properties, *Carbohydrate Polymers*, 78, 894–901.

15. V. T. P. Vinod, R. B. Sashidhar, A. A. Sukumar. (2010), Competitive adsorption of toxic heavy metal contaminants by gum Kondagogu (Cochlospermum gossypium): A natural hydrocolloid, *Colloids and Surfaces B: Biointerfaces*, 75, 490–495.

16. S. Shinoj, R. Visvanathan, S. Panigrahi, M. Kochubabu. (2011), Oil palm fiber (OPF) and its composites: A review, *Industrial Crops and Products*, 33, 7–22.

17. M. S. Sreekala, M. G. Kumaran, S. Thomas. (1997), Oil palm fibers: Morphology, chemical composition, surface modification, and mechanical properties, *Journal of Applied Polymer Science*, 66, 821–835.

18. P. H. F. Pereira, N. F. Souza, H. L. Ornaghi Jr., M. Rosa de Freitas. (2020), Comparative analysis of different chlorine-free extraction on oil palm mesocarp fiber, *Industrial Crops and Products*, 150, 112305.

19. K. Obi Reddy, K. Raja Narender Reddy, J. Zhang, J. Zhang, A. Varada Rajulu. (2013), Effect of alkali treatment on the properties of century fiber, *Journal of Natural Fibers*, 10, 282–296.

20. K. Raja Narender Reddy, D. K. N. Rao, K. Gopala Kishan Rao, K. K. Kar. (2012), Studies on woven century fiber polyester composites, *Journal of Composite Materials*, 46, 2919–2933.

21. N. Lopattananon, K. Panawarangkul, K. Sahakaro, B. Ellis. (2006), Performance of pineapple leaf fiber–natural rubber composites: The effect of fiber surface treatments, *Journal of Applied Polymer Science*, 102, 1974–1984.

22. O. Velazquez-Meraz, J. E. Ledezma-Sillas, C. Carre~no-Gallardo, W. Yang, N. M. Chaudhari, H. A. Calderon, I. Rusakova, F. C. Robles Hernandez, J. M. Herrera-Ramirez. (2019), Improvement of physical and mechanical properties on bio-polymer matrix composites using morphed grapheme, *Composites Science and Technology*, 184, 107836.

23. A. Atiqah, M. Jawaid, S. M. Sapuan, M. R. Ishak, O. Y. Alothman. (2018), Thermal properties of sugar palm/glass fiber reinforced thermoplastic polyurethane hybrid composites, *Composite Structures*, 202, 954–958.

24. J. Gassan, A. K. Bledzki. (1999), Possibilities for improving the mechanical properties of jute/epoxy composites by alkali treatment of fibres, *Composites Science and Technology*, 59, 1303–1309.

25. S. Krishnasamy, S. M. K. Thiagamani, C. M. Kumar, R. Nagarajan, R. M. Shahroze, S. Siengchin, S. O. Ismail, P. Indira Devim. (2019), Recent advances in thermal properties of hybrid cellulosic fiber reinforced polymer composites-review, *International Journal of Biological Macromolecules*, 141, 1–13.

26. N. Mohd Nurazzi, A. Khalina, S. M. Sapuan, R. A. Ilyas, S. Ayu Rafiqah, Z. M. Hanafee. (2020), Thermal properties of treated sugar palmyarn/glass fiber reinforced unsaturated polyesterhybrid composites, *Journal of Material Research and Technology*, 9, 1606–1618.

Chapter 14

Biomedical study of femur bone fracture and healing

Ashwani Kumar and Arun Kumar Singh Gangwar
Technical Education Department Uttar Pradesh Kanpur

Avinash Kumar
Indian Institute of Information Technology Design
& Manufacturing Kancheepuram Chennai

Chandan Swaroop Meena
CSIR-Central Building Research Institute Roorkee

Varun Pratap Singh
University of Petroleum and Energy Studies Dehradun

Nitesh Dutt
College of Engineering Roorkee

Arbind Prasad
Katihar Engineering College Katihar

Yatika Gori
Graphic Era University Dehradun

CONTENTS

DOI: 10.1201/9781003344810-14

14.1 INTRODUCTION

The objective of this chapter is to perform the biomedical study of femur bone using FEA. In previous studies, researchers performed only modal and structural analyses of femur bone at different boundary conditions, but in the present study, structural, modal, scale-up, scale-down, and crack analyses and crack healing using plates were performed. Modeling of femur bone was done using SolidWorks considering the drawing dimensions of CT scanned femur bone, and this model of femur bone was also scaled down (90%) and scale up (110%) of original bone dimension to consider anthropometrics factor. There are four different types of cells present in bone tissue. Every cell has definite function in the repairing and restructuring of human bone [1].

14.2 INTERNAL FIXATION FOR FRACTURE

Nowadays, physicians have started performing surgical procedures allowing them to set the bones at designated place (repositioning) and stabilize the bone internally for fractured bones [2]. For replacement of joints, mostly cobalt and chrome implants are used. Plates are used for fixation of internal fractured bone to hold the broken parts of bone together for faster healing with the help of screws. These plates may be kept intact after healing or can be removed in some cases depending upon the location and type of fracture [2]. In an external fixation, a bar is used from outside of body and metal pins or screws are used in to the bone through small incisions into the skin. By this way, the broken bone is held together until the bones are not healed properly to wear the load static and dynamic. It is very different from casts and splints, which are purely external support [3]. CT-based finite element analysis (CTFEA) is used to find the risk of fracture in femur bone and to identify the location where the chances of fracture are more [4]. We know that the bone healing is greatly affected by the process used to stabilize the fractured joint [5–6]. Experimentally, it has been found that fractures mainly occurred in the neck-head region due to lower mass density [7].

In human body, the bone tissue has a unique property to regenerate itself, while the other body tissue may not have this property. Biomechanical behavior and performance of implants are also affected by the principle of fixation of joint for healing purpose [8]. Hydroxyapatite $Ca_{10}(PO_4)_6(OH)_2$ is one of the minerals of natural hard tissues. When implant material is added or coated with hydroxyapatite, it forms biocompatible and bioresorbable implants, which also promotes restructuring of fractured bone [9]. In composite materials, fibers provide the structural strength, while the matrix protects the fiber from external environment and from damage that leads to the thermal stability of the composite [10].

14.3 CURRENT STATUS OF RESEARCH

A lot of research articles and papers have been published in the field of vibration and structural analysis of femur bone and different methods of healing of fractured femur bone, among which some of important studies are discussed below:

Paddan and Griffin [11] studied that how vibration of seat is transmitted to head and harmful effect of whole-body vibration was studied. Holmlund et al. [12] studied the mechanical impedance in operator at various working conditions while different sitting postures in vertical direction. Tiemessen et al. [13] worked for improving the human comfort by finding methods to reduce whole-body vibration.

Ingólfsson et al. [14] performed a brief literature survey on lateral vibrations of footbridges induced by pedestrians and suggested an improved design of footbridges with less vibration and cost. They mainly studied the synchronous lateral excitation (SLE) phenomenon. Lings and Leboeuf-Yde [15] did the literature review (1992–1999) and found that lower back pain and whole-body vibration are interrelated. They also suggested methods to reduce whole-body vibration as well as lower back pain. Valentini [16] studied in simulation of the human spine vibration with the help of innovative numerical dynamic model. The simulation result was compared with the literature result. Hight et al. [17] did compare the analytical results obtained from beam-type FEA model and the experimental results from human tibia vibration analysis. So, it is necessary to calculate the stiffness of boundary condition in order to generate correct frequency response. Pelker and Saha [18] studied the effect of the dynamic loading on femur bone with stress wave. They studied the traveling wave phenomenon for a single compressive pulse in fresh bone.

Huiskes and Chao [19] studied the biomechanics of femur bone. Finite element analysis (FEA) tool was used to study and analyze complicated structured geometry. Khalil et al. [20] performed two different methods in order study the femur bone. While considering the real femur bone between pelvis and tibia, natural frequencies for both free-free and fixed-fixed boundary conditions are considered. Yu et al. [21] studied the knee joint structure. Kumar and Parhi [22] studied the identification of cracks, places of stress concentration, and maximum stress points during different loading conditions. Vijayakumar and Madheswaran [23] found different possible causes of fracture in femur bone and their effect on physical and mechanical properties. Chandramohan and Ravikumar [24] studied the effect of various factors on humeral bone shaft. For this, they reduced the geometry of the humeral shaft bone to a cylinder and two spheres mounted to its two ends.

Wirtz [25] studied the physical and mechanical properties of real femur bone experimentally. It has been seen that several mechanical properties have not been correlated to these main criteria; further experimental study will be required in future. Chethan et al. [26] did a static structural analysis of different loads on femur bone ranging from 1 to 8 kN. It has been found that long femur bone has better load-carrying capability as compared to short femur bone, which fails about nine times of body weight. Sharma [27] studied the biodynamic response of femur bone due to variation in the cup radius. They performed FEA to get fracture points and model frequencies of model. They validated the simulation and experimental results. Jia et al. [28] focused on the supporting plate weight reduction used as bone implants by considering different grades of available biomaterials. Rajapakse and Chang [29] performed an MRI-guided FEA technique in order to perform fracture strength analysis of hip. In future, this technology can be used to manage hip fracture risk analysis. Esmaeili et al. [30] performed the modeling of femur bone using a PLA-HA nanocomposite material that has properties close to bone material.

Ong et al. [31] suggested a new technique SHM with the existing technique for monitoring femur bone healing. Reina-Romo et al. [32] highlighted how mechanical vibration affects the study of femur bone. At different boundary conditions, natural frequencies and mode shapes were generated and stress analysis and deformation at different frequencies verified. Satapathy et al. [33] studied the different methods of healing the fractured bone by providing the different grades of materials for implant. Adachi et al. [34] studied the new bone formation. The mechanical simulation method was applied for the study of bone formation and scaffold surfaces. Kim et al. [35] studied various types of healing method used for long bone fracture conditions. For fractured bone structure stabilization, bone plates were used with fastening screws. Chiu et al. [36] studied different vibration-based healing methods, while the fixation is done internally in the fractured femur bone. Gupta and Tse [37] did a FEA of femur bone using Abaqus software in order to find the natural frequencies and mode shapes for fixed-fixed boundary condition.

Masood et al. [38] studied that when pressure was applied on the upper side of femur bone while epicondyle was restrained, then the maximum deformations occur on the upper side of the femur bone and minimum deformation occurs on the lower side of the femur bone. Nareliya and Kumar [39] studied the biomechanical analysis of femur bone under physiological conditions, as most of the body weight is taken by femur bone during normal weight-bearing activities. Fanisam et al. [1] studied the reason of femur bone fracture and the different types of methods for healing and replacement of bone implants. Gupta and Tse [37] studied that mode shapes are essential to find the behavior of any structure that has external exposure. Francis and Kumar [40] studied the patient-specific model generation from CT scan data. In their article, the authors studied the deformation in the femur bone at different inclination angles in male patients of different age groups when load is half-body weight applied on head of right proximal femur of male patients. Kumar et al. [41] studied the modal analysis of hand-arm vibration using FEA, and they performed the optimization gearbox using FEA, which is a technique used for femur bone [42]. Kumar et al. [43] performed the static structural analysis of cortical bone and also studied the performance of automobile objects using FEA boundary conditions, which were used for femur bone analysis [44]. Kumar et al. [45] used the FEA method for performing the analysis on cracked bone and used the FEA model for various parameter variation studies of gear [46]. Gangwar et al. [47] investigated the biomechanical aspects of femur bone. Patil et al. [48] performed the tribological study using pin-on-disk experimental method; this method is helpful for the tribological analysis of materials for orthopedic applications and they also used ANN for sensor [49] that can be applied for biomechanical study of bones. Kumar et al. [50] used the FEA model with grid independency test, which is helpful for bone analysis. Gangwar et al. [51] investigated the biomechanical response of femur bone. Patil et al. [52] used modeling influence property on tube material, which was used for scale-up and scale-down analyses. Structural and modal analysis method [53,54] is useful for dynamic response analysis of bones. Kumar et al. [55] found out the natural frequencies of femur bone, which were used for finding crack propagation and healing purpose. The critical review of femur bone has been performed, and it is observed that there is lot of scope to conduct new research studies considering biomechanical aspects of femur bone.

14.4 BOUNDARY CONDITIONS

The femur bone structure has been designed using SolidWorks [56] (Figure 14.1). The biomechanical analysis of femur bone has been done using ANSYS based on FEA. Femur bone design is a complex procedure having bone shaft, neck, and tissues. For simplification, only bone shaft and neck have been considered in designing. FEA is based on nodes and elements. For bone properties, Young's modulus, Poisson's ratio, and bone density were

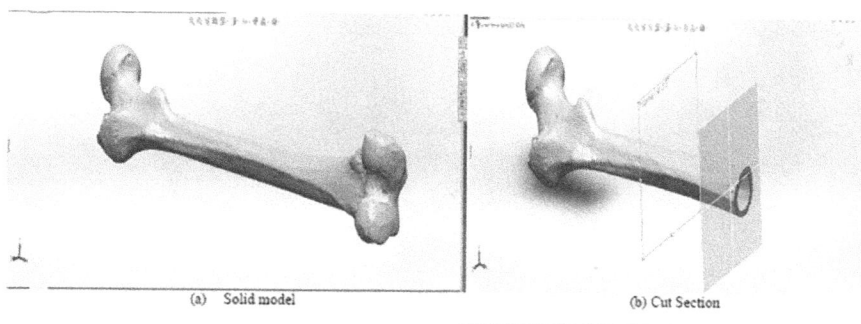

(a) Solid model

(b) Cut Section

Figure 14.1 Design of femur bone model using SolidWorks.

considered. These are the critical parameters that govern the FEA results. The mechanical properties of femur bone are the following: Young's modulus: 7.585 GPa, Poisson's ratio: 0.35, and bone density: 866 kg/m³ (Wirtz [25]); for modal analysis, two boundary conditions will be applied, i.e., free-free and fixed-fixed boundary conditions. Free-free boundary conditions show natural frequency of femur bone. In natural form, femur bone is constrained between pelvis and tibia. Sudden loading, high vibration excitation, and road accidents are few reasons for femur bone fracture [10].

14.5 RESULTS AND DISCUSSION

In order to perform FEA, first we designed the 3D CAD model of femur bone. In the previous literature for femur bone drawing, dimensional data are taken from frozen bone, or from wet femur bone. But in this case, geometrical data of femur bone are taken from CT scanned real femur bone. In order to make the analysis more realistic, scaling of model is also done 90% in lower side and 110% in upper side so that all people should be considered in analysis; it makes the study more global. To make the study more realistic, bone material is selected. Modeling of femur bone is done on SolidWorks software [56]. Figure 14.2 shows four different models of femur bone geometry. In order to optimize the parameter base, the heights

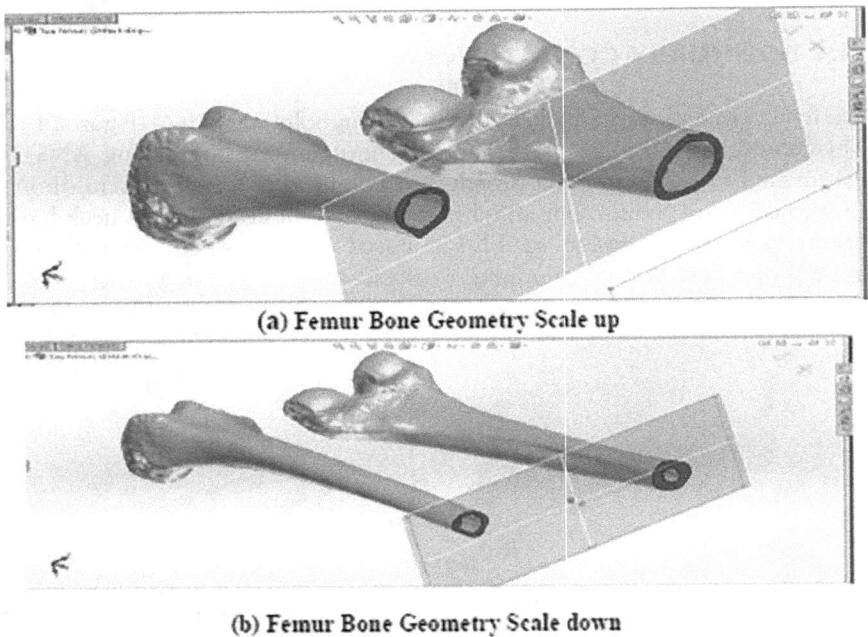

(a) Femur Bone Geometry Scale up

(b) Femur Bone Geometry Scale down

Figure 14.2 Femur bone geometry: (a) scale-up model and (b) scale-down model.

of triangles are also adjusted in such a way that the number. of triangles is to be reduced without compromising the quality of analysis results. The FEA-based meshed model of femur bone has 15,463 nodes and 8507 elements. ANSYS software [57] was used for modal and structural analyses. Figure 14.2 shows the scale-up and scale-down models of femur bone for considering geographical differences in geometry design.

Figure 14.3 shows that a uniform pressure of 750 Pa was applied on the femoral head shown in red contour. In the first case, pressure was applied on the upper side of femur bone while epicondyle was restrained (displacement boundary condition applied). During pressure application, the condyles and patellar surface were in constraint position. The duration of pressure application is 2.5 seconds. Figure 14.4 shows that a uniform pressure of 750 Pa was applied on femoral head shown in red hues. During pressure application, the condyles and patellar surface were in constraint position, as shown in Figure 14.4. The duration of pressure application is 2.5 seconds. In this case where pressure is applied at one end while restrained on the other end, bone is behaving as a cantilever beam. The main purpose of this study is to examine the strength of femur bone during sudden impact or accident conditions.

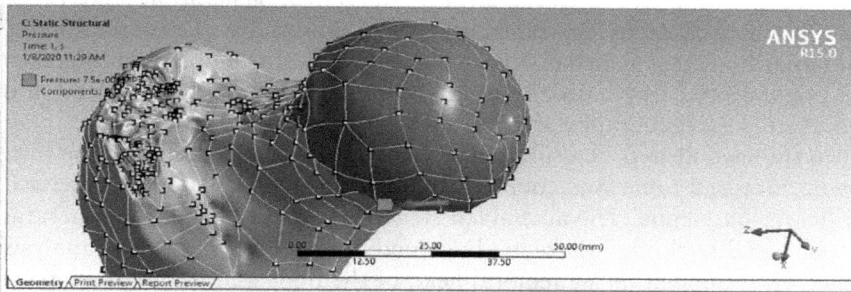

Figure 7 Pressure force application on femur bone head

Figure 14.3 Pressure force application on femur bone head.

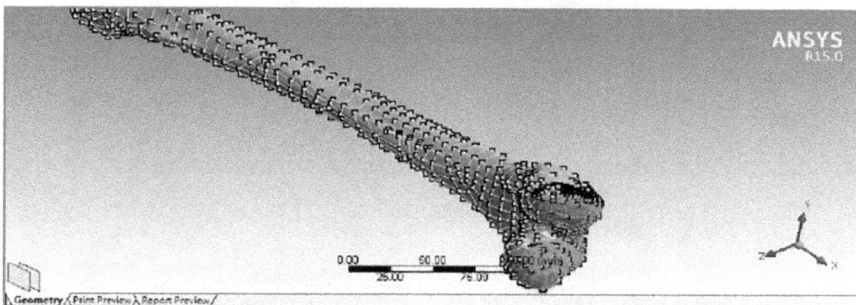

Figure 14.4 Load and pressure application on femur bone.

Based on these boundary conditions, the structural analysis was performed. For static analysis, average human body weight is considered as 76 kg ($76 \times 9.81 = 745.56$ N). So, 750 N load is applied on spherical heads of femur bone. From the static analysis results, it has been found that the maximum stress and displacement are 0.52381 MPa and 0.22 mm, respectively.

Drawing data are taken from CT scan in order to generate the 3D model of the femur bone structure using SolidWorks. Due to complex shape and structure of femur bone, which consists of bone shaft, neck, and tissues, we used FEA to study the biomechanical behavior of femur bone. In order to simplify the design, only bone shaft and neck are taken. In the FEA of femur bone, we consider the modulus of elasticity as 7.585 GPa, Poisson's ratio as 0.35, and bone density as 866 kg/m^3. This mechanical parameter greatly affects the FEA results (Wirtz [25]). As we know that the femur bone is held between the pelvis and tibia, using fixed-fixed condition gives more accurate results because it gives the natural frequencies for constrained femur bone and mode shape for analysis.

14.5.1 Structural analysis results

Structural analysis, modal analysis, and crack generation and crack-rectifying analysis are the central theme of this study. The original model of femur bone was scaled down and scaled up for the global representation of population. The length and width of femur bone vary with variation in continents and geographical conditions.

In the second step, fractured femur bone was analyzed, and in the third step, fractured bone was coupled with the prosthetic plate and screws of different biometals. The assembled structure was analyzed for structural, modal, and buckling failure loading conditions. During buckling analysis, the load is applied to the femoral head of the bone and the bottom end of femur bone is fixed in the static analysis. The purpose is to find out the load at which the femur bone fails due to buckling. Therefore, loads of different intensities are applied to the femoral head of the femur bone. Figure 14.5

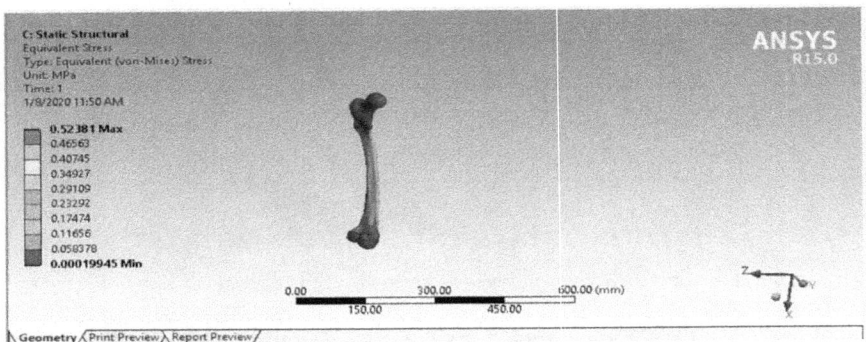

Figure 14.5 Von Mises stress variation in femur bone.

shows the von Mises stress induced in femur bone. In order to prevent the failure of femur bone due to buckling, the von Mises stress in the bone material should be less than the permissible stress.

The maximum induced von Mises stress in bone is 0.52381 MPa, which is within permissible range. The magnitudes of max. total deformations were 0.22 mm. The maximum stresses were on the lower end of femur bone. The maximum stress using von Mises criterion was 0.52381 MPa. In all three cases, it has been observed that maximum deformations are at the point where pressure is applied and deformations decrease as we go away from the area of application of pressure. Maximum stresses are located at restraint end and decrease toward free end. In structural analysis, von Mises stress, maximum stress, elastic strain, and deformation were calculated. The maximum von Mises stress was at the left corner of femur shaft as 0.46–0.52 MPa (Figure 14.5). Maximum stress variation is only 0.32 MPa (Figure 14.6). The elastic strain corresponding to the applied pressure is within range. The lower portion of femur bone has a very small area shown in red hues (Figure 14.7). It was concluded that at 750 Pa pressure and load condition, the designed femur bone is safe and the applied bone material properties are sufficient to withstand the loading and sudden impact.

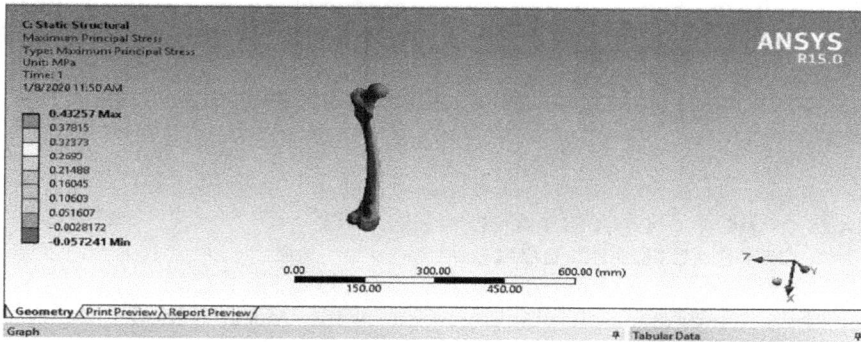

Figure 14.6 Maximum stress variation in femur bone.

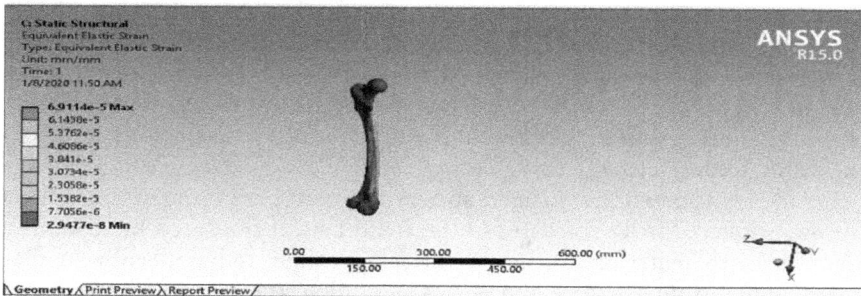

Figure 14.7 Elastic strain generation in femur bone.

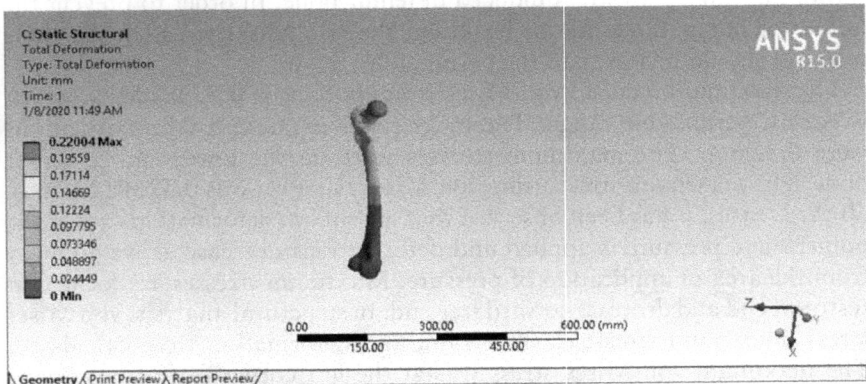

Figure 14.8 Deformation under applied loading conditions.

Figure 14.8 shows the total deformation generated due to pressure application. It was observed that femur bone head is the most prone area that is subjected to fracture conditions. There is a maximum deformation of 0.22 mm at bone head. In practical orthopedic cases, it is observed that the maximum fracture occurs at bone head area. So the results obtained from FEA are accurate from practical point of view. Results show that higher deformation occurs at the head of femur and the lowest occurs at the lower end. The results show that higher weight provides higher total displacement.

14.6 CRACK ANALYSIS AND HEALING OF FRACTURED BONE

The first step of crack analysis is generating the fractured model of femur bone. The first ten natural frequencies and mode shapes have been investigated using modal analysis. The natural frequency of fractured femur bone varies from 28.83 to 2087.2 Hz. It was observed that there is a change in the natural frequency due to crack generation. The original model of femur bone has a frequency in range of 64.06–3010.5 Hz. The difference of first and last natural frequency 35.23 and 923.3 Hz. A supporting plate having corrosion resistance properties has been investigated. The following mechanical properties of the implant material are used in the analysis shown in Table 14.1.

Figure 14.9 shows that using a supporting plate, the hairline crack area is now protected from fracture. In the treatment of fractured bone, equivalent strength material is selected for femur bone. It has been seen that mostly 316L stainless steel and Ti-6Al-4V alloy are used as human bone implants by orthopedic surgeons. Figure 14.9 shows the frequency variation

Table 14.1 Mechanical properties of implants

S. No.	Material used	Young's modulus (GPa)	Poisson's ratio	Yield strength (MPa)	Density (kg/mm³)
1	Stainless steel 316L	110	0.24	666	7.9
2	Ti-6Al-4V	200	0.30	800	4.4

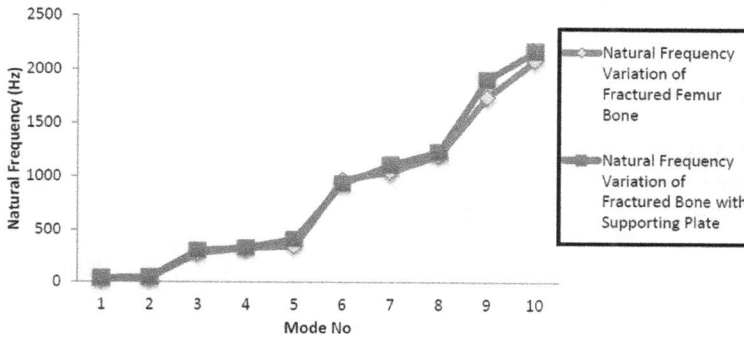

Figure 14.9 Frequency variation of cracked femur bone.

of fractured femur bone and support plate femur bone. There is increment in natural frequency of femur bone with support plate of 87.6 Hz. The first natural frequency is increased by 5.6 Hz.

14.7 CONCLUSIONS AND FUTURE SCOPE

In this research, the modal analysis and structural strength analysis have been done at different conditions of femur bone; also, varying boundary conditions were applied for better FEA results and the following observations have been made:

- From the results, it is identified that the maximum von Mises stress is 0.5231 MPa at the lower end of femur bone shaft and the minimum stress is 0.000199 MPa in all areas of femur bone. The maximum principal stress is 0.43257 MPa at lower side of femur shaft, and the minimum principal stress is −0.057241 MPa having compressive nature. The maximum deformation due to loading is 0.22 mm at femur bone head, 0.195 mm below head, and 0.12224 mm at the shaft area. So it is concluded that the area of bone failure is femur bone head and bone shaft.
- The natural frequency of the original femur bone varies from 64.062 to 3010.5 Hz, that of the scale-down model varies from 0 to 1935 Hz,

and that of the scale-up model varies from 0 to 1582.9. Fractured femur bone modal analysis was performed for studying the variation in the natural frequency of crack and non-crack bone.

- For fracture rectification, different grades of materials for support plate were analyzed. Titanium alloy materials are best suited in conclusion because they show the same strength as the original femur bone and have no buckling failure condition. They show good physical and mechanical properties.

REFERENCES

1. Fanisam, M. B. N., Mitesh, P., & Nitin, P. (2017). Finite element analysis of femur bone. *International Journal of Advanced Engineering Research and Applications (IJA-ERA)*, 3(4), 215–231.
2. Kumar, K. N., Griya, N., Shaikh, A., Chaudhry, V., & Chavadaki, S. (2020). Structural analysis of femur bone to predict the suitable alternative material. *Materials Today: Proceedings*, 26, 364–368.
3. Kalaiyarasan, A., Sankar, K., & Sundaram, S. (2020). Finite element analysis and modeling of fractured femur bone. *Materials Today: Proceedings*, 22, 649–653.
4. Bhandari, A., Gangil, B., Ahmad, F., & Bisht, T. (2020, August). Finite element analysis based on mechanical vibration characteristics of femur bone. In *2020 International Conference on Advances in Computing, Communication & Materials (ICACCM)* (pp. 131–135). IEEE.
5. Sternheim, A., Traub, F., Trabelsi, N., Dadia, S., Gortzak, Y., Snir, N., & Yosibash, Z. (2020). When and where do patients with bone metastases actually break their femurs? A CT-based finite element analysis. *The Bone & Joint Journal*, 102(5), 638–645.
6. Wang, J., Ma, J. X., Lu, B., Bai, H. H., Wang, Y., & Ma, X. L. (2020). Comparative finite element analysis of three implants fixing stable and unstable subtrochanteric femoral fractures: Proximal Femoral Nail Antirotation (PFNA), Proximal Femoral Locking Plate (PFLP), and Reverse Less Invasive Stabilization System (LISS). *Orthopaedics & Traumatology: Surgery & Research*, 106(1), 95–101.
7. Rathor, S., Jena, J., Uddanwadikar, R., & Apte, A. (2021). Finite element analysis of type I and type II fracture with PFN implant—A comparative study. In Kalamkar, V., Monkova, K. (eds.) *Advances in Mechanical Engineering*, Lecture Notes in Mechanical Engineering (pp. 243–251). Springer, Singapore. DOI: 10.1007/978-981-15-3639-7_29.
8. Gujar, R. A. & Warhatkar, H. N. (2021). In vitro estimation of fracture load and strain in sheep femur bone: Experimental approach. *Materials Today: Proceedings*, 44(5), 3792–3797.
9. Gómez-Vallejo, J., Roces-García, J., Moreta, J., Donaire-Hoyas, D., Gayoso, Ó., Marqués-López, F., & Albareda, J. (2021). Biomechanical behavior of an hydroxyapatite-coated traditional hip stem and a short one of similar design: Comparative study using finite element analysis. *Arthroplasty Today*, 7, 167–176.

10. Gee, A., Bougherara, H., Schemitsch, E. H., & Zdero, R. (2021). Biomechanical design using in-vitro finite element modeling of distal femur fracture plates made from semi-rigid materials versus traditional metals for post-operative toe-touch weight-bearing. *Medical Engineering & Physics*, 87, 95–103.

11. Paddan, G. S. & Griffin, M. J. (1998). A review of the transmission of translational seat vibration to the head. *Journal of Sound and Vibration*, 215, 863–882.

12. Holmlund, P., Lundstrok, R., & Lindberg, M. L. (2000). Mechanical impedance of the human body in vertical direction. *Journal of Applied Ergonomics*, 31, 415–422.

13. Tiemessen, I. J., Hulshof, C. T. J., & Frings-Dresen, M. H.W. (2007). An overview of strategies to reduce whole-body vibration exposure on drivers: A systematic review. *International Journal of Industrial Ergonomics*, 37, 245–256.

14. Ingólfsson, E. T., Georgakis, C. T., & Jönsson, J. (2012). Pedestrian-induced lateral vibrations of footbridges: A literature review. *Journal of Engineering Structures*, 45, 21–52.

15. Lings, S. & Leboeuf-Yde, C. (2000). Whole-body vibration and low back pain: A systematic, critical review of the epidemiological literature 1992–1999. *International Archives of Occupational and Environmental Health*, 73, 290–297.

16. Valentini, P. P. (2012). Modeling human spine using dynamic spline approach for vibrational simulation. *Journal of Sound and Vibration*, 331, 5895–5909.

17. Hight, T. K., Piziali, R. L., & Nagel, D. A. (1980). Natural frequency analysis of a human tibia. *Journal of Biomechanics*, 13, 139–147.

18. Pelker, R. R. & Saha, S. (1983). Stress wave propagation in bone. *Journal of Biomechanics*, 16, 481–489.

19. Huiskes, R. & Chao, E. Y. S. (1983). A survey of finite element analysis in orthopedic biomechanics: The first decade. *Journal of Biomechanics*, 16, 385–409.

20. Khalil, T. B., Viano, D. C., & Taber, L. A. (1981). Vibrational characteristics of the embalmed human femur. *Journal of Sound and Vibration*, 75, 417–436.

21. Yu, P. P., Tseng, J. G., Huang, M. Y., & Huang, B. W. (2017). Injury assessment via stress analysis of the human knee joint.

22. Kumar, P. B. & Parhi, D. R. (2017). Vibrational characteristics and stress analysis in a human femur bone. *Materials Today: Proceedings*, 4(9), 10084–10087.

23. Vijayakumar, R. & Madheswaran, M. (2017, March). Modal analysis of femur bone using finite element method for healthcare system. In *2017 Conference on Emerging Devices and Smart Systems (ICEDSS)* (pp. 224–228). IEEE.

24. Chandramohan, D. & Ravikumar, L. (2019). Free vibrational analysis of cortical/hard cancellous bone by using of FEA. *Materials Today: Proceedings*, 16, 744–749.

25. Wirtz, D. C. (2000). Critical evaluation of known bone material properties to realize anisotropic FE simulation of the proximal femur. *Journal of Biomechanics*, 33, 1325–1330.

26. Chethan, K. N., Bhat, S. N., Zuber, M., & Shenoy, S. B. (2018). Patient-specific static structural analysis of femur bone of different lengths. *The Open Biomedical Engineering Journal*, 12(1), 108–114.

27. Sharma, N. K. (2017). Finite element analysis of humerus bone for cup radious variations. *Materials Today: Proceedings*, 4(9), 9450–9455.

28. Jia, D., Li, F., Zhang, C., Liu, K., & Zhang, Y. (2019). Design and simulation analysis of Lattice bone plate based on finite element method. *Mechanics of Advanced Materials and Structures*, 28(13), 1311–1321. DOI: 10.1080/15376494.2019.1665759.

29. Rajapakse, C. S. & Chang, G. (2018). Micro-finite element analysis of the proximal femur on the basis of high-resolution magnetic resonance images. *Current Osteoporosis Reports*, 16(6), 657–664.

30. Esmaeili, S., Aghdam, H. A., Motififard, M., Saber-Samandari, S., Montazeran, A. H., Bigonah, M., Sheikhbahaei, E., & Khandan, A. (2019). A porous polymeric–hydroxyapatite scaffold used for femur fractures treatment: Fabrication, analysis, and simulation. *European Journal of Orthopaedic Surgery & Traumatology*, 1–9.

31. Ong, W. H., Chiu, W. K., Russ, M., & Chiu, Z. K. (2016). Integrating sensing elements on external fixators for healing assessment of fractured femur. *Structural Control and Health Monitoring*, 23(12), 1388–1404.

32. Reina-Romo, E., Rodríguez-Vallés, J., & Sanz-Herrera, J. A. (2018). In silico dynamic characterization of the femur: Physiological versus mechanical boundary conditions. *Medical Engineering & Physics*, 58, 80–85.

33. Satapathy, P. K., Sahoo, B., Panda, L. N., & Das, S. (2018, March). Finite element analysis of functionally graded bone plate at femur bone fracture site. In *IOP Conference Series: Materials Science and Engineering* (Vol. 330, No. 1, p. 012027). IOP Publishing.

34. Adachi, T., Osako, Y., Tanaka, M., Hojo, M., & Hollister, S. J. (2006). Framework for optimal design of porous scaffold microstructure by computational simulation of bone regeneration. *Biomaterials*, 27(21), 3964–3972.

35. Kim, S. H., Chang, S. H., & Jung, H. J. (2010). The finite element analysis of a fractured tibia applied by composite bone plates considering contact conditions and time-varying properties of curing tissues. *Composite Structures*, 92(9), 2109–2118.

36. Chiu, W. K., Vien, B. S., Russ, M., & Fitzgerald, M. (2019). Vibration-based healing assessment of an internally fixated femur. *Journal of Nondestructive Evaluation, Diagnostics and Prognostics of Engineering Systems*, 2(2), 021003. DOI: 10.1115/1.4043276 (11 pages).

37. Gupta, A. & Tse, K. M. (2013, December). Finite element analysis on vibration modes of femur bone. In *International Conference on Advances in Mechanical Engineering (AME)*, NCR, India, Dec (pp. 10–13).

38. Masood, M. S., Ahmad, A., & Mufti, R. A. (2013). Unconventional modeling and stress analysis of femur bone under different boundary condition. *International Journal of Scientific & Engineering Research*, 4(12), 293–296.

39. Nareliya, R. & Kumar, V. (2012). Finite element application to femur bone: A review. *Journal of Biomedical and Bioengineering*, 3(1), 57–62.

40. Francis, A. & Kumar, V. (2012). Computational modeling of human femur using CT data for finite element analysis. *International Journal of Engineering Research & Technology*, 1(6), 1–7.

41. Kumar, A., Mamgain, D.P., Jaiswal, H., & Patil, P. (2015). Modal analysis of hand arm vibration (humerus bone) for biodynamic response using varying boundary conditions based on FEA. *Advances in Intelligent Systems and Computing*, 308, 169–176. DOI: 10.1007/978-81-322-2012-1_18.

42. Kumar, A. & Patil, P. P. (2016). FEA simulation and RSM based parametric optimization of vibrating transmission gearbox housing. *Perspectives in Science*, 8, 388–391. DOI: 10.1016/j.pisc.2016.04.085.

43. Kumar, A., Behmad, S. I., & Patil, P. (2014). Vibration characterization and static analysis of cortical bone fracture based on finite element analysis. *Engineering and Automation Problems*, No 3, 115–119.

44. Kumar, A. & Patil, P. P. (2016). FEA simulation based performance study of multi-speed transmission gearbox. *International Journal of Manufacturing, Materials, and Mechanical Engineering*, 6(1), 57–67. DOI: 10.4018/IJMMME.2016010103.

45. Kumar, A., Jaiswal, H., Garg, T., & Patil, P. (2014). Free vibration modes analysis of femur bone fracture using varying boundary conditions based on FEA. *Procedia Materials Science*, 6, 1593–1599. DOI: 10.1016/j.mspro.2014.07.142.

46. Patil, P. P. & Kumar, A. (2016). Dynamic structural and thermal characteristics analysis of oil lubricated multi speed transmission gearbox: Variation of load, rotational speed and convection heat transfer. *Iranian Journal of Science and Technology Transactions of Mechanical Engineering (ISTM)*, pp. 1–11. DOI: 10.1007/s40997-016-0063-z.

47. Gangwar, A. K. S., Rao, P. S., & Kumar, A. (2021). Bio-mechanical design and analysis of femur bone. *Materials Today: Proceedings*, 44(Part 1), 2179–2187. DOI: 10.1016/j.matpr.2020.12.282.

48. Patil, P., Gori, Y., Kumar, A., & Tyagi, M. R. (2021). Experimental analysis of tribological properties of polyisobutylene thickened oil in lubricated contacts. *Tribology International*, 159, 106983, 1–7. DOI: 10.1016/j.triboint.2021.106983.

49. Patil, P., Sharma, S., Saini, A., & Kumar, A. (2014). ANN modelling of Cu type omega vibration based mass flow sensor. *Procedia Technology*, 14, 260–265. DOI: 10.1016/j.protcy.2014.08.034.

50. Kumar, A., Rana, S., Gori, Y., & Sharma, N. K. (2021). Thermal contact conductance prediction using FEM based computational techniques. In *Advanced Computational Methods in Mechanical and Materials Engineering*, (pp. 183–220). DOI: 10.1201/9781003202233-13, ISBN: 9781032052915.

51. Gangwar, A. K. S., Rao, P. S., Kumar, A., & Patil, P. P. (2019). Design and analysis of femur bone: BioMechanical aspects. *Journal of Critical Reviews*, 6(4), 133–139.

52. Patil, P. P., Sharma, S. C., Jaiswal, H., & Kumar, A. (2014). Modeling influence of tube material on vibration based EMMFS using ANFIS. *Procedia Materials Science*, 6, 1097–1103. DOI: 10.1016/j.mspro.2014.07.181.

53. Kumar, A. & Patil, P. P. (2016). Modal analysis of heavy vehicle truck transmission gearbox housing made from different materials. *Journal of Engineering Science and Technology*, 11(2), 252–266.

54. Kumar, A., Joshi, H., & Patil, P. P. (2014). Vibration based failure analysis of heavy vehicle truck transmission gearbox casing using FEA. In *International Conference on Mechanical Engineering*, pp. 251–259. ISBN: 9789-3510-72713.

55. Kumar, A., Gori, Y., Rana, S., Sharma, N. K., & Yadav, B. (2022). FEA of humerus bone fracture and healing. In Kumar, A., Ram, M. and Singla Y.K. (eds.) *Advanced Materials for Biomechanical Applications* (1st ed.) CRC Press. DOI: 10.1201/9781003286806.

56. SOLIDWORKS 17 for Designing of Femur Bone

57. ANSYS 15.0 Academic, Structural analysis Guide.

Chapter 15

Bio-based environmentally benign polymeric resorbable materials for orthopedic fixation applications

Arbind Prasad

Katihar Engineering College Katihar

Gourhari Chakraborty

National Institute of Technology Andhra Pradesh

Ashwani Kumar

Technical Education Department Uttar Pradesh Kanpur

CONTENTS

15.1 INTRODUCTION

The fracture of the bone is increasing gradually due to many reasons such as sudden jerk felt by the person, imbalanced movement during sports, falls, car accidents, and low density of bones. The lifestyle of the people can also be the factor related to calcium deficiency [1,2]. The metallic internal

DOI: 10.1201/9781003344810-15

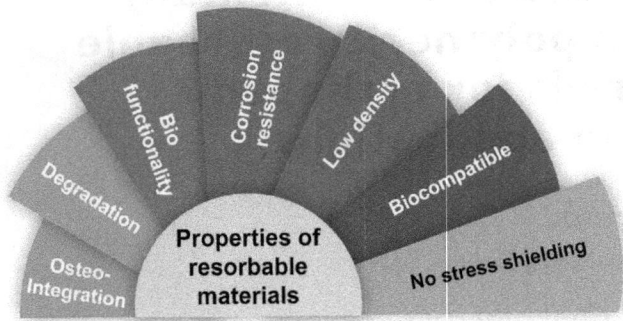

Figure 15.1 Properties of resorbable materials for biomedical applications.

fixation devices have lot of limitations such as stress shielding, palpability, leaching of ions, corrosion, and heavy in weight [3,4]. The underlying bone near metallic internal fixations also gets damaged due to severe stress shielding. The bio-based resorbable polymers have many properties and must be chosen as alternatives in place of metallic fixations. Figure 15.1 shows the various properties related to resorbable polymers [5–7].

The worldwide interest in bio-based polymers has accelerated in the recent years due to the desire and need to find non-fossil fuel-based polymers. Bio-based polymers are materials which are produced from renewable resources. Biodegradable polymers are defined as materials whose physical and chemical properties undergo deterioration and completely degrade when exposed to microorganisms, carbon dioxide (aerobic process), methane (anaerobic process), and water (aerobic and anaerobic processes). Once the bone gets healed, then again, the patient has to visit for extraction of metallic implants, which is non-desirable for the suffered patients. Therefore, resorbable polymers are increasingly being used since they do not require second surgical event. The resorbable polymer-based fixation devices and scaffolds should permit cell adhesion and encourage new bone formation [8]. It should also degrade at the rate at which the rate of healing of fracture bone takes place. The researchers have used various nanofillers such as nano-hydroxyapatite, chitosan, and other bio-based bioactive materials, which leads to the generation of bone-like structure and also maintains the porosity and increases surface area and adequate space for regeneration of extracellular matrix [9,10].

15.2 BONE AND BONE FRACTURE STATICS

Bone is a natural composite material, which involves organic phase and inorganic phase. In organic phase, calcium is embedded into it. Bone by weight contains around 30% extracellular matrix, 60% mineral, and 10%

water [11]. The bone matrix is essentially collagen, which is answerable for the tensile strength. The mineral part of bone is calcium phosphate, which provides compressive strength to the tissue. There are two kinds of bone tissues: cortical (hard) and cancellous (trabecular). The cortical bone has a Young's modulus ranging from 17 to 20 GPa and compressive strength in the scope of 131–224 MPa, while Young's modulus and compressive strength for trabecular bones are 50–100 and 5–10 MPa, respectively [12–17]. As per the endocrine society, more than 10 million US adults have osteoporosis and many more have vitamin deficiency. When bony tissues fail due to trauma or disease, additional support is required to take over their mechanical function. For example, in spinal diseases causing degeneration, instability, and/or severe deformations, spinal fusion of the segments may be needed. Metals and/or alloys have proven to be successful, although drawbacks do exist. In spinal surgery, among others, permanent materials such as metals (and non-resorbable polymers) remain susceptible to long-term complications such as migration, wear, and late foreign body reaction and infection [18].

15.3 RESORBABLE POLYMERS IN SCAFFOLDS AND IMPLANTS

The scaffolds are the temporary 3D structure that is similar to bone architecture in order to provide a support to regenerate the bone. The scaffolds based on resorbable polymers should have a 3D environment, high elasticity, cell affinity, and also sufficient mechanical strength in order to exhibit good performance [19]. Figure 15.2 shows the progress in the materials for

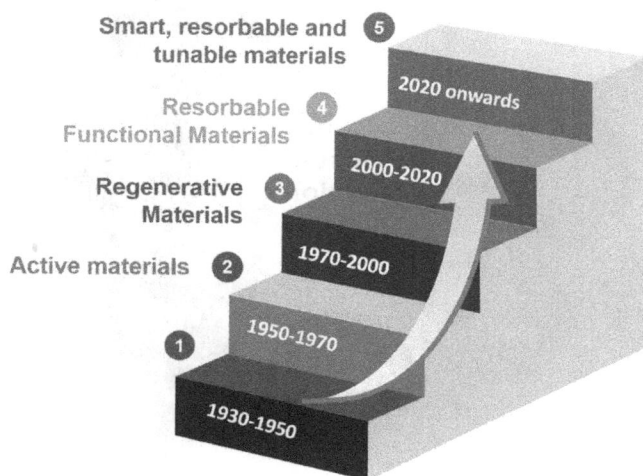

Figure 15.2 Progress in the development of materials for biomedical applications.

biomedical applications. From the year 2020 onward, researchers are engaging themselves in the area of smart materials, self-healing materials, and tunable resorbable materials so that the requirement of the huge demand of the orthopedic fixation devices could be fulfilled and also approachable to all needy persons of the society [20].

15.4 BONE FIXATION IMPLANTS

The bone fixation implants are of various types such as screws, plates, staples, and Steinmann pins. These implants are widely used in joint replacement, spine implants, and bioresorbable tissue fixations. Figure 15.3 shows the widely used bone tissue fixation devices. A screw converts all the forces that arise out of bone movement into compression and distributes this compression evenly throughout the surface of injured bones [6,21,22]. It is due to this compression that a bone stays in place and heals faster. The plate is affixed with screws to properly align the bone and aid in the healing process.

The stabilization of the fracture in the bone is also required until natural healing processes have restored sufficient strength so that the implant can be removed. If the method of fixation is not proper, then the interfaces can result in osteolysis and loosening [23,24]. The researchers are in the process of developing nanomaterials-modified implants, which have improved mechanical and tribological properties such as high wear and corrosion resistance,

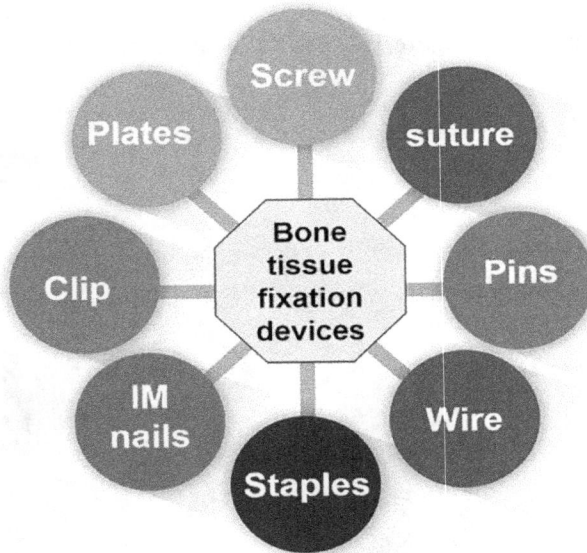

Figure 15.3 Widely used bone tissue fixation devices.

high fatigue strength, high tensile strength, and good fracture toughness [25]. The improvement in biological properties leads to good cell material interaction, enhanced tissue integration, osteoconduction, and multifunctional properties such as antimicrobial and antibacterial properties [26].

15.5 HYDROLYTIC DEGRADATION OF RESORBABLE POLYMERS

Hydrolytic degradation is the autocatalytic bond cleavage reaction of polymer which converts polymer into small fragments. Hydrolytic degradation of resorbable polymers is one of the important properties that determine the applicability as biomedical products such as orthopedic implants, fixation elements, suture, and drug delivery. Hydrolytic degradation can be of two types: (i) surface erosion and (ii) bulk erosion (shown in Figure 15.4). In case of orthopedic implants, hydrolytic degradation causes decrement of

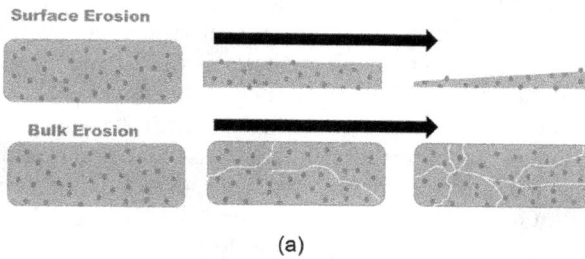

(a)

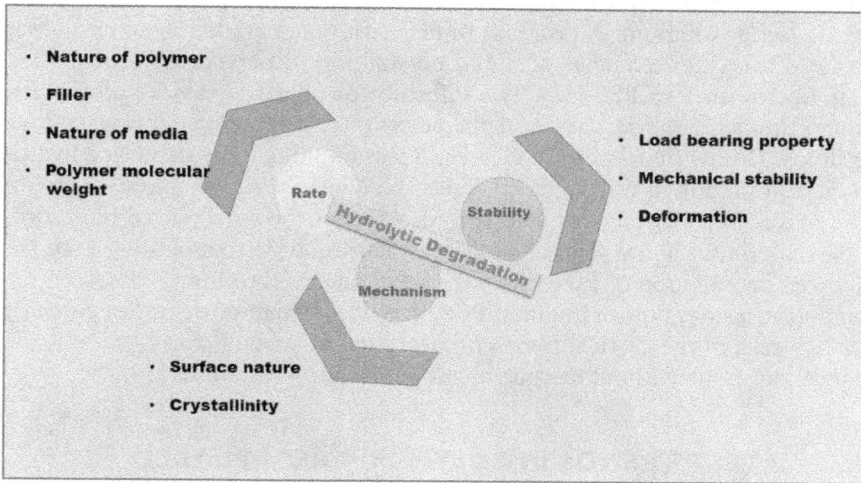

(b)

Figure 15.4 (a) Hydrolytic degradation types and (b) parameters associated with hydrolytic degradation.

the load-bearing property of the particular product. Degradation also indicates the resorbable nature of the polymer. Similarly, for drug delivery, tissue culture, and suture applications, the overall effectivity of product is dependent on the targeted property and in vivo degradation of the same. Polymer processing route, filler properties and loading, temperature, crystallinity, and polymer molecular weight are prime factors that control the degradation of biomedical implants [27,28]. Kobielarz et al. investigated the degradation behavior of laser-modified poly(lactic-co-glycolic acid) (PLGA) implants under *in vitro* condition. The impact on mechanical properties along with degradation was also recorded in the work. PLGA specimens were made into dumbbell shape through compression molding technique, and prior to hydrolytic degradation, some of the specimens were subjected to CO_2 laser ablation. It was observed that tensile strength decreased with the increase in the exposure time in water for the specimens. After the first stage of degradation, it was observed that for modified PLGA specimens, percentage reduction in tensile strength was dependent on the type of surface treatment, whereas after 12 weeks, the reduction was more than 45% and it was independent of surface nature of the specimen [29]. In another study, the lasting strength of poly(L-lactide)-based bioresorbable vascular scaffolds was investigated by Ramachandran et al. It was observed that crimping develops a variation in microstructure that provides strength and resists hydrolysis, which opens up the application domain for bioresorbable materials for vascular scaffolds. The degradation behavior is dependent on blend composition for resorbable polymeric blends [30]. Oosterbeek et al. investigated the change in the mechanical property of poly(L-lactide) (PLLA) and poly(L-lactide-co-ε-caprolactone) blend of different compositions under hydrolytic degradation media (phosphate buffer solution). A decrease in pH with the degradation of blend was noticed for all different blends, and crystallinity observed to be increasing due to exposure to PBS [31]. The influence of filler properties and loading alters the degradation nature of the composite. In case of microcrystalline cellulose (MCC)-reinforced PLA, weight loss found to increase during hydrolytic degradation in water, which is possibly due to the hydrophilic nature of the MCC [32]. Polyglycolic acid (PGA) is one of the widely used bioresorbable materials that are semi-crystalline in nature. In vitro and in vivo studies showed degradation of PGA can vary between 4 and 6 months based on the composition and type of implant. PGA was observed to be degraded partially in 12 weeks in the cortical bone and degraded to a significant extent also in cancellous bone without causing any inflammatory responses [33].

15.6 LATEST TRENDS IN POLYMERIC RESORBABLE MATERIALS FOR BIOMEDICAL APPLICATIONS

Polymeric resorbable materials because of their easy processability, biocompatibility, and tunable mechanical property are becoming lucrative materials for biomedical product manufacturing. PLA because of its biocompatibility and biodegradability has become one of the major clinical materials. PLA-based composites are in use for orthopedics, tissue engineering, drug delivery, etc. [34–36]. Ahuja et al. developed a PLA-based cardiovascular stent. In this work, inclusions of 5% of polycaprolactone (PCL) and magnesium were carried out in PLA matrix through extrusion technique in the form of tube. This component was found to be significantly effective upon vascularization only at 8 weeks compared to pure PLA [37].

In medical implants and theranostic systems also, PLA was observed to be effective. PLA is also very much effective in scaffold fabrication [38]. Grigoriev et al. fabricated spongious scaffolds using different molecular weight PLLA and PDLLA. It was observed that there is no cytotoxicity for the porous scaffolds and cell adhesion study has shown cell attachment to the scaffolds for SHED cells. PLA/Mg composite is found to be a promising material for bone replacement with comparable mechanical property and degradability. PLA/Mg composite with spherical particles after 7 days and 28 days of immersion maintains more than 90% and 60% of its mechanical properties, respectively [39]. PGA is another promising resorbable polymer widely used for different biomedical applications. Different forms of PGA were utilized for different biomedical applications. In an osteoblast investigation, PGA-PLA blend reinforced with chitosan and hydroxyapatite is coated over Ti6Al4V alloy with a diameter of 12 mm and thickness of 3 mm.

The growth of osteoblast cells increased due to the addition of chitosan and hydroxyapatite in matrix PLA-PGA [40]. In case of scaffold fabrication, PGA is utilized in different ways such as melt foaming technique [41]. PGA-PCL with beta-tricalcium phosphate was also successfully utilized for scaffold fabrication by Kumar et al. [42]. The use of copolymers is also significantly high in biomedical applications. Lactide and glycolide copolymer was used and reinforced with hydroxyapatite for bone tissue investigation by Lytkina et al. [43]. The incorporation of hydroxyapatite in PLGA copolymer has increased the strength and biocompatibility of PLGA. Poly(N-(2-hydroxypropyl)methacrylamide) (HPMA)-based copolymer was also used for deferent orthopedic implants by different groups [44]. Poly(L-lactide-co-ε-caprolactone) (PLCL) having flexible and biodegradable properties became one of the prime ingredients of biomedical implants [45]. Different fillers such as clay-reinforced copolymer-based composites are also utilized for the enhancement of the effectivity of biomedical implants [46].

15.7 CHALLENGES

Resorbable material-based biomedical products have emerged as an effective replacement for the conventional materials. Even though resorbable materials have lots of advantages, some limitations restrict extensive applications in real field (as shown in Figure 15.5).

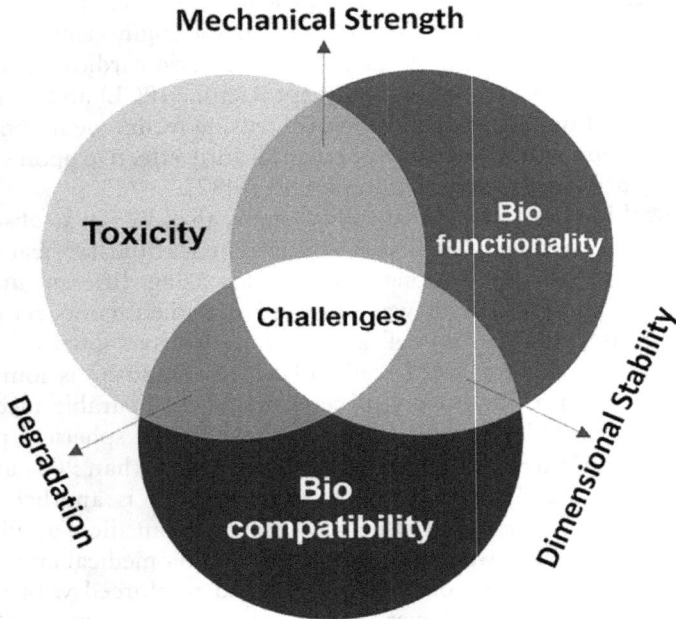

Figure 15.5 Challenges associated with resorbable material-based biomedical products.

- In case of orthopedic applications, the mechanical property with respect to degradation needs to be maintained up to initial support time.
- In some of the resorbable polymers, degradation is very fast, which leads to inadequate bone recovery.

15.8 APPLICATIONS OF RESORBABLE MATERIALS BASED IN OTHER BIOMEDICAL APPLICATIONS

Resorbable materials have versatile applications in the biomedical field. In previous Sections 15.3 and 15.6, the applications of resorbable materials in implants, bone fixation, and scaffolds are discussed. In this section, some of the major biomedical applications of resorbable materials (as shown in Figure 15.6) are discussed in brief.

15.8.1 Suture

The application of bio-based degradable polymers and copolymers for the preparation of surgical sutures has increased remarkably. PLA, PCL, and PGA are some of the resorbable polymers majorly used for the preparation of suture [47–49].

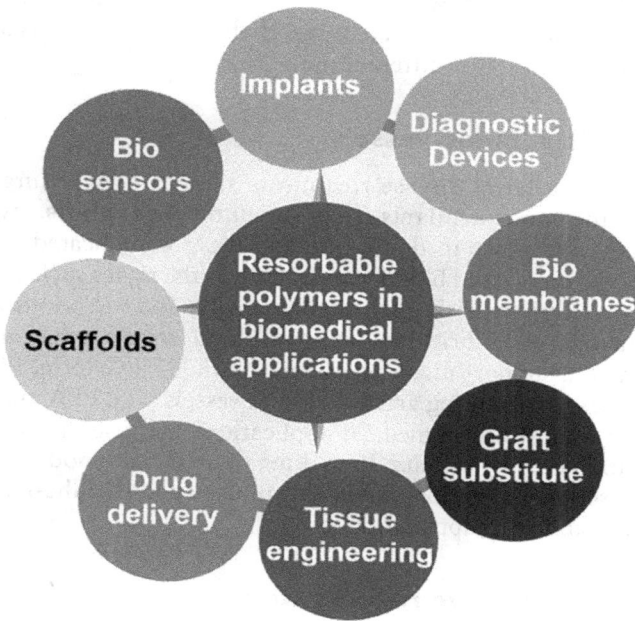

Figure 15.6 Different biomedical applications of resorbable materials.

15.8.2 Drug delivery

Resorbable polymeric gel and coating material are majorly used for drug delivery applications. The release behavior of drug depends on the resorbable polymer, nature of cross-linking, pH, and temperature of the targeted area. Herrero-Herrero et al. fabricated PLA-PCL nanofibers through electrospinning technique and observed that the release behavior of bovine serum albumin was dependent on fiber diameter [50]. Injectable gel made up of resorbable polymer PLGA-PLA was synthesized by Zhang et al. [51]. PLA-based gels are used for different drug loading and release by Upadhyay et al. for anti-TB drug release and by Romano Perinelli et al. for drug delivery to endometrial carcinoma [52,53].

15.8.3 Tissue culture

Electrospun nanofiber-based bags/materials/mats prepared from resorbable polymers have a large surface-to-volume ratio and in some cases have a porous structure with exceptional pore interconnectivity applicable for the development of cells for tissue engineering [54]. Sharma et al. fabricated electrospun nanofibrous mats from the PLA-PCL blend [55]. The mats were found to be bead-free and turned out to be suitable for further cell adhesion study. Trapani et al. observed for resorbable implants a significantly higher collagen I/III ratio, which was detected from statistical analysis in fascial tissue samples culture [56]. Different resorbable polymer blends and copolymers are also utilized for different tissue culture studies.

15.8.4 Artificial blood vessels

In present days, arterial disease treatments such as bypass surgery, stent placement, and anticoagulants require autologous grafts, which are less available, morbidity in donor site and more complicated operations. Resorbable polymer-based blood vessels address the issues such as low compliance, poor elasticity, risk of thrombogenicity, and infectious complications. Dastagir et al. fabricated artificial blood vessels using an in vitro technique with a support made up of spider silk [57]. Gelatin, PCL, collagen, etc., are used in making artificial blood vessels [58]. PLA and PHA are applicable in almost all biomedical applications because of their superior properties and biocompatibility. In making of artificial blood vessels, PLA- and PHA-based nanocomposites are also in use and cell adhesion behavior shows the possibility of application [59].

15.8.5 Artificial nerve regeneration

Peripheral nerve injury (PNI) is clinically intractable; however, it is common and accounts for almost 3% of all injuries worldwide. Nerve guidance conduit (NGC) tissue-engineered nerve grafts (TENGs) are some of the promising alternatives to nerve autograft for cells and growth factors and enhance nerve regeneration [60,61]. Resorbable polymers such as collagen and PCL are used for making nerve grafts [62]. Afrash et al. fabricated polycaprolactone/chitosan electrospun fibers for peripheral nerve regeneration. Along with improved surface and mechanical property, improvement in PC12 cell attachment and proliferation was also observed. This indicates the possibility of the biodegradable polymers in this application area [63].

In addition to above-mentioned applications, resorbable materials are also used as biosensor for biomolecules such as glucose and glycine [64–66].

15.9 CONCLUSIONS

The application of resorbable materials in the field of biomedical is in the developing stage. Orthopedic implants and bone fixation elements need biocompatibility and balanced in vivo degradation. Both magnesium-based and polymeric resorbable materials showed promising applicability. In other biomedical applications such as tissue engineering, surgical suture, drug delivery, artificial blood vessels, and artificial nerve grafts, the utilization of resorbable materials, particularly biodegradable polymers, blends, and copolymers, has increased. The incorporation of fillers such as hydroxyapa-tite, carbon materials, clays, and metallic fillers further improved the effectiv-ity of such polymers. However, some challenges are also discussed and need to be focused in future research, which are as follows:

- Dimensional stability and mechanical property of resorbable poly-mer-based implants.
- In situ drug loading in orthopedic implants, which can reduce the postoperative complexities.
- Stimuli-responsive suture and nerve regeneration materials function-ality of which can be further tuned by applying external simulates such as pH, magnetic field, or electric field.
- In case of artificial blood vessel research, more pressure-withstanding ducts or vessels need to be focused.

REFERENCES

1. Sahoo, N. G., Pan, Y. Z., Li, L., & Bin He, C. (2013). Nanocomposites for bone tissue regeneration. *Nanomedicine*, 8(4), 639–653, doi: 10.2217/nnm.13.44.
2. Prasad, A., Sankar, M. R., & Katiyar, V. (2017). State of art on solvent casting particulate leaching method for orthopedic scaffoldsfabrication. *Materials Today Proceedings*, 4(2), 898–907, doi: 10.1016/j.matpr.2017.01.101.
3. Prasad, A., Devendar, B., Sankar, M. R., & Robi, P. S. (2015). Micro-scratch based tribological characterization of Hydroxyapatite (HAp) fabricated through fish scales. *Materials Today Proceedings*, 2(4–5), 1216–1224, doi: 10.1016/j.matpr.2015.07.034.
4. Mulchandani, N., Prasad, A., & Katiyar, V. (2019). *Resorbable Polymers in Bone Repair and Regeneration*. In Valentina Grumezescu, Alexandru Mihai Grumezescu (Eds.), *Materials for Biomedical Engineering*, 87–125, Elsevier Inc. ISBN 9780128184158, doi: 10.1016/B978-0-12-818415-8.00004-8.
5. Middleton, J. C. & Tipton, J. (2000). Synthetic biodegradable polymers as orthopedic devices. *Biomaterials*, 21(23), 2335–2346, doi: 10.1016/S0142-9612(00)00101-0.
6. Friis, E. A., Decoster, T. A., & Thomas, J. C. (2017). *Mechanical Testing of Fracture Fixation Devices*. In Elizabeth Friis (Ed.), *Mechanical Testing of Orthopaedic Implants*, 131–141, Woodhead Publishing. ISBN 9780081002865, doi: 10.1016/B978-0-08-100286-5.00007-X.
7. Monmaturapoj, N., et al., (2017). Properties of poly(lactic acid)/hydroxyapa-tite composite through the use of epoxy functional compatibilizers for bio-medical application. *Journal of Biomaterials Applications*, 32(2), 175–190, doi: 10.1177/0885328217715783.
8. Dutra Messias, A., Aragones, A., & Aparecida de Rezende Duek, E. (2009). PLGA-hydroxyapatite composite scaffolds for osteoblastic-like cells. *Key Engineering Materials*, 396–398, 461–464, doi: 10.4028/www.scientific.net/KEM.396-398.461.

9. Prasad, A. (2021). Bioabsorbable polymeric materials for biofilms and other biomedical applications: Recent and future trends. *Materials Today Proceedings*, 44, 2447–2453, doi: 10.1016/j.matpr.2020.12.489.

10. Gupta, A., et al., (2017). Multifunctional nanohydroxyapatite-promoted toughened high-molecular-weight stereocomplex poly(lactic acid)-based bionanocomposite for both 3D-printed orthopedic implants and high-temperature engineering applications. *ACS Omega*, 2(7), 4039–4052, doi: 10.1021/acsomega.7b00915.

11. Kokubo, T., Kim, H.-M., & Kawashita, M. (2003). Novel bioactive materials with different mechanical properties. *Biomaterials*, 24(13), 2161–2175, doi: 10.1016/S0142-9612(03)00044-9.

12. Prasad, A., Bhasney, S., Katiyar, V., & Ravi Sankar, M. (2017). Biowastes processed hydroxyapatite filled poly (lactic acid) bio-composite for open reduction internal fixation of small bones. *Materials Today Proceedings*, 4(9), 10153–10157, doi: 10.1016/j.matpr.2017.06.339.

13. Castellani, A., et al., (2011). Acta Biomaterialia Bone – implant interface strength and osseointegration: Biodegradable magnesium alloy versus standard titanium control. *Acta Biomaterials*, 7(1), 432–440, doi: 10.1016/j.actbio.2010.08.020.

14. Kumar, A., Mamgain, D. P., Jaiswal, H., & Patil, P. (2015). Modal analysis of hand arm vibration (humerus bone) for biodynamic response using varying boundary conditions based on FEA. *Advances in Intelligent Systems and Computing*, 308, 169–176, doi: 10.1007/978-81-322-2012-1_18.

15. Kumar, A., Behmad, S. I., & Patil, P. (2014). Vibration characterization and static analysis of cortical bone fracture based on finite element analysis. *Engineering and Automation Problems*, No 3, 115–119.

16. Kumar, A., Jaiswal, H., Garg, T., & Patil, P. (2014). Free Vibration Modes Analysis of Femur Bone Fracture using varying boundary conditions based on FEA. *Procedia Materials Science*, 6, 1593–1599, doi: 10.1016/j.mspro.2014.07.142.

17. Gangwar, A. K. S., Rao, P. S., & Kumar, A. (2021). Bio-mechanical design and analysis of femur bone. *Materials Today: Proceedings*, 44(Part 1), 2179–2187, doi: 10.1016/j.matpr.2020.12.282.

18. Buijs, G. J. J., Stegenga, B., & Bos, R. R. M. R. M. (2006). Efficacy and safety of biodegradable osteofixation devices in oral and maxillofacial surgery: A systematic review. *Journal of Dental Research*, 85(11), 980–989, doi: 10.1177/154405910608501102.

19. Henkel, J., et al., (2013). Bone regeneration based on tissue engineering conceptions – A 21st century perspective. *Bone Research*, 1(3), 216–248, doi: 10.4248/BR201303002.

20. Prasad, A. (2021). State of art review on bioabsorbable polymeric scaffolds for bone tissue engineering. *Materials Today Proceedings*, 44, 1391–1400, doi: 10.1016/j.matpr.2020.11.622.

21. Burns, A. E. (1995). Biofix fixation techniques and results in foot surgery. *Journal of Foot and Ankle Surgery*, 34(3), 276–282, doi: 10.1016/S1067-2516(09)80060-4.

22. Gangwar, A. K. S., Rao, P. S., Kumar, A., & Patil, P. P. (2019). Design and analysis of femur bone: BioMechanical aspects. *Journal of Critical Reviews*, 6(4), 133–139.

23. Perren, S. M. (2002). Evolution of the internal fixation of long bone fractures: The scientific basis of biological internal fixation: Choosing a new balance between stability and biology. *Journal of Bone and Joint Surgery*, 84(8), 1093–1110, doi: 10.1302/0301-620X.84B8.13752.

24. Kumar, A., Gori, Y., Rana, S., Sharma, N. K., & Yadav, B. (2022). FEA of humerus bone fracture and healing. *Advanced Materials for Biomechanical Applications* (1st ed.) CRC Press, doi: 10.1201/9781003286806.

25. Nainar, S. M., Vicki, W. V., Begum, S., & Ansari, M. N. M. (2014). A review on bioscaffolds for tissue engineering application. *Scholars Journal of Engineering and Technology*, 2, 184–192.

26. Besinis, A., et al., (2015). Review of nanomaterials in dentistry: Interactions with the oral microenvironment, clinical applications, hazards, and benefits. *ACS Nano*, 9(3), 2255–2289, doi: 10.1021/nn505015e.

27. Rosli, N. A., Karamanlioglu, M., Kargarzadeh, H., & Ahmad, I. (2021). Comprehensive exploration of natural degradation of poly (lactic acid) blends in various degradation media: A review. *International Journal of Biological Macromolecules*, 187, 732–774.

28. Elsawy, M. A., Kim, K. H., Park, J. W., & Deep, A. (2017). Hydrolytic degradation of polylactic acid (PLA) and its composites. *Renewable and Sustainable Energy Reviews*, 79, 1346–1352.

29. Kobielarz, M., Tomanik, M., Mroczkowska, K., Szustakiewicz, K., Oryszczak, M., Mazur, A., & Filipiak, J. (2020). Laser-modified PLGA for implants: In vitro degradation and mechanical properties. *Acta of Bioengineering and Biomechanics*, 22, 179–197.

30. Ramachandran, K., Di Luccio, T., Ailianou, A., Kossuth, M. B., Oberhauser, J. P., & Kornfield, J. A. (2018). Crimping-induced structural gradients explain the lasting strength of poly l-lactide bioresorbable vascular scaffolds during hydrolysis. *Proceedings of the National Academy of Sciences*, 115(41), 10239–10244.

31. Oosterbeek, R. N., Kwon, K. A., Duffy, P., McMahon, S., Zhang, X. C., Best, S. M., & Cameron, R. E. (2019). Tuning structural relaxations, mechanical properties, and degradation timescale of PLLA during hydrolytic degradation by blending with PLCL-PEG. *Polymer Degradation and Stability*, 170, 109015.

32. Ishak, W. H. W., Rosli, N. A., & Ahmad, I. (2020). Influence of amorphous cellulose on mechanical, thermal, and hydrolytic degradation of poly (lactic acid) biocomposites. *Scientific Reports*, 10(1), 1–13.

33. Low, Y. J., Andriyana, A., Ang, B. C., & Zainal Abidin, N. I. (2020). Bioresorbable and degradable behaviors of PGA: Current state and future prospects. *Polymer Engineering & Science*, 60(11), 2657–2675.

34. Gigante, A., Setaro, N., Rotini, M., Finzi, S. S., & Marinelli, M. (2018). Intercondylar eminence fracture treated by resorbable magnesium screws osteosynthesis: A case series. *Injury*, 49, S48–S53.

35. Diekmann, J., Bauer, S., Weizbauer, A., Willbold, E., Windhagen, H., Helmecke, P., ... Ezechieli, M. (2016). Examination of a biodegradable magnesium screw for the reconstruction of the anterior cruciate ligament: A pilot in vivo study in rabbits. *Materials Science and Engineering: C*, 59, 1100–1109.

36. Valiño-Cultelli, V., Varela-López, Ó., & González-Cantalapiedra, A. (2021). Preliminary clinical and radiographic evaluation of a novel resorbable implant of Polylactic Acid (PLA) for Tibial Tuberosity Advancement (TTA) by Modified Maquet Technique (MMT). *Animals*, 11(5), 1271.

37. Ahuja, R., Kumari, N., Srivastava, A., Bhati, P., Vashisth, P., Yadav, P. K., ... Bhatnagar, N. (2020). Biocompatibility analysis of PLA based candidate materials for cardiovascular stents in a rat subcutaneous implant model. *Acta Histochemica*, 122(7), 151615.

38. Da Silva, D., Kaduri, M., Poley, M., Adir, O., Krinsky, N., Shainsky-Roitman, J., & Schroeder, A. (2018). Biocompatibility, biodegradation and excretion of polylactic acid (PLA) in medical implants and theranostic systems. *Chemical Engineering Journal*, 340, 9–14.

39. Grigoriev, T. E., Bukharova, T. B., Vasilyev, A. V., Leonov, G. E., Zagoskin, Y. D., Kuznetsova, V. S., ... Paltsev, M. A. (2018). Effect of molecular characteristics and morphology on mechanical performance and biocompatibility of pla-based spongious scaffolds. *BioNanoScience*, 8(4), 977–983.

40. Supelano, N. M., Amador, A. S., Duran, H. E., & Ballesteros, D. P. (2018). Dielectric properties of PLA-PGA-Chitosan–Hydroxyapatite composites. *Journal of Materials and Environmental Sciences*, (9), 2956–2963.

41. Zhang, J., Yang, S., Yang, X., Xi, Z., Zhao, L., Cen, L., ... Yang, Y. (2018). Novel fabricating process for porous polyglycolic acid scaffolds by melt-foaming using supercritical carbon dioxide. *ACS Biomaterials Science & Engineering*, 4(2), 694–706.

42. Kumar, A., Mir, S. M., Aldulijan, I., Mahajan, A., Anwar, A., Leon, C. H., ... Yu, X. (2021). Load-bearing biodegradable PCL-PGA-beta TCP scaffolds for bone tissue regeneration. *Journal of Biomedical Materials Research Part B: Applied Biomaterials*, 109(2), 193–200.

43. Lytkina, D., Berezovskaya, A., Korotchenko, N., Kurzina, I., & Kozik, V. (2017, November). Preparation of composite materials based on hydroxyapatite and lactide and glycolide copolymer. In *AIP Conference Proceedings* (Vol. 1899, No. 1, p. 020015). AIP Publishing LLC.

44. Wei, X., Li, F., Zhao, G., Chhonker, Y. S., Averill, C., Galdamez, J., ... Wang, D. (2017). Pharmacokinetic and biodistribution studies of HPMA copolymer conjugates in an aseptic implant loosening mouse model. *Molecular Pharmaceutics*, 14(5), 1418–1428.

45. Haim Zada, M., Kumar, A., Elmalak, O., Mechrez, G., & Domb, A. J. (2019). Effect of ethylene oxide and gamma (γ-) sterilization on the properties of a PLCL polymer material in balloon implants. *ACS Omega*, 4(25), 21319–21326.

46. Murugesan, S., & Scheibel, T. (2020). Copolymer/clay nanocomposites for biomedical applications. *Advanced Functional Materials*, 30(17), 1908101.

47. Liu, S., Wu, G., Chen, X., Zhang, X., Yu, J., Liu, M., ... Wang, P. (2019). Degradation behavior in vitro of carbon nanotubes (CNTs)/poly (lactic acid) (PLA) composite suture. *Polymers*, 11(6), 1015.

48. Budak, K., Sogut, O., & Sezer, U. A. (2020). A review on synthesis and biomedical applications of polyglycolic acid. *Journal of Polymer Research*, 27(8), 1–19.

49. Liu, S., Yu, J., Li, H., Wang, K., Wu, G., Wang, B., ... Zhang, M. (2020). Controllable drug release behavior of polylactic acid (PLA) surgical suture coating with ciprofloxacin (CPFX)—Polycaprolactone (PCL)/Polyglycolide (PGA). *Polymers*, 12(2), 288.

50. Herrero-Herrero, M., Gómez-Tejedor, J. A., & Vallés-Lluch, A. (2018). PLA/PCL electrospun membranes of tailored fibres diameter as drug delivery systems. *European Polymer Journal*, 99, 445–455.

51. Zhang, C., Yang, L., Wan, F., Bera, H., Cun, D., Rantanen, J., & Yang, M. (2020). Quality by design thinking in the development of long-acting injectable PLGA/PLA-based microspheres for peptide and protein drug delivery. *International Journal of Pharmaceutics*, 585, 119441.

52. Upadhyay, S., Khan, I., Gothwal, A., Pachouri, P. K., Bhaskar, N., Gupta, U. D., ...Gupta, U. (2017). Conjugated and entrapped HPMA-PLA nano-polymeric micelles based dual delivery of first line anti TB drugs: Improved and safe drug delivery against sensitive and resistant Mycobacterium tuberculosis. *Pharmaceutical Research*, 34(9), 1944–1955.

53. Perinelli, D. R., Cespi, M., Bonacucina, G., & Palmieri, G. F. (2019). PEGylated polylactide (PLA) and poly (lactic-co-glycolic acid)(PLGA) copolymers for the design of drug delivery systems. *Journal of Pharmaceutical Investigation*, 49(4), 443–458.

54. Wu, T., Ding, M., Shi, C., Qiao, Y., Wang, P., Qiao, R., ... Zhong, J. (2020). Resorbable polymer electrospun nanofibers: History, shapes and application for tissue engineering. *Chinese Chemical Letters*, 31(3), 617–625.

55. Sharma, D., Saha, D., & Satapathy, B. K. (2021). Structurally optimized suture resistant polylactic acid (PLA)/poly (ε-caprolactone)(PCL) blend based engineered nanofibrous mats. *Journal of the Mechanical Behavior of Biomedical Materials*, 116, 104331.

56. Trapani, V., Bagni, G., Piccoli, M., Roli, I., Di Patti, F., & Arcangeli, A. (2020). Analysis of resorbable mesh implants in short-term human muscular fascia cultures: A pilot study. *Hernia*, 24(6), 1283–1291.

57. Dastagir, K., Dastagir, N., Limbourg, A., Reimers, K., Strauß, S., & Vogt, P. M. (2020). In vitro construction of artificial blood vessels using spider silk as a supporting matrix. *Journal of the Mechanical Behavior of Biomedical Materials*, 101, 103436.

58. Wang, D., Xu, Y., Li, Q., & Turng, L. S. (2020). Artificial small-diameter blood vessels: Materials, fabrication, surface modification, mechanical properties, and bioactive functionalities. *Journal of Materials Chemistry B*, 8(9), 1801–1822.

59. Sun, J., Shen, J., Chen, S., Cooper, M. A., Fu, H., Wu, D., & Yang, Z. (2018). Nanofiller reinforced biodegradable PLA/PHA composites: Current status and future trends. *Polymers*, 10(5), 505.

60. Shintani, K., Uemura, T., Takamatsu, K., Yokoi, T., Onode, E., Okada, M., & Nakamura, H. (2017). Protective effect of biodegradable nerve conduit against peripheral nerve adhesion after neurolysis. *Journal of Neurosurgery*, 129(3), 815–824.

61. Zhang, X., Qu, W., Li, D., Shi, K., Li, R., Han, Y., ... Chen, X. (2020). Functional polymer-based nerve guide conduits to promote peripheral nerve regeneration. *Advanced Materials Interfaces*, 7(14), 2000225.

62. Samadian, H., Farzamfar, S., Vaez, A., Ehterami, A., Bit, A., Alam, M., ... Salehi, M. (2020). A tailored polylactic acid/polycaprolactone biodegradable and bioactive 3D porous scaffold containing gelatin nanofibers and Taurine for bone regeneration. *Scientific Reports*, 10(1), 1–12.

63. Afrash, H., Nazeri, N., Davoudi, P., Majidi, R. F., & Ghanbari, H. (2021). Development of a bioactive scaffold based on NGF containing PCL/chitosan nanofibers for nerve regeneration. *Biointerface Research in Applied Chemistry*, 11, 12606–12617

64. Chakraborty, G., Pugazhenthi, G., & Katiyar, V. (2019). Exfoliated graphene-dispersed poly (lactic acid)-based nanocomposite sensors for ethanol detection. *Polymer Bulletin*, 76(5), 2367–2386.

65. Chakraborty, G., Dhar, P., Katiyar, V., & Pugazhenthi, G. (2020). Applicability of Fe-CNC/GR/PLA composite as potential sensor for biomolecules. *Journal of Materials Science. Materials in Electronics*, 31(8), 5984–5999.

66. Chakraborty, G., Katiyar, V., & Pugazhenthi, G. (2021). Improvisation of Polylactic acid (PLA)/Exfoliated graphene (GR) Nanocomposite for Detection of Metal ions (Cu^{2+}). *Composites Science and Technology*, 213, 108877.

Index

For Product Safety Concerns and Information please contact our EU
representative GPSR@taylorandfrancis.com
Taylor & Francis Verlag GmbH, Kaufingerstraße 24, 80331 München, Germany